Essential Public Health
Theory and Practice

How can society most effectively prevent disease and promote health? This is the challenge addressed by this textbook.

Public health has been defined as the art and science of preventing disease, prolonging life and promoting health through the organised efforts of society. The 'science' is concerned with making a diagnosis of a population's health problems, establishing their cause, and determining effective interventions. The 'art' is to address these problems creatively. The aim of this book is to capture both the art and the science of the field.

Essential Public Health – Theory and Practice is divided into two major sections. The first part provides a toolkit of skills the practitioner must acquire, including coverage of all the disciplines underpinning public health. Part two describes the challenges faced, and explains how to go about the task. This section takes a life-course approach, considering the challenges of child public health, before moving on to the health of adults and older people. The section concludes with consideration of health inequalities, quality measurement techniques and global public health before examining opportunities to improve public health for the future.

This will be essential reading for these training in health care, social care and related disciplines such as environmental health. It includes a CD containing interactive, self-assessment questions and exercises to test understanding.

Stephen Gillam is Director of Undergraduate Public Health Teaching, Department of Public Health and Primary Care at the Institute of Public Health, University of Cambridge and a GP in Luton/ Visiting Professor at the University of Luton.

Jan Yates is a Public Health Specialist with experience of public health practice in Primary Care Trusts and acute hospital and mental health settings. She is a qualified teacher.

Padmanabhan Badrinath is a Consultant in Public Health Medicine in Suffolk Primary Care Trust and an Affiliated Clinical Lecturer, Department of Public Health and Primary Care at the Institute of Public Health, University of Cambridge.

Essential
Public Health

Theory and Practice

Stephen Gillam, Jan Yates
Padmanabhan Badrinath

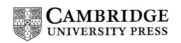

CAMBRIDGE UNIVERSITY PRESS
Cambridge, New York, Melbourne, Madrid, Cape Town, Singapore, São Paulo

Cambridge University Press
The Edinburgh Building, Cambridge CB2 8RU, UK

Published in the United States of America by Cambridge University Press, New York

www.cambridge.org
Information on this title: www.cambridge.org/9780521869720

First published 2007

Printed in the United Kingdom at the University Press, Cambridge

A catalogue record for this publication is available from the British Library

ISBN   978-0-521-86972-0 hardback
ISBN   978-0-521-68983-0 paperback

Contents

Contributors

JENNY AMERY
Department for International Development
1 Palace Street
London SW1E 5HE

CAROL BRAYNE
Institute of Public Health
Addenbrooke's Hospital
Hills Road
Cambridge CB2 2SR

RACHEL CROWTHER
327 Woodstock Road
Oxford OX2 7NX

JOHN DANESH
Department of Epidemiology and Medicine
University of Cambridge

TONY JEWELL
Welsh Assembly Government
Cathays Park
Cardiff CF10 3NQ

RICHARD LEWIS
Health Policy
King's Fund
11–13 Cavendish Square
London WC1 0NS

DAVID PENCHEON
Eastern Region Public Health Observatory
Institute of Public Health
Addenbrooke's Hospital

Hills Road
Cambridge CB2 2SR

CHRISSIE PICKIN
Health Promotion and Chronic Disease Prevention
Department of Human Services
Victorian State Government
Melbourne VIC 3000
Australia

VEENA RODRIGUES
School of Medicine, Health Policy and Practice
University of East Anglia
Norwich NR4 7TJ

LINCOLN SARGEANT
Institute of Public Health
Addenbrooke's Hospital
Hills Road
Cambridge CB2 2SR

NICHOLAS STEEL
School of Medicine Health Policy and Practice
University of East Anglia
Norwich NR4 7TJ

SARAH STEWART-BROWN
Division of Health in the Community
Warwick Medical School, LWMS
The University of Warwick
Coventry CV4 7AL

Foreword

Myriad challenges face international health today, from the prospect of hundreds of millions of tobacco-related deaths in the twenty-first century, to the devastation of sub-Saharan Africa by AIDS, to the rise of cardiovascular and metabolic diseases in many countries still laid low by ancient communicable diseases. The tide of the tobacco epidemic is turning in Britain and in some other industrialised countries, but in these places further progress depends on greater use of proven life-saving interventions (such as those in the prevention of vascular diseases) as well as on appropriate responses to challenges posed by ageing populations, unhealthy lifestyles and major – but comparatively neglected – sources of disability such as mental and musculoskeletal diseases.

The editors of this book have produced a lucid and thoughtful account of critical perspectives and tools that will enable students and practitioners to understand and tackle such prevailing problems in public health. This book's appeal to health-care professionals from many different backgrounds should help to advance the interdisciplinary approach to health promotion and disease prevention that the editors themselves wisely advocate.

John Danesh
Professor of Epidemiology and Medicine
University of Cambridge

Public health knowledge and practice is derived from a number of different academic fields. This makes the specialty very stimulating but immediately confronts the student with a dilemma: breadth versus depth. This book strikes the right balance between the need for coverage of several relevant disciplines with the detail required to understand specific public health challenges. We all need to use the frameworks described here to locate our learning and practice.

The three-domains model of public health practice described in the introduction has utility for all health workers – and we need to reflect on the location of information we use at the intersection of the three domains. Modern information technology provides assistance to health practitioners, e.g. through search engines and internet resources, but the growth in information and specialised knowledge characteristic of modern health systems can be overwhelming. For practitioners dedicated to improving public health there is always a 'population of interest'. For example, for the health visitor deprived families in her locality, for the general practitioner a practice population, for the director of public health a whole population and for the paediatrician or children's lead manager a subset of that population.

The community diagnostic model and the life-course structure is welcome. This book is written to assist learning for students from many disciplines studying public health. They will benefit from the clarity of the authors' approach, the wisdom distilled here and the recognition of our global and local public health challenges.

Tony Jewell
Chief Medical Officer, Wales

Acknowledgements

The authors would like to thank the following for their contribution: Sian Rees, Ian Sullivan, Sue Halliday, Peter Bradley, Ibrahim Abubakar, and John Powles. Thanks for encouragement and ideas are also due to family, friends, colleagues and – of course – our students.

Introduction

Historical background

Until recently it was a commonly held view that improvements in health were the result of scientific medicine. This view was based on experience of the modern management of sickness by dedicated health workers able to draw on an ever-growing range of diagnostics, medicines and surgical interventions. The demise of epidemics and infectious disease (until the manifestation of AIDS – acquired immunodeficiency syndrome), the dramatic decline in maternal and infant mortality rates and the progressive increase in the proportion of the population living into old age coincided in Britain with the development of the NHS (National Health Service, established in 1948). Thereafter, good quality medical care was available to most people when they needed it at no immediate cost. Clearly there have been advances in scientific medicine with enormous benefit to humankind, but have they alone or even mainly been responsible for the dramatic improvements in mortality rates evident in developed countries in the last 150 years? What lessons can we learn from how these improvements have been brought about?

Public health has been defined as *'the science and art of preventing disease, prolonging life and promoting health through the organised efforts of society'* [1]. In Europe and North America four distinct phases of activity in relation to public health over the last two hundred years can be identified. The first phase began in the industrialised cities of Northern Europe in response to the appalling toll of death and disease among working class people who were living in abject poverty. Large numbers of people had been displaced from the land by landlords seeking to take advantage of the agricultural revolution. They had been attracted to growing cities as a result of the industrial revolution and produced massive changes in population patterns and the physical environment in which people lived [2].

The first Medical Officer of Health in the UK, William Duncan, was appointed in Liverpool. Duncan surveyed housing conditions in the 1830s and discovered that one third of the population was living in the cellars of back-to-back houses with

Essential Public Health, eds. Stephen Gillam, Jan Yates and Padmanabhan Badrinath.
Published by Cambridge University Press. © Cambridge University Press 2007.

earth floors, no ventilation or sanitation and as many as 16 people to a room. It was no surprise to him that fevers were rampant. The response to similar situations in large industrial towns was the development of a public health movement based on the activities of medical officers of health, sanitary inspectors and supported by legislation.

The public health movement, with its emphasis on environmental change, was eclipsed in the 1870s by an approach at the level of the individual, ushered in by the development of the 'germ theory' of disease and the possibilities offered by immunisation and vaccination. Action to improve the health of the population moved on first to preventive services targeted at individuals, such as immunisation and family planning, and later to a range of other initiatives including the development of community and school nursing services. The introduction of school meals was part of a package of measures to address the poor nutrition among working-class people, which had been brought to public notice by the poor physical condition of recruits to the army during the Boer War at the turn of the twentieth century.

This second phase also marked the increasing involvement of the state in medical and social welfare through the provision of hospital and clinic services. It was in turn superseded by the therapeutic era dating from the 1930s with the advent of insulin and sulphonamides. Until that time there was little that was effective in doctors' therapeutic arsenals. The beginning of this era coincided with the apparent demise of infectious diseases on the one hand and the development of ideas about the welfare state in many developed countries on the other. Historically it marked a weakening of departments of public health and a shift of power and resources to hospital-based services.

By the early 1970s, the therapeutic era was itself being challenged by those, such as Ivan Illich (1926–2002), who viewed the activities of the medical profession as part of the problem rather than the solution. A catholic priest, he came to view the medical establishment as a major threat to health and produced the most radical critique of industrialised medicine so far [3]. His argument is simply summarised. Death, pain and sickness are part of human experience and all cultures have developed means to help people cope with them. Modern medicine has destroyed these cultural and individual capacities, through its misguided attempts to deplete death, pain and sickness. Such 'social and cultural iatrogenesis' has shaped the way that people decipher reality. People are conditioned to 'get' things rather than 'do' them. 'Well-being' has become a passive state rather than an activity.

The most influential body of work belonged to Thomas McKeown (1911–88). He demonstrated that dramatic increases in the British population could only be accounted for by a reduction in death rates, especially in childhood. He estimated that 80 to 90% of the total reduction in death rates from the beginning of the eighteenth century to the present day had been caused by a reduction in those deaths due to infection – especially tuberculosis (TB), chest infections and water- and food-borne diarrhoeal disease [4].

Most strikingly, with the exception of vaccination against smallpox (which was associated with nearly 2% of the decline in the death rate from 1848 to 1971), immunisation and therapy had an insignificant effect on mortality from infectious diseases until well into the twentieth century. Most of the reduction in mortality from TB, bronchitis, pneumonia, influenza, whooping cough and food- and water-borne diseases had already occurred before effective immunisation and treatment became available. McKeown placed particular emphasis on raised nutritional standards as a consequence of rising living standards. This thesis was challenged in turn by those who stress the importance of public health measures [5].

The birth of a new public health movement dated from the 1970s [6]. This approach brought together environmental change and personal preventive measures with appropriate therapeutic interventions, especially for older and disabled people. Educational approaches to health promotion have proved disappointingly ineffective. Contemporary health problems are therefore seen as being societal rather than solely individual in their origins, thereby avoiding the trap of 'blaming the victim'.

The intriguing truth is that the role of knowledge as a determinant of health is as yet ill defined (Chapter 1). Scientific advances in our understanding of how to improve health are embodied in the evolving panoply of medical interventions – new drugs, vaccines, diagnostics, etc. These new insights are, in turn, assimilated more informally by health professionals and the general public. How to harness new knowledge more effectively, for example, through the exploitation of new information technologies and marketing techniques, is a topic of growing interest to students of public health [7].

In any event, what are needed to address society's health problems are rational health-promoting public policies with a sound basis in epidemiology: the study of the distribution and determinants of disease in human populations. That is where this book begins.

Health care's contribution in context

Health professionals have long lived with the ambiguities of their portrayal in literature and the media: on the one hand as compassionate modern miracle-workers, on the other as self-interested charlatans. The implications of McKeown and Illich's work were largely ignored by clinicians. However, powerful counter-arguments have been mounted in their defence.

Attempts have been made to estimate the actual contribution of medical care to life extension or quality of life [8]. Estimating the increased life expectancy attributable to the treatment of a particular condition involves a three-step procedure:

- calculating increases in life expectancy resulting from a decline in disease-specific death rates
- estimating increases in life expectancy when therapy is provided under optimal conditions (using the results of clinical trials, using life tables), and
- estimating how much of the decline in death rates can be attributed to medical care provided in routine practice.

Bunker credits five of the thirty years' increase in life expectancy since 1900, and half the seven years of increase since 1950 to clinical services (preventive as well as therapeutic). In other words, compared with the large improvements in life expectancy gained from advancing public health in the first half of the century, the contribution of medical care was relatively small. It is now a more significant determinant of life expectancy. The continuing inequalities in health by social class point to further potential for improvement. The net effect of social class on the life expectancy of the whole population is three years, of which about a third can be charged against the use of tobacco and possibly a third against poorer access to medical care. Bunker estimates that the population would gain up to $2^{1}/_{2}$ years of life expectancy if everyone assumed the lifestyle of the fittest.

There are thus three main approaches to improving the health of the population as a whole and national policy must take into account their strengths and limitations. Firstly, investment in medical care can be increased and its quality improved (chapter 16). This may make the most predictable contribution to reducing death and suffering but, as we have seen, its impact is limited. Secondly, health promotion and changing lifestyles to prevent disease has obvious potential (chapter 4). However, the impact of educational programmes is less predictable. Thirdly, the redistribution of wealth and resources addresses the material determinants of health inequalities (chapter 14). Though tackling fundamental causes, this approach is of still more uncertain benefit.

Domains of public health

Public health in the NHS has undergone dramatic changes in recent years. All health professionals require some generalist understanding in this field. Rather fewer will need more advanced skills in support of aspects of their jobs (health visitors, general practitioners, commissioning managers, for example). This group also includes non-medical professions such as environmental health and allied agencies such as charities and voluntary groups. A small number of individuals specialise in public health but this group is expanding. Directors of public health increasingly hail from non-medical backgrounds.

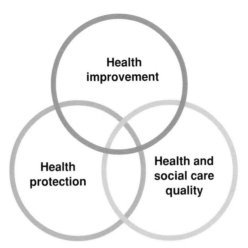

Health improvement
•Improving and promoting health
•Reducing inequalities
•Tackling broader determinants such as employment and housing
•Family/community health
•Education
•Lifestyle/health education

Health protection
•Clean air, water and food
•Infectious disease surveillance and control
•Protection from radiation, chemicals and poisons
•Preparedness and disaster response
•Environmental health hazards
•Prevent war and social disorder

Health and social care quality
•Health systems policy and planning
•Quality and standards
•Evidence-based healthcare
•Clinical governance
•Efficiency
•Research, audit and evaluation

Nowadays public health is seen as having three domains: health improvement, health protection and health and social care quality (Figure 1). All these domains are covered within this book. Each has its own chapter and examples from all three are used to demonstrate how the skills underpinning public health are put into practice. The disciplines that underpin public health include medicine and other clinical areas, epidemiology, demography, statistics, economics, sociology, psychology, ethics, policy and management. Public health specialists typically work with many other disciplines whose activities impact on the population's health. These might, for example, include health service managers, environmental health officers or local political representatives.

The science of public health is concerned with using these disciplines to make a diagnosis of a population's, rather than an individual's, health problems, establishing the causes and effects of those problems, and determining effective interventions. The art of public health is to create and use opportunities to implement effective solutions to population health and health-care problems. This book intends to capture both the art and the science.

Throughout their careers health-care and allied professionals are presented with opportunities to help prevent disease and promote health. Doctors and

Fig. 1 Three domains of public health.

Table 1. Parallels between activities of health professionals and public health workers

Individual	Population
Examination of a patient	Community health surveys
Drawing up diagnostic possibilities	Assessing health-care needs: setting priorities
Treatment of a patient	Preventive programmes, service organisation
Continuing observation	Continuing monitoring and surveillance
Evaluation of treatment	Evaluation of programmes/services

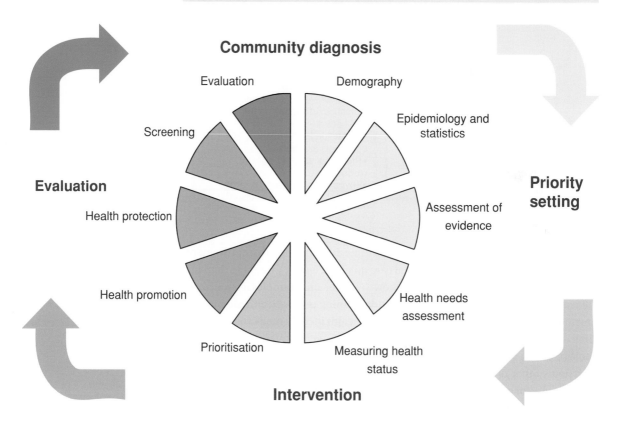

Fig. 2   Public health toolkit.

nurses need to look beyond their individual patients to improve the health of the population. Later in their careers, many will be involved in health-service management. Health professionals with a clear understanding of their role within the wider context of health and social care can influence the planning and organisation of services. They can help to ensure that the development of health services really benefits patients. This book seeks to develop for its readers a 'public health perspective' asking such questions as:

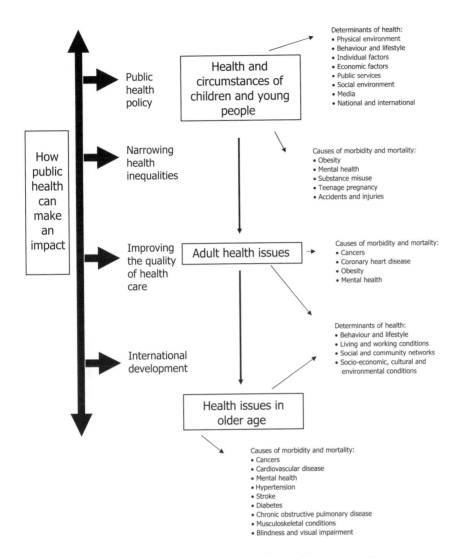

Fig. 3 The challenges of public health – using a life-course model.

- What are the basic causes of this disease and can it be prevented?
- What are the most cost-effective approaches to its clinical management?
- Can health and other services be better organised to deliver the best models of practice such as health-care delivery?
- What strategies could be adopted at a population level to ameliorate the burden of this disease?

As we have seen, population approaches to health improvement can be portrayed as in opposition to clinical care. This dichotomy is overstated and, in many respects, clinical and epidemiological skills serve complementary functions. There are parallels between the activities of health professionals caring for individuals and public health workers tending populations (Table 1).

Structure of this book

Following this introductory chapter, the book falls into two main sections. Public health practice should be about change. The first section of the book takes readers round a four-stage cycle (see Figure 2). This begins with the assessment of a population's health needs and how priorities are agreed. Interventions are defined and evaluated for their impact on those same needs. At the centre of this cycle can be seen the toolkit of public health skills a practitioner needs to acquire. These are added to at each stage of the cycle. The foremost of these disciplines is epidemiology, the subject of a companion book in this series.

The second half of the book will consider the main challenges that public health practitioners are facing. We use a life-course approach to this, considering first the challenges of child public health before moving on to the health of adults and older people. Next, we consider the impact of working in public health on the narrowing of health inequalities, policy development, improving the quality of health care and on international development. Figure 3 demonstrates how these public health challenges are connected. The final chapter examines future challenges.

We begin by examining the factors shaping the growth of populations: the science of demography.

REFERENCES

1. Public Health in England. Report of the Committee of Inquiry into the Future Development of the Public Health Function. Department of Health, London, 1988.
2. C. Hamlin, The history and development of public health in developed countries. In R. Detels, J. McEwen, R. Beaglehole and H. Tanaka (eds.), *Oxford Textbook of Public Health*, 4th edn, vol. 1, (The Scope of Public Health), Oxford, Oxford University Press, 2002, ch. 1.2, pp. 21–37.
3. I. Illich, *The Limits to Medicine. Medical Nemesis: The Expropriation of Health*, London, Penguin, 1976.
4. T. McKeown, *The Modern Rise of Population*, London, Edward Arnold, 1976.
5. S. Szereter, The importance of social intervention in Britain's mortality decline. 1850–1914: a re-interpretation of the role of public health. In B. Davey, A. Gray and C. Seale (eds.), *Health and Disease: A Reader*. Milton Keynes, Open University Press, 1995.
6. J. Ashton, Public health and primary care: towards a common agenda. *Public Health* **104**, 1990, 387–98.
7. National Social Marketing Centre for Excellence, *Social Marketing. Pocket Guide*, 1st edn, London, Department of Health, 2005.
8. J. Bunker, The role of medical care in contributing to health improvement within society. *International Journal of Epidemiology*, **30**, 2001, 1260–3.

Part 1

The public health toolkit

Demography

Key points

- Demography is the scientific study of human populations.
- It is important to understand the structure of a population in order to plan health and public health interventions; population structures can be represented as population pyramids.
- Population growth or decline depends upon fertility, mortality and migration.
- The concept of demographic, epidemiological and health transitions helps explain dramatic shifts in population structure and patterns of disease that have taken place in most countries.
- The measurement of demographic statistics is difficult and modelling is used to provide comparable data across the world.

Introduction

Demography is the scientific study of human populations. It involves analysis of three observable phenomena: changes in population size, the composition of the population and the distribution of populations in space. Demographers study five processes: fertility, mortality, marriage, migration and social mobility. These processes determine populations' size, composition and distribution. Basic understanding of demography is essential for public health practitioners because the health of communities and individuals depends on the dynamic relationship between the numbers of people, the space which they occupy and the skills they have acquired. The main sources of demographic information vary between countries and they are well developed in the western hemisphere.

Essential Public Health, eds. Stephen Gillam, Jan Yates and Padmanabhan Badrinath.
Published by Cambridge University Press. © Cambridge University Press 2007.

Fig. 1.1   Population pyramid for India, 2000. Source: US Census Bureau, International Data Base.

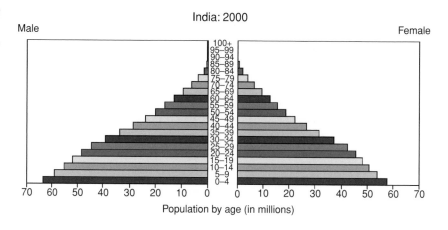

Fig. 1.2   Population pyramid for the UK, 2000. Source: US Census Bureau, International Data Base.

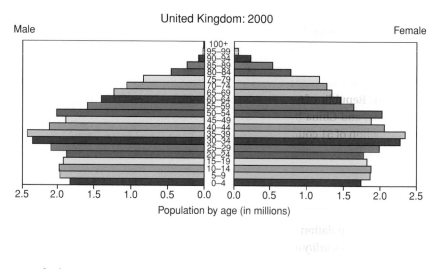

Population structure

Understanding the structure of a population in terms of the numbers and proportions of men and women and different age groups informs the planning of preventive and health care interventions. One way of depicting the structure of a population is a population pyramid. This is a graphical way of presenting population data by sex and age group. Pyramids provide a simple way to compare population structures across countries and can provide an indication of the state of development of each country. As an illustration, Figures 1.1 and 1.2 show the data for India and the UK. India is typical of a developing country with a broad base tapering at the top. In developed countries such as the UK, the pyramid generally shows a bulge in the middle and has a narrower base.

Use the two pyramids above to describe in words the population structure of India and the UK.

In India there are larger numbers of young people and, as age increases, the population within each age band decreases. This tapering shape is typical of a developing country where fertility is high but mortality in childhood is high and fewer people live to older ages. In the UK there is a bulge in the numbers of people around 25–54 years. Fertility has recently been lower but more people survive into middle age.

Population trends

World population trends available from the United Nations (UN) show that while the population at the global level continues to increase, that of more developed regions as a whole is hardly changing. Virtually all population growth is occurring in the less-developed regions with rapid population growth being a characteristic of the 50 least developed countries. The population is projected to triple between 2005 and 2050 in many countries including Afghanistan, Liberia, Mali, Niger and Uganda. During 2005–2050 the following nine countries are expected to account for half of the world's projected population increase: India, Pakistan, Nigeria, the Democratic Republic of Congo, Bangladesh, Uganda, the United States of America, Ethiopia and China (in order of size of contribution to population growth). The population of 51 countries including Germany, Italy, Japan, the Baltic States and most of the former Soviet Union is expected to be lower in 2050 than in 2005.

Reasons for population trends

These overall population trends are underpinned in the main by distinct changes in *fertility* and *mortality* across the globe. *Migration* also plays a part when large numbers of people move from one country to another.

Fertility

Fertility refers to the actual bearing of children, the child-bearing performance of a woman, couple or population. As a simple measure of fertility the crude birth rate of a population can be used (with either live or all births as the numerator and person-time at risk as the denominator). A more sophisticated measure of fertility is the general fertility ratio (the number of births per 1,000 women of child-bearing age, generally 15–44 or 49 years) but this requires more detailed population data and may not always be available. At a further level of complexity fertility rates may be standardised to account for differences in the age structures of populations and this is termed the total fertility rate. Total fertility rate is defined as the number of children that would be born per woman if she were to live to the end of her child-bearing years and bear children at each age in accordance with prevailing age-specific fertility rates. The total fertility rate for the world is estimated to be 2.59 children per woman but is 1.66 in the UK and 6.07 in Congo demonstrating the difference between countries.

In more developed regions people bear insufficient children to replace those people who die and this trend, termed below replacement fertility, is expected to continue to 2050. Conversely, fertility is still high in most of the least developed countries; it is expected to show some decline but still remain higher than the rest of the world. Fertility is influenced by various factors. In the developing countries these include universality of marriage, lower age at marriage, low level of literacy, poor standard of living, limited use of contraceptives and traditional ways of life.

Mortality

Mortality describes the death rates due to a range of causes. The ways in which mortality is measured are detailed in Chapter 7. Trends in mortality have been shifting over time and still vary across the globe. Most people nowadays live longer on average than the wealthiest people did a century ago. Despite these gains there remains a huge preventable burden of premature death and disease worldwide. The dramatic reduction in death rates over the last two centuries can be explained by changes in the social and economic determinants of health and to a lesser extent by public health interventions. 'High tech' medical interventions, if narrowly defined, explain only a small amount. Medical interventions can be defined more broadly to include technologies such as oral rehydration solutions that are widely used both by professionals and lay people. These have certainly had more impact in recent decades especially on child mortality in low-income countries.

There are approximately 50 million deaths worldwide each year, over half of which occur in people aged less than 60 years. Four out of five deaths occur in low-income countries. A quarter of all deaths occur in children under five; almost all of these deaths occur in low-income countries. There are striking differences in the pattern of death between high- and low-income regions (see Chapter 17). Communicable diseases are responsible for over 40% of deaths in low-income regions but non-communicable diseases account for a rising proportion of deaths also.

While child mortality rates are falling slowly in most countries, the relative gap between high- and low-income countries has worsened. In low-income countries, children still die of the infectious diseases that have plagued populations for centuries. Over 60% of the deaths in children under five years are accounted for by just three broad causes: vaccine-preventable diseases (three million), diarrhoea (2.7 million) and respiratory infection (1.7 million). These deaths are the direct result of poverty and malnutrition and the vast majority can be prevented through low-cost, social policy and public health interventions. Progress on the

Millennium Development Goals is described in Chapter 17. In wealthy countries, child mortality is dominated by sudden infant death syndrome, congenital disorders and injury. These too are increasingly preventable.

The maternal mortality rate (actually the ratio of pregnancy-related deaths to live births) has reduced dramatically over the last two centuries, especially in the developed world, as a result of reforms of obstetric practice and the reduction in puerperal sepsis. By contrast, over 700 mothers die for every 100,000 births in sub-Saharan Africa where the lifetime risk of maternal death is about one in twenty. In western Europe, less than 10 mothers die for every 100,000 births and the lifetime risk of a maternal death is about one in 10,000. The provision of extended family-planning services, the availability of safe abortion and improved services for antenatal and obstetric care illustrate the importance in this area of technical interventions.

Adults make up about one half of the world's population and 70% of all deaths occur in adults. About half of these deaths are premature. The chance of an adult dying prematurely varies about ten fold among countries. Differences in the risk of adult death between regions are largely explained by variation in non-communicable disease death rates and death rates from injury. The death rates from heart disease, diabetes and smoking-related illness are increasing globally. The assessment of the relative importance of cause of death depends upon the indicator used. When potential years of life lost (YLL – see Chapter 7) before the age of 65 years are used, conditions that affect younger adults such as injuries, tuberculosis and maternal mortality assume greater importance. As mortality rates from cardiovascular disease have declined, the proportion of deaths due to cancer has increased and now exceeds the former in many wealthy countries. Reasons for changing patterns of mortality are discussed further below.

Migration

Recent United Nations' estimates suggest that, worldwide, nearly 200 million people live outside the country of their birth with an imbalance across the globe and 60% of migrants living in developed countries.

There are benefits and risks to increasing migration which can:
- increase educational levels, or decrease them as young people take up unskilled positions abroad or those educated abroad fail to return home.
- have a positive effect on income (for example, through remittances as migrants send funds home to families). Migration may also increase socio-economic inequity as some individuals, communities or countries benefit more than others; or it may have a negative effect on an economy by potentially reducing external competitiveness.
- increase poverty and inequity within countries where rural to urban migration is high (for example China). In rural areas the poorest cannot afford to move and those who move into cities tend to be the more educated.

- increase personal vulnerability due to the potential for illegal migration and 'human trafficking'. For example, women recruited as domestic labour may be vulnerable to sexual exploitation.
- lead to racism and isolation.
- lead to a reduction in the human capital needed to deliver key services at home. For example, only 9 of the 47 sub-Saharan African countries have the World Health Organisation (WHO) recommended level of physicians (20 doctors per 10,000 people).
- lead to population structural imbalances, for example as those unable to move such as the elderly concentrate in one place.

Information on migration may be derived from censuses, surveys and other administrative record systems. However, these vary in accuracy across the world.

Migration that increases population sizes or alters patterns of infectious diseases may result in changing needs for health care. Public health professionals need to ensure that local health services are culturally sensitive and accessible to migrants (e.g. through appropriate translation services).

Life expectancy

The decline in death rates has led to major improvements in life expectancy and life expectancy is a key determinant of future population patterns. Life expectancy at birth is the average number of additional years a person could expect to live if current mortality trends were to continue for the rest of that person's life. An important tool, the demographic life table, is used to estimate life expectancy. This uses data on age specific mortality rates for a specific year to estimate the lifetime experience of a hypothetical cohort (group) of individuals born that year. It assumes that the current mortality rates continue throughout the lifetime of the cohort and, while this is not completely accurate, it does allow the average life expectancy to be calculated. Life tables are an extremely powerful means of summarising the mortality experience in a way which can be compared across populations, and they are also the basis for population projections which predict population growth over time. More complex life tables can be used to estimate the proportion of deaths attributable to different causes, and measures of morbidity can also be introduced to provide estimates of healthy life expectancy.

Global life expectancy at birth is estimated to have risen from 47 years in 1950–1955 to 65 years in 2000–2005. This is expected to keep on increasing to reach 75 years in 2045–2050. However, patterns of mortality vary across countries. In eastern Europe mortality has been increasing since the late 1980s and in 2000–2005 life expectancy was in the region of 67.9 years: lower than the 1960–1965 level of 68.6 years. The Russian Federation and the Ukraine are particularly affected by rises in mortality resulting partly from the spread of HIV (human immunodeficiency virus), vascular disease and injury.

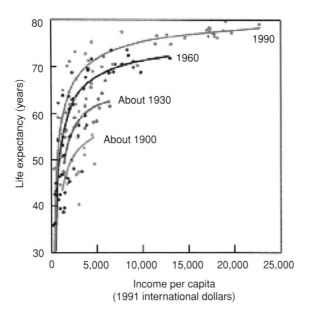

Fig. 1.3 The changing relationship between life expectancy and income during the twentieth century [1].

Life expectancy at birth has increased in most countries since 1950 but there are huge disparities evident between high- and low-income countries. Sub-Saharan Africa, with the advent of HIV/AIDS (acquired immunodeficiency syndrome) has shown a major reversal in life expectancy, and in some countries of central and eastern Europe life expectancy at birth has also been declining over the past decade. This is attributed in part to economic and industrial disruption following dissolution of the Soviet Union, and increasing death rates from heart disease, injuries and alcohol-related illness.

The primary outcome of fertility decline combined with increases in life expectancy, is population ageing; the increasing share of older people in a population relative to the younger persons. Globally the number of persons aged 60 years or over is expected almost to triple, increasing from 672 million in 2005 to nearly 1.9 billion by 2050.

As longevity increases, the health experience of older people assumes greater importance both socially and economically. The proportion of people 60 years and over is higher in wealthy countries but more older people live in low-income countries. Projections suggest a four-fold expansion in the global population of older people during the first quarter of this century. The health and social policy challenges this raises are described in Chapter 13.

Preston and colleagues [1] have investigated the relationship between life expectancy and income during the twentieth century (Figure 1.3). The positions of the dots show the relationship between a single country's income and its life expectancy. The different colours refer to the specified years. With the passage of time the level of life expectancy attainable at a given income has increased. Why?

The most fundamental cause is likely to be the advance of knowledge working in two main ways [2]. This knowledge may be formally embodied as medical techniques and interventions. Simultaneously, knowledge informs the actions of both health professionals and the general public. These actions need then to be reinforced by appropriate social policies (Chapter 5). The history of tobacco control provides perhaps the best contemporary illustration [3].

Health transitions

The health transition is a framework for explaining the spectacular shifts in population structure and patterns of disease that have taken place in most countries [4]. It describes the ways in which the world's health needs have changed and will continue to change. The demographic transition describes the change in birth and death rates from high fertility and high mortality rates in more traditional societies to low fertility and low mortality rates in so-called modern societies. The epidemiological transition refers to the long-term changes in the patterns of sickness and disability that have occurred as societies have changed their demographic, economic and social structures. As originally described, the epidemiological transition consists of three stages [5]:

- The era of pestilence and famine when life expectancy was low. The major causes of death were malnutrition, infectious disease, complications of pregnancy and childbirth.
- The era of receding pandemics which in western Europe began in the eighteenth century and lasted until the early years of the twentieth century with the great influenza pandemic of 1918–20.
- The era of non-communicable diseases characterised by low fertility rates, population growth and in particular cardiovascular disease and cancer among other so-called degenerative or chronic disease.

A fourth stage has also been proposed [6]:

- The age of delayed degenerative diseases where, as preventive and interventional advances are made, degenerative diseases are postponed. Here the patterns of mortality remain similar to those in the third stage but are shifted progressively toward older ages; rapid improvements in survival are concentrated among the population in older ages.

Of course, the way this transition has evolved in different countries is highly variable; low-income countries today are not merely replicating the experience of wealthier countries. For example, population growth, poverty, environmental degradation and the demographic trap (constant rapid population growth due to high fertility and low mortality) may prevent the transition from high mortality/fertility to low mortality/fertility in some sub-Saharan African countries. The poorest in developing countries may be experiencing a triple burden

Box 1.1 Three instances of health in transition:

- The burden of mental illnesses, such as depression, alcohol dependence and schizophrenia has been seriously underestimated by traditional approaches that take account of deaths and not disability.
- Adults under 70 years of age in sub-Saharan Africa today face a higher probability of death from a non-communicable disease than adults of the same age in established market economies.
- By 2020 tobacco is expected to kill more people than any single disease, even HIV/AIDS.
  Source: World Health Organisation

of communicable disease, non-communicable disease and socio-behavioural illness.

The major factors responsible for the health transition are health determinants, demographic changes and therapeutic interventions. Historically, social and economic development, improving nutritional status, sanitary systems and increased literacy among women have been of major importance. Thomas McKeown proposed that improved nutrition beginning in the eighteenth century, together with improvements in water supply and sanitation services and the reduction in birth rates, propelled the health transition (see Introduction). Effective medical measures came too late to make a significant contribution. For example, it has been estimated that only 3.5% of the total decline in mortality in the USA between 1900 and 1973 could be ascribed to medical measures introduced for the major infections (see Chapter 15). On the other hand, targeted public health interventions including vaccination and improved child health care have had major benefits. These general developments have interacted with more specific public health measures directed towards the control of both infectious and non-communicable disease.

The universal ageing of the population as a result of declining fertility and, to a lesser extent, declining death rates has resulted in the emergence of non-communicable diseases in adulthood with a long latent period. The absolute number of people with these diseases has increased inexorably, even as age- and cause-specific death rates have declined.

Factors that tend to reduce the risk of dying once disease has become established include effective health services and higher education levels. The most effective health services are not necessarily those most technologically advanced but rather those which are readily accessible. Historically speaking, the contribution of health services has been small because until recently most medical interventions were ineffective. In low-income countries, however, the therapeutic component has been of greater importance contributing to the major decline in child mortality seen over the past few decades. While its impact on adult mortality has been smaller, health services are nevertheless important in the relief of suffering. Future gains in health status are most likely to derive from more effective public health measures.

By focussing on the important social and economic causes of changing death rates, the concept of health transition offers potential for understanding health trends and thus improving health in all countries. However, it does not explain all differences in death rates between countries or necessarily predict changes associated with modernisation (as the recent deterioration in life expectancy in some eastern European countries illustrates). Furthermore, the theory does not easily account for marked declines in mortality rates from major non-communicable disease such as heart disease and stroke. In other words, although health transition theory provides a useful descriptive tool, it requires more elaboration to be of much predictive value.

Disease and disability

While mortality is important for the study of demography it does not provide a complete picture to inform public health action. Premature and potentially preventable death represents the most important challenge for public health but death rates alone as an indicator of health status fail to account for the full burden of disease. A more comprehensive indicator promoted by the World Bank combines losses from premature death with loss of healthy life resulting from disability (see Chapter 13) to calculate the disability-adjusted life year (DALY). The calculation of DALYs involves multiple assumptions and has many limitations. In some regions and for many diseases, the necessary data on disease incidence and duration are unavailable. Nevertheless, DALYs provide a broader measure of the global impact of disease. They help highlight inexpensive and effective ways to reduce dramatically the burden of communicable disease which accounts for 35% of the world total. Tackling the remaining 65% requires more complex policy approaches.

Healthy-life expectancy rises with increasing life expectancy. However, the percentage of life expected to be lived in healthy states declines. Overall disability rises with age and disability onset becomes more compressed around the average age. Prevalence levels of disability are greater in low socio-economic groups than in higher socio-economic groups. Major inequalities in health are apparent when the population is categorised by social class, income, occupation, education and ethnicity (Chapter 14). Several possible explanations for these have been advanced: misclassification of social class, particularly in women and the retired; downward 'drift' because of ill health; inequalities in the distribution of major risk factors for disease; inequalities in the distribution of income. An important reason for inequalities in health appears to be the distribution of wealth within a country. In countries where income distribution is relatively equal, health inequalities are less than in countries where there are gross disparities in wealth [7]. In short, health inequalities may reflect social policies that neglect the needs of poor people.

Methodological issues in demography

The accuracy with which demographic statistics are collected across the world varies greatly. In order to compare the measures discussed in this chapter data are needed on the numbers of people (population 'stock'), births, deaths, disease and migration. It is a necessary element of demography to collect these data in the best possible way, assess their accuracy and, where necessary, deal with gaps or inaccuracy through estimation.

The data on population stock often come from censuses. While the United Nations has worked to improve comparability across the world there will still be variations. As well as numbers of people censuses may be used to collect data on age, sex, ethnicity, residence, fertility, health and other factors. Censuses are costly to administer and, although crucial in providing the denominator for many demographic and health measures, carry some inherent problems:

- Not all countries carry them out.
- They may not be carried out at the same intervals (decennially is recommended).
- Data become less accurate as time since census elapses.
- Under-enumeration may occur due to, for example, non-response (e.g. of older people), mobility of population (e.g. seasonal migrants).
- Data accuracy may be poor, e. g. for people reporting a digit preference for stating their age (30, 35, 40), inaccurate reporting of marital status or overstatement of age by the elderly.
- Inaccurate assignment of people to geographical areas (e.g. deaths in hospital all reported as from one town but residence being from a much wider area).

Attempts to reduce these inherent errors include validation surveys where intensive efforts are made to contact a sample of respondents to check data.

Vital registration systems collect data on births and deaths. In many countries this is compulsory, which helps ensure data completeness. In much of the developing world however, birth and death need not be registered so these data can be seriously incomplete. Even with well-established systems inaccuracies are inevitable as they rely heavily on the quality of information and coding being high. In particular, there may be problems with the accuracy of the recording of cause of death. For example, with the increasing age at death of much of the population it is increasingly likely that people die with multiple pathologies; which to state as primary cause of death may be an arbitrary decision. Variations have occurred over time as fashions change, knowledge increases and deaths in countries with well-established systems are better defined (for example, death from bronchopneumonia rather than old age).

Where demographic data are systematically absent an alternative is the application of population surveys, which sample a proportion of the population. For example, the Demographic and Health Surveys (DHS) Project is a worldwide research project to provide data and analysis on the population, health and nutrition of women and children in developing countries.

We have seen the importance of fertility in determining population trends but fertility is very difficult to estimate accurately. Estimates of fertility depend, to varying degrees, on the availability of data on births, maternal age and deaths. As we have seen these are of variable accuracy and completeness and this leads to a range of measures being used and potential problems with comparability.

Measuring mortality is similarly problematic. As with fertility, crude measures are possible (number of births or deaths per unit population) but these are highly dependent upon the age structure of the population, so are not comparable. With mortality, age-specific death rates are preferable but not always possible due to data deficiencies. Standardisation is a technique used to apply standard population age-specific mortality rates (for example, the national or regional rates) to the population under study to give an expected number of deaths. This is then used in a ratio with the observed deaths to give a standardised mortality ratio (SMR), which is a useful summary (i.e. an SMR over 100 suggests the mortality experience of this population is worse than that of the standard population).

Life tables also rely on accurate demographic data but when there are insufficient data available to construct them they can be modelled with limited mortality rates estimated from global averages. These modelled life tables can then be used to estimate age-specific mortality rates, which are extremely useful in areas where vital registration systems are poor.

Measuring migration can also present particular difficulties. Differences in the size of administrative regions may mean that a short move would count as a migration in one country and a huge move not count in another. Comparability is therefore problematic especially if boundaries change. It may also be difficult to distinguish temporary migration (e.g. a move to university) from a permanent one. If censuses are taken then an estimate of migration can be made by determining the difference in population between two censuses not accounted for by natural increases or depletion. This is termed the 'balancing equation' and estimates net migration (or errors in the data).

Conclusion

It can be seen that the field of demography requires a detailed understanding of a variety of data sources and robust methods to analyse their accuracy and deal with consequent levels of uncertainty. However, demography provides the public health practitioner with some of the most fundamental measures with which to assess the health of a population.

FURTHER READING AND SOURCES OF DATA

World Health Organisation: www.who.int/en/

WHO Annual World Health Reports: www.who.int/whr/en/

J. B. McKinlay, S. M. McKinlay and R. Beaglehole, A review of the evidence concerning the impact of medical measures on recent mortality and morbidity in the United States. *International Journal of Health Services* **19**(2), 1989, 181–208.

National statistics for the USA, UK and other countries: www.census.gov/, www.statistics.gov.uk/

United Nations Department of Economic and Social Affairs. Population Division: www.un.org/esa/population/

UNICEF State of the World's Children Reports: www.unicef.org/sowc/

S. H. Preston, P. Heuveline and M. Guillot, *Demography: Measuring and Modeling Population Processes*. London, Blackwell, 2000

Demographic and Health Surveys: www.measuredhs.com/

E. Grundy, Demography and public health. In *Oxford Textbook of Public Health* R. Detels, J. McEwen, R. Beaglehole and H. Tanaka (eds.) (Oxford, Oxford University Press) 2002, pp. 807–28.

REFERENCES

1. S. H. Preston, The changing relation between mortality and level of economic development. *Population Studies* **29**, 1975, 231–48.
2. J. Powles, personal communication.
3. S. Glanz and E. Balbach, *Tobacco War: Inside the California Battles*. Berkeley University, California Press, 2000.
4. R. Beaglehole and R. Bonita, *Public Health at the Crossroads. Achievements and Prospects*, Cambridge, Cambridge University Press, 1997.
5. A. R. Omran, The epidemiologic transition. *Milbank quarterly*, **49** (1), 1971, 509–38.
6. S. J. Olshansky and A. B. Ault, The fourth stage of the epidemiologic transition: the age of delayed degenerative diseases. *Milbank quarterly* **64**(3), 1986, 355–91.
7. R. G. Wilkinson, *Unequal Societies: the Afflictions of Inequality*, London, Routledge, 1996.

2

Epidemiology

Key points

- Epidemiology concerns the study of the distribution and determinants of disease and health-related states.
- The uses of epidemiology include:
  - determination of the major health problems occurring in a community;
  - monitoring health and disease trends across populations;
  - making useful projections into the future and identify emerging health problems;
  - describing the natural history of new conditions, e.g. who gets the disease, who dies from it, and the outcome of the disease;
  - estimating clinical risks for individuals;
  - evaluating new health technologies, e.g. drugs or preventive programmes;
  - investigating epidemics of unknown aetiology.

Introduction

At the core of epidemiology is the use of quantitative methods to study diseases in human populations and how they may be prevented. Thus epidemiology can be defined as the 'study of distribution and determinants of health related states and events in the population and the application of this science to control health problems'[1]. It is important to note that epidemiology concerns not only the study of diseases but of all health-related events. For example, we can study the epidemiology of breast feeding or drug misuse. Rational health-promoting public policies require a sound basis in epidemiology.

The epidemiological analysis of a disease from a population perspective is vital in order to be able to organise and monitor effective preventive, curative and

Essential Public Health, eds. Stephen Gillam, Jan Yates and Padmanabhan Badrinath.
Published by Cambridge University Press. © Cambridge University Press 2007.

rehabilitative services. All health professionals and health-service managers need an awareness of the principles of epidemiology. They need to go beyond questions relating to individuals such as 'What should be done for these patients now?', to challenging fundamentals such as 'Why did *this* person get *this* disease at *this* time?,' 'Is the prevalence of the disease increasing and, if so, why?' and 'What are the causes or risk factors for this disease?'

In the following pages we look briefly at the origins of epidemiology and then examine some of its key concepts including:

- disease variation
- the concept of a population
- measures of disease frequency – rates
- quantifying differences in risk
- types of epidemiological study
- how to interpret the results of epidemiological studies.

The history of epidemiology

The origins of modern epidemiology can be traced back to the work of English reformers and French scientists in the first half of the nineteenth century. However, writers of the Hippocratic School in the fourth century BC, who stressed the effects of physical factors such as air, geographical location and water on health and disease[2], are often claimed as prototypic epidemiologists. The Hippocratic corpus underpinned one of two explanatory theories of disease that competed until modern times. Poisonous particles generated by the decomposition of organic matter (miasma) were held responsible for many diseases. Though eventually discredited, the notion of miasma led to important public health interventions – better-ventilated housing and the provision of sanitation. By contrast, contagion theory, which ultimately underpinned germ theory, had its origins in the ancient practice of isolating diseased people.

John Graunt laid the basis of health statistics and epidemiology with his analyses of the weekly bills of mortality in the seventeenth century. Using these data, Graunt described the patterns of mortality and fertility and seasonal variations charting the progress of epidemics, most famously in the plague years. In 1747, James Lind, a British naval surgeon, undertook a study testing his hypothesis of the cause of scurvy and the clinical trial was born (see Box 2.1).

Building on the ideas of Graunt, William Farr institutionalised epidemiology in Victorian England. He developed a system of vital statistics that was to form the basis of disease classification now in its tenth revision. The International Classification of Diseases and Related Health Problems (commonly known by the abbreviation ICD) is designed to promote international comparability in the

Box 2.1 James Lind

In 1747 Lind took twelve seamen with scurvy and, in addition to their normal diet, gave each of six pairs a different dietary supplement for six days. The two seamen given oranges and lemons made an almost complete recovery from which Lind inferred that citric acid fruits could prevent scurvy. It was not until 1795 that the British naval authorities accepted his results and included limes in the diet of sailors. Such delays in disseminating evidence were much later to provide the rationale for the evidence-based medicine (EBM) movement (Chapter 3). Only in 1920 were alternative theories eliminated and consensus reached that scurvy was a dietary deficiency.

collection, processing, classification and presentation of morbidity and mortality statistics. Over a long career Farr developed methods for studying the distribution and determinants of human diseases.

Twentieth-century epidemiologists have added to the body of knowledge on disease patterns and their causes in the population by meticulously studying large sections of the population with respect to particular conditions or risk factors. Examples of landmark studies are given later in the chapter.

Time, place, person – disease variation

Epidemiologists seek answers to the following questions:
- How does the pattern of this disease vary over *time* in this population? A decline in disease is as worthy of investigation as a rise.
- How does the *place* in which the population lives affect the disease? International differences in disease patterns mainly, although not wholly, reflect the fact that populations are at different stages in their demographic and epidemiological transitions. International variations are reducing as these transitions take place, just as migrant populations' disease patterns tend to converge towards those of the populations they join.
- How do the *personal characteristics* of people in the population affect the disease's pattern? We can ask 'What is the relative importance of genetic and environmental influences in bringing about population differences in disease?' In large populations, genetic makeup is relatively stable. Changes in disease frequency in large populations over short periods of time are almost wholly due to environmental factors. In individuals as opposed to populations, genetic makeup is profoundly important in shaping risk of disease, for genetic variation between individuals is great. Disease is, of course, caused by the interaction of the genome and the environment [3].

Fig. 2.1   The iceberg of disease.

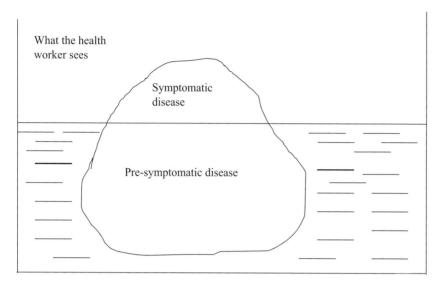

What the health
worker sees

Symptomatic
disease

Pre-symptomatic disease

This is often summarised by describing health states and determinants in terms of 'time, place and person'.

The concept of a population

Epidemiology and public health policy depend on the notion of *population*. Traditionally, health systems have been designed around a population of people with health problems, those who contact the service. Public health specialists, however, have responsibility for the whole population, those who are at risk of health problems and have them at early stages. This can be seen as the submerged part of the disease 'iceberg' (Figure 2.1). People with symptomatic disease can be further subdivided into those with symptoms not seeking medical help, symptomatic but self-treating and those who are symptomatic but accessing informal care. Even among the symptomatic only some people seek formal health care. Below the surface there are a large number who may have latent, pre-symptomatic, undiagnosed disease. However, not all people without symptoms can be described as in perfect health. Many people may have risk factors that make them more prone to various diseases: for example smoking, sedentary lifestyle and obesity which puts them at increased risk of coronary heart disease.

Firstly, we need to define clearly the population we are interested in. This might vary in size from an entire country to a small community. It may also be restricted by the disease in question, e.g. to those suffering from coronary heart disease. When the population is defined we can then consider how the pattern of disease varies. This will allow us to plan services based on the pattern of disease in the population as a whole and not just among users of the service. Secondly, we can then deliver modified services to sub groups of the population who differ in terms of their needs and are not making effective use of existing services (e.g. home-less, non-native-language-speaking). Thirdly, by using knowledge of population trends and health status we anticipate the need for future services.

Populations may be *stable* or *dynamic*. A stable population is known as a cohort (a group of people with common characteristics). The population is defined at the start of the follow-up period and gradually diminishes in size as its members cease to be at risk of becoming a case (e.g. they die). In contrast, a dynamic population is one in which there is turnover of membership while it is being observed. People enter and leave the population at different times.

Epidemiological variables

Disease patterns are influenced by the interaction of factors (variables) at social, environmental and individual levels. Consideration of these factors aids in the depiction, analysis and interpretation of differences in disease patterns within and between populations. Age, sex, economic status, social class, occupation, country of residence or birth and racial or ethnic classifications may be used to show variations in health status. Most variables used in epidemiology are markers for complex, underlying phenomena that cannot be measured easily. For example, we might measure obesity levels in a population as a marker of the risk of heart disease.

A good epidemiological variable should:

- have an impact on health in individuals and populations
- be measurable
- differentiate populations in their experience of disease and health
- differentiate populations in some underlying characteristics relevant to health, e.g. income or behaviour
- generate testable aetiological hypotheses
- help to develop health policy, plan and deliver health care, prevent and control disease.

For each of the qualities listed above, consider whether age can be considered a useful epidemiological variable
See Table 2.1.

Once we have identified that a disease varies according to such factors as age or social class we can begin to consider how the factor exerts an effect. For example, it is well known that the occurrence of heart disease is more common in men than women. Some of the possible explanations for this include differences in lifestyle factors, occupations and levels of co-existing diseases. Refer to the exercise in the CD for a detailed discussion of this topic.

Table 2.1. Age as a useful epidemiological variable

Criteria for a good epidemiological variable	Criteria in relation to the factor age
Impact on health in individuals and population	Age is a powerful influence on health as chronological age is related to the general health of the individual
Be measurable accurately	In most populations age is measurable to the day, but in some it has to be guessed, as people are not aware of their exact birth day
Differentiate populations in their experience of disease or health	Large differences by age are seen for most diseases or their determinants
Generate testable aetiological hypotheses, and/or	It is hard to test hypotheses because there are so many underlying differences between populations of different ages
Help in developing health policy, and/or Help to plan and deliver health care and/or Help to prevent and control disease	Age differences in disease patterns could affect health policy and planning of services. Knowing the age structure of a population is critical to good planning. By understanding the age at which diseases start, preventive and control programmes can be targeted at appropriate age groups

Geographical differences in epidemiological variables can also provide important clues to the causes of disease. Figure 2.2 shows the distribution of blood pressure in two populations in two different continents.

Referring to Figure 2.2, answer the following questions.
a. **In what ways do the shapes of the distributions differ in the two populations?**
b. **Roughly, what percentage of the Kenyans and London civil servants have hypertension (assuming a systolic blood pressure over 150 mm Hg is hypertension)?**
c. **Is there any suggestion from the above figure that the cause of high blood pressure in an individual Kenyan nomad and a London civil servant is likely to differ?**
d. **What are the possible causes of the different distribution of blood pressure in the two populations?**

a. The shape of the distributions of blood pressure is similar – a so-called 'normal' distribution.
b. Five per cent nomads and about 20% of civil servants.
c. No, the cause of high blood pressure in individuals is not presented in the data.
d. Nomads' blood pressures are more normally distributed and the Londoners' distribution has shifted rightwards. The causes of the rightward shift

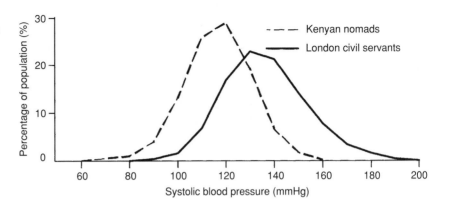

Fig. 2.2 The distribution of blood pressure values in Kenyan nomads and London civil servants [4].

probably include dietary factors, obesity, insufficient exercise, stress and genetic factors.

Measures of disease frequency – rates

One measure of disease frequency is a count of the number of cases of a disease occurring in a population. However, the number of cases alone is not particularly informative. Account must also be taken of the size of the population and usually the length of time over which its members were observed. This gives rise to a comparison between the number of cases in the population and the size of the population, often expressed as a rate.

The numerator of a rate is the number of 'cases' but defining people as cases can be difficult. For some diseases (e.g. rabies) case definition is clear; for others (such as hypertension) the disease shows a spectrum of severity and arbitrary criteria must be imposed to distinguish diseased from non-diseased.

The denominator of a rate is the 'population at risk' and this too must be carefully defined.

In calculating the pregnancy rate what would be the appropriate denominator?

The ideal denominator for this rate is dependent upon the culture of the population being measured. In some cases it is married women in the 15–44 or 15–49 year age groups as these are the only women at risk of becoming pregnant. However, in some cultures this would not be the case and the denominator would not be restricted to married women. This leaves us with a problem if pregnancy rates are compared across populations, as the denominators do not match. When comparing rates across populations it is important to ensure that the same measures are taken as numerators and denominators.

Prevalence

A measure of the burden of disease in a population is the *prevalence*. This is the number of cases of disease in a population at a given time and it is frequently used in planning the allocation of health-service resources. Generally, we use the term prevalence to mean a *point prevalence* which is defined as follows:

$$\text{Point prevalence} = \frac{\text{Number of diseased persons in a defined population at one point in time}}{\text{Number of persons in the defined population at the same moment in time}} \quad (2.1)$$

Point prevalence is a proportion and does not involve time. *Period prevalence* is the number of cases of disease during a specified time (e.g a week, month or year). When the period is long the denominator is usually the number of persons at the mid point of the time period (e.g. the mid-year population).

$$\text{Period prevalence} = \frac{\text{Number of diseased persons in a defined population during a specified period of time}}{\text{Number of persons in the defined population over the same period of time}} \quad (2.2)$$

Incidence

When researching the aetiology of diseases, measures of disease *incidence* are of primary interest. Cases of incident disease in a defined period of time are those which first occur during that time. There are two ways of expressing disease incidence: risk (or cumulative incidence) and incidence rate but in most situations these give very similar results.

Risk is defined as the number of cases of a disease that occur in a defined period of time as a proportion of the number of people in the population at the beginning of the period. Deaths in the population may be measured rather than the number of cases:

$$\text{Risk in defined period of time} = \frac{\text{Number of persons who become diseased (or die) during the period}}{\text{Number of persons in the population at the beginning of the period}} \quad (2.3)$$

Risk may also be known as cumulative incidence. It describes the way that populations as a whole experience disease. However, it may also be thought of as the risk an individual has of developing the disease in the specified period of time. Risk is the possibility of harm. In epidemiology, the association between risk of disease and both individual and social characteristics (risk factors) provides the starting point for analysing the causes of disease.

Incidence rate is defined as the number of new cases (or deaths) occurring in a defined period of time in a defined population. The sum of the periods of time for each individual when he or she is disease-free but may develop the disease is the denominator and is known as the person–time at risk.

$$\text{Incidence rate} = \frac{\text{Number of persons who have become diseased}}{\text{Person–time at risk}} \qquad (2.4)$$

Figure 2.3 shows two populations, A and B, which are observed for ten years. Over time members of the populations die. The length of time each person spends alive (and therefore at risk of death) is shown by the bars on the charts. For population A the person–time at risk, the incidence rate and the risk at ten years can be calculated:

- Person–time at risk – 10 people with $4 + 3 + 2 + 10 + 1 + 2 + 3 + 4 + 2 + 4$ years at risk. Person–time at risk $= 35$ person years.
- Incidence rate at ten years $= 9$ people who died/35 person years at risk $= 0.257$ people per year (number of cases is 9 as one person remains alive at the end of the period).
- Risk at 10 years $= 9$ people who died /10 people at the start of the period $= 0.9$ people per year.

Calculate these for population B
- Person–time at risk – 10 people with $4 + 6 + 4 + 8 + 2 + 1 + 6 + 10 + 5 + 6$ years at risk. Person–time at risk $= 52$ person years.
- Incidence rate $= 9/52 = 0.173$ people per year.
- Risk at 10 years $= 9/10 = 0.9$ people per year.

So far we have calculated incidence rates in stable populations (cohorts). The same calculations can be done for dynamic populations. Figure 2.4 shows how incidence might look in a dynamic population.

From Figure 2.4 calculate a. the person–time at risk at the end of year 7; b. incidence rate after 7 years; and c. the risk of the condition in year 3.
a. Person–time at risk $= 3 + 4 + 5 + 3 + 5 + 2 + 4 + 3 + 3 + 6 = 38$ person years.
b. Incidence rate $= 8/38 = 21.1\%$ (2 people remain at risk at the end of the period and are not counted in the numerator for incidence rate).
c. Risk in year 3 $= 9/10 = 90\%$ (only person 6, of the 10 people present in this year, does not have the disease).

Sometimes direct measurement of person–time at risk is not possible. This is true for mortality rates where we do not know when each individual became at risk or stopped being at risk. Instead, as with estimates of period prevalence, an estimate of the person–time at risk is taken to be the population at the mid-point of the calendar period of interest $\times$ the length of the period (usually a year).

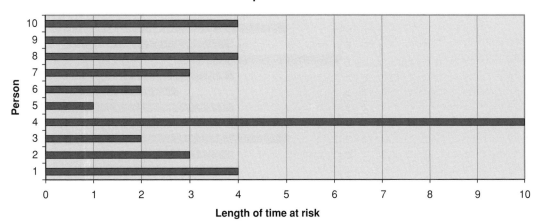

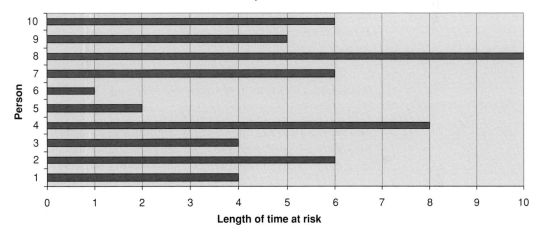

Fig. 2.3   Populations at risk of death.

For example, the all-cause mortality rate for females in England and Wales for 2005 is defined as:

$$\text{Mortality rate per year} = \frac{\begin{array}{c}\text{Number of female deaths from all causes} \\ \text{in England and Wales in 2005}\end{array}}{\begin{array}{c}\text{Estimate of 2005 mid-year female population} \\ \text{of England and Wales}\end{array}} \quad (2.5)$$

Relationship between prevalence, incidence and duration of disease

Figure 2.5 shows the prevalent population as the circle on the right and people entering this as incident cases from the non-diseased population on the left. So, in a fixed population, prevalence rate is approximately equal to the incidence

Fig. 2.4   Incidence in dynamic
populations.

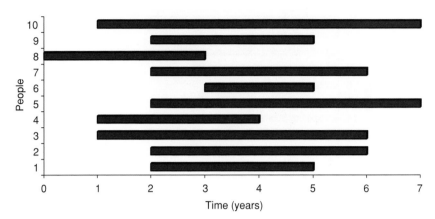

Incidence in dynamic populations

rate (the number of people entering the prevalent population in a defined
period of time) multiplied by the duration of the disease (how long they stay
there):

Prevalence = Incidence rate × Period of follow-up   (2.6)

This means that for conditions with a long duration (e.g. diabetes or heart disease)
prevalence is a good estimate of the burden of disease but for conditions with a
short duration (e.g. influenza) incidence is a better measure.

An exercise on incidence and prevalence

**10,000 miners were recruited to a study. At baseline 50 were found to have
lung cancer and were excluded from follow-up. The remainder
underwent six monthly reviews for five years. At the end of five years, 9
miners had developed lung cancer.**
a. What was the prevalence of lung cancer at baseline?
b. What was the risk of developing lung cancer over five years?
c. What is the approximate incidence rate of lung cancer among miners?
d. Why is it only an approximation?
   a. Prevalence at baseline = 50/10,000 = 0.5%.
   b. Risk or cumulative incidence over five years = 9/9950 = 0.905 per 1,000.
   c. Incidence rate = 9/(9950 × 5) = 0.181 per 1000 person years.
   d. It is assumed that each person contributed a full five years of follow-up to the
       denominator, hence the rate is likely to be underestimated.

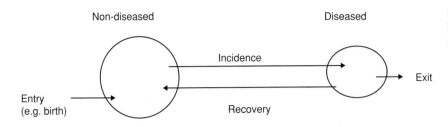

Fig. 2.5 The relationship between prevalence and incidence.

Case fatality and survival rates

The terms case fatality and survival rate are often used to compare the killing power of diseases. The case fatality rate is actually a form of risk, which measures the proportion of people with a disease (e.g. cancer) who die within a defined period of diagnosis. If we assume that all cases either die or survive the case fatality rate is related to the survival rate from a disease:

Probability (survival) + Probability (death)-1   (2.7)

The case fatality and survival rates are not true rates, as they do not measure the rate per unit of time at risk at which death occurs; they are probabilities. The case fatality rate is simply the ratio of deaths to cases.

Quantifying differences in risk

When epidemiologists seek to explain health experiences they often compare the rates of diseases across populations. These may be populations with different risk factors for disease, or populations who are being treated differently for a disease they already have. In order to do this it is helpful to use measures which summarize the difference between the two populations.

Relative risks

Relative risk tells us how much more at risk one population is compared to another. For example, we might want to compare how many children with meningitis die if they are treated using antibiotics alone with how many die if they are given steroids as well. To begin we must define the risk in both populations. There are two main ways of summarising these risks, as either a proportion (a risk as defined earlier in this chapter) or as an odd. For example, if 320 children developed meningitis during one year and 32 died, this can be expressed as a proportion: 32/320 (10%) – i.e. 15 children die for every 152 who get meningitis; or it can be expressed as the odds of dying: 32/288 – i.e. 32 children die for every 288 with meningitis who survive. Then, to compare the risk in two groups we can calculate the ratio between the risk measured in one group and the risk

Table 2.2. A 2 × 2 table for calculating relative risks of giving up smoking

	Given nicotine gum	No nicotine gum
Gave up smoking	1149	893
Did not give up	5179	7487
Total	6328	8380

measured in the other group (i.e. divide the risk in one group by the risk in the other group).

Now a note on epidemiological terminology which can be incredibly confusing. A ratio can be calculated from both the measures of risk defined above. If we use the ratio between the proportions it is known as the *Relative Risk*; if we use the ratio between the odds it is called the *Odds Ratio*. Both the Relative Risk and the Odds Ratio are measures of relative risk in a general sense. Reading epidemiological texts, you will come across the term 'risk ratio' – used as a synonym for the Relative Risk or with reference to both the Relative Risk and Odds Ratio. In this book we use 'relative risk' as an overarching term referring to the ratio of either two risks or two odds, Relative Risk (note capitals) to mean the ratio of two risks and Odds Ratio to mean the ratio of two odds.

Example

In a trial of nicotine gum a group of smokers were given gum and a control group were not. Out of 6328 smokers who were given nicotine gum, 1149 stopped smoking. Out of 8380 smokers in the control group, 893 stopped. So the numbers who did not give up smoking are 6328 − 1149 = 5179 and 8380 − 893 = 7487 respectively.

These figures can be shown on a 2 × 2 table (Table 2.2) which often helps to support calculating relative risks.

The Relative Risk = risk of stopping smoking in nicotine-gum group/risk of stopping smoking in the control group. The Odds Ratio = odds of stopping smoking in the nicotine-gum group/odds of stopping smoking in the control group. NB We can see here that the word 'risk' can be applied to an outcome which we want (i.e. stopping smoking) as well as to an outcome we want to avoid such as death. Therefore:

Relative Risk = 1149/6328 893/8380 = 1.70

Odds Ratio = 1149/5179 893/7487 = 1.86.

This can be put into words such that we can say someone who uses nicotine gum is 1.7 times more likely to give up smoking as someone who does not. Or the odds

Table 2.3. A 2 × 2 table for calculating relative risks for higher prevalence of smoking

	Given nicotine gum	No nicotine gum
Gave up smoking	3000	2000
Did not give up	5179	7487
Total	6328	8380

of someone stopping smoking if they use nicotine gum are 1.86 times greater than if they don't.

Relative risks can be used as a measure of the *strength of association* between a risk factor and an outcome (e.g. smoking and lung cancer) or a measure of the effectiveness of an intervention in causing an outcome (e.g. nicotine gum and stopping smoking). Odds Ratios are calculated in case control studies because in case–control studies we can only derive the odds of exposure among cases (those with the condition of interest) and the odds of exposure in controls (those without the condition of interest). Relative Risks can be calculated in cohort studies (see later) and, in instances when the condition under study is rare, Odds Ratio = Relative Risk. This approximation is useful as it helps us interpret studies simply and assumes that an Odds Ratio quoted is an approximation of a Relative Risk, but it must be remembered that this only holds for rare conditions. The following example illustrates this point.

In the nicotine-gum example from earlier the Relative Risk and the Odds Ratio are similar (1.70 and 1.86), but imagine that the prevalence of stopping smoking was much higher (Table 2.3):

Calculating the Relative Risk and Odds Ratio now we find:

Relative Risk = 3000/6328 2000/8380 = 4.4

Odds Ratio = 3000/5179 2000/7487 = 2.1.

The Relative Risk is now much greater than the Odds Ratio and we cannot assume that an Odds Ratio quoted in a study for a very common outcome would be the same as a Relative Risk.

Relative risks are also useful in epidemiology as they provide a single summary statistic where no difference (i.e. no association between a risk factor and an outcome or no effect of an intervention) will give a Relative Risk of one. A Relative Risk greater than one suggests there is an association between the risk factor or intervention and the outcome. So if the outcome is something we want (such as cure or reduced mortality) a Relative Risk greater than one is good but if we want less of the outcome (such as death) then a Relative Risk below one is good.

The Relative Risk of death due to lung cancer among smokers is 15.34 compared to non-smokers. The same study found that the Relative Risk in smokers for coronary heart disease (CHD) was 1.45. What is your interpretation of these findings?

Smokers are 15.34 more likely to die of lung cancer compared to non-smokers. This risk is very high and there is a strong association between smoking and lung cancer. However, for CHD the risk is much smaller as smokers are at only 1.45 times higher risk of dying due to CHD compared to non-smokers.

Absolute risk reduction

The *absolute risk reduction* (ARR) is the difference in the absolute risk (rates of adverse events) between study and control populations:

Absolute risk reduction (ARR)

    = Risk in exposed (experimental event rate, EER)

    − Risk in unexposed (control event rate, CER)   (2.8)

The ARR is a measure of the absolute effect of exposure and is a guide to individual needs and benefits. It may be estimated in cohort studies but not in case-control studies (see below).

When to use relative risk and when to use absolute risk

In general, relative risks are more useful for expressing the population impact of a risk factor or intervention and absolute risks are more useful when considering individual needs and benefits. For example, if the risk of recurrence of a cancer goes from 5% down to 2.5% after treatment with a new drug, the relative risk reduction is 50% (50% of 5% is 2.5%) but the absolute risk reduction is only 2.5% (5% minus 2.5% = 2.5%). So, any one individual, with a small risk to begin with, reduces their risk by a small absolute amount. However, across a population this may be a significant risk reduction.

In a clinical trial the event rate in the control group is 40 per 100 patients, and the event rate in the treatment group is 30 per 100 patients. Calculate the Relative Risk and ARR in this trial.

Relative Risk = 40/100 ÷ 30/100 = 1.33, ARR = 40% − 30% = 10%.

Number needed to treat (NNT)

The *number needed to treat* is another summary measure that is helpful in making decisions over which interventions are effective. The NNT is the number of people who (on average) need to receive a treatment to produce one additional successful outcome. If, for example, NNT for a treatment is 10, the practitioner would have to give the treatment to ten patients to prevent one patient from having the adverse outcome over the defined period, and each patient who received the treatment would have a 1 in 10 chance of being a beneficiary.

For example, if the NNT for the use of nicotine chewing gum in helping people stop smoking for at least one year is 14, we need to treat 14 smokers by giving them nicotine gum, for one extra person to stop smoking.

Calculation of NNT

If a disease has a death rate of 100% without treatment and treatment reduces that mortality rate to 50%, the ARR is $100/100 - 50/100 = 0.5$. How many people would we need to treat to prevent one death? In this example treating 100 patients with the otherwise fatal disease results in 50 survivors. This is equivalent to one out of every two treated, an NNT of 2.

Alternatively, the NNT to prevent one adverse outcome equals the inverse of the absolute risk reduction, i.e. $NNT = 1/ARR$.

Example

Out of 6328 smokers who were given nicotine gum, 1149 stopped smoking. Out of 8380 smokers in the control group, 893 stopped smoking. What is the NNT?

$NNT = 1/ARR = 1/(1149/6328 - 893/8380) = 1/(0.182 - 0.107) = 1/0.075 = 13.3$. The NNT gives more information than relative risk because it takes into account the baseline frequency of the outcome. The question below illustrates this.

A drug reduces the risk of dying from a heart attack by 40% (Relative Risk = 0.60). In terms of relative risk this drug has the same 'clinical effectiveness' for everyone. Calculate the NNT if it is given to people with a 1 in 10 annual risk of dying from a heart attack and to people with a 1 in 100 risk.

For a risk of 1/10
The original risk is 1/10 (0.1) and with the drug $0.6 \times 1/10 = 0.06$
So the ARR is $0.1 - 0.06 = 0.04$
And the NNT $= 1/0.04 = 25$

For a risk of 1/100
The original risk is 1/100 (0.01) and with the drug $0.6 \times 1/100 = 0.006$
So the ARR is $0.01 - 0.006 = 0.004$
And the NNT $= 1/0.004 = 250$

So we can see that the NNT is much higher when the risk of the condition (incidence rate) is lower. If the drug causes serious side effects in 1 in 100 people then we would probably not use it for people with a low risk but it would still be an effective treatment for people with high baseline risk. So the NNT helps us estimate how likely the treatment is to help an individual patient.

Measures of population impact

So far we have considered how we measure the rates of disease or risk factors in populations and how we measure the effects of risk factors or interventions in populations exposed to them compared to unexposed populations. Another useful measure when looking at the health of populations or individuals is a measure of what proportion of death or disease can be attributed to specific causes. For individuals the *attributable risk* (AR) is usually expressed as a percentage.

$$AR = \frac{(\text{Incidence in exposed} - \text{Incidence in unexposed}) \times 100}{\text{Incidence in exposed}} \qquad (2.9)$$

This is the rate of disease occurrence or death ('risk') in a group that is exposed to a particular factor, which can be attributed to that factor. For example, in deciding whether or not to indulge in a dangerous sport such as rock climbing, the attributable risk of injury (i.e. the risk due solely to the rock climbing and not other causes) must be weighed against the pleasures of participation.

For populations the *population attributable risk*

= attributable risk

     × prevalence of exposure to risk factor in population; or: (2.10)

     Population attributable risk = Rate in population – Rate in unexposed

The population attributable risk tells us what proportion of a population's disease or death experience is due to a particular cause and can indicate the potential impact of control measures in a population (i.e. what proportion of disease would be eliminated in a population if its disease rate were reduced to that of unexposed persons). Population attributable risk is, therefore, particularly relevant to decisions in public health. The following exercises examine the risks attributable to smoking at a population level.

A classic study of smoking and mortality[5, 6]

The British Doctors' Study was set up in 1951 to investigate the relationship between smoking habits and mortality. A total of 59,600 members of the medical profession in the United Kingdom were asked to fill in a simple questionnaire on smoking habits

Complete replies were received from 34,440 men – that is, about 69% of the male doctors who were alive when the questionnaire was sent. Further inquiries about changes in smoking habit were made in 1957, 1966, 1971 and 1991; i.e. after 6, 15, 20 and 40 years.

Of the initial respondents in 1951, 17% were classified as non-smokers. In the first twenty years of follow-up (1951–71) a total of 10,000 deaths occurred in the 34,440 men, 441 of which were from lung cancer and 3191 from ischaemic heart disease (IHD); see Table 2.4.

Table 2.4. The British Doctors Study [6]. Death rate for men by cause of death and cigarette smoking habit

Cause of death	Death rate per 1000	
	Smokers	Non-smokers
Lung cancer	0.9	0.07
IHD	4.87	4.22

Table 2.5. Exercise on relative risk and population attributable risk [6].

	Annual death rates per 100,000 from lung disease
Heavy smokers	224
Non-smokers	10
Total population	74

a. Calculate relative risks (as Relative Risks) and attributable risk for the data in Table 2.4 relative to non-smokers?
b. (i) Which disease is most strongly related to cigarette smoking?
   (ii) Which disease has the largest number of deaths statistically attributable to cigarette smoking?

a. The Relative Risks are 12.86 (0.9/0.07) for lung cancer and 1.15 (4.87/4.22) for IHD. The attributable risk is 92% ([0.9 − 0.07] 10.9 × 100) for lung cancer and 13.3% ([4.87 − 4.22] 14.87 × 100) for CHD

b. (i) The data shows that 92% of lung cancer is attributable to smoking and 13.3% of CHD. In CHD both Relative Risk and AR are not very high suggesting not much of the disease could be prevented as compared to lung cancer.
   (ii) Ischaemic heart disease.

From Table 2.5, calculate the Relative Risk and population attributable risk of lung disease associated with smoking.

Relative Risk for heavy smokers   224/10 = 22.4
Compared to non-smokers
Population attributable risk   74 − 10 = 64 deaths per 100,000 person years

Summary

Table 2.6 summarises the concepts explained so far in the epidemiological description of disease (or risk factors) by time, place and person.

> ### Box 2.2 Descriptive studies
>
> Population (correlation or ecological studies)
> > Individual
> > > Case reports
> > > Case series
> > > Cross-sectional surveys
>
> Analytical studies
> > Observational studies
> > > Case–control studies
> > > Cohort studies
> > Interventional studies
> > > Clinical trials
> > > Community trials

Types of epidemiological study

We now move on to consider how various epidemiological study designs help answer questions about health and health care.

Epidemiologists seek answers to the following questions:

- Description. What is the extent of disease or risk factors in this population?
- Prognosis. How does this disease progress, what is its natural history?
- Aetiology. What are the causes of disease? What risk factors increase the chance of becoming diseased?
- Prevention/treatment. How well does an intervention work to prevent or treat a condition?

Different types of study will help us answer the different questions above. Epidemiological studies can be divided into descriptive and analytical studies and they can be further subdivided.

Hennekens and Buring[1] classified epidemiological design strategies as shown in Box 2.2.

Descriptive studies help us to describe the health status of populations whereas *analytical* studies, which are observational in nature, are employed to test hypotheses or establish aetiology. Interventional studies provide us with information on what works to prevent or treat a disease.

Table 2.6. Summary of concepts

Concept	Definition	Comment
Dynamic population	Population in which person–time experience can accumulate from a changing group of individuals	Ideal in cohort studies as every one contributes to the denominator
Static population	Fixed population with no loss to follow up	Difficult to achieve as people tend to drop out of studies
Period prevalence	The number of existing cases of an illness during a period or interval, divided by the average population	A problem may arise with calculating period prevalence rates because of the difficulty of defining the most appropriate denominator
Point prevalence	The prevalence of a condition in a population at a given point in time	Prevalence data provide an indication of the extent of a condition and may have implications to the provision of services needed in a community
Incidence	Number of new cases	Used in cohort studies
Risk	Risk can be thought of as a probability of developing disease given a set of factors	Preventive measures try and address risk factors
Incidence rate	The proportion of new cases of the target disorder in the population at risk during a specified time interval. It is usual to define the disorder, the population, and the time, and is reported as a rate	Can be calculated in cohort studies
Relative Risk	Incidence among exposed/incidence among unexposed	Important in aetiological enquiries
Risk ratio	Another term for relative risk	Important in aetiological enquiries
Odds Ratio	Ratio of odds of exposure in cases and controls	Used for studying rate diseases
Absolute risk reduction	The absolute arithmetic difference in rates of unwanted outcomes between experimental and control participants in a trial, calculated as the experimental event rate (EER) minus the control event rate (CER)	Inverse of this provides numbers needed to treat (see below)
Number needed to treat (NNT)	The inverse of the absolute risk reduction or increase and the number of patients that need to be treated for one to benefit compared with a control NNT = 1/ARR	The ideal NNT is 1, where everyone has improved with treatment and no-one has with control. Broadly, the higher the NNT, the less effective is the intervention
Attributable risk	The rate of disease occurrence or death ('risk') in a group that is exposed to a particular factor, which can be attributed to that factor Attributable risk = (Incidence in exposed – Incidence in unexposed) × 100/incidence in exposed	This suggests the amount of disease that might be eliminated if the factor under study could be controlled or eliminated
Population attributable risk	What proportion of a population's disease or death experience is due to a particular cause Population attributable risk = Rate in population – Rate in non-exposed Or Population attributable risk = attributable risk × prevalence of exposure to risk factor in population	This provides an estimate of the amount by which the disease could be reduced in the population if the suspected factor is eliminated or modified

Descriptive studies

These studies attempt to describe patterns of diseases within and between populations. They seek to answer the question 'What is the extent of disease or risk factors in this population?' They often use routinely collected data to identify relationships between the prevalence of disease and other variables such as time, place and personal characteristics. Data collection can take place at the level of the population or individual.

Population studies

Here variables are measured at population or group level. These are also called correlation or ecological studies. In these studies the unit of analysis is an aggregate of individuals and information is collected on this group rather than on individual members. The statistical relationship between exposure and outcome is calculated using the correlation coefficient. The correlation between exposure and outcome can be positive or negative. An example of a population study would be an analysis of the childhood immunisation coverage at ward level using the Index of Multiple Deprivation. Here both deprivation (exposure) and immunisation coverage (outcome) are measured at ward level. However, there are two problems with this approach. Firstly, the observed association may be due to confounding factors (see below). Secondly, beware of the so-called '*ecological fallacy*'. Observations made at population or aggregate levels may not be true at an individual level. For example, it may not be true that all children living in deprived communities are unvaccinated and all those living in affluent wards are fully vaccinated. Ecological studies generate hypotheses but cannot be used to test them.

Individual studies

These are *case reports, case series* and *cross-sectional studies*. A case report describes the medical details of one case of disease. For example, this is helpful in the post-marketing surveillance of licensed drugs when rare adverse outcomes not found in original studies may be seen. Case series (descriptions of several patients) can also be useful in generating hypotheses for further testing.

In cross-sectional studies both exposure and outcome are measured at individual and population level at the same point in time. Classical examples are the health and lifestyle surveys undertaken in various populations. In the Health Survey for England various health determinants and health-status indicators are measured on a sample of the English population (see Chapter 7). The major disadvantage of this design is that it cannot determine whether the outcome preceded the exposure or was due to the exposure as both are measured simultaneously. Hence this design is not suitable to test hypotheses.

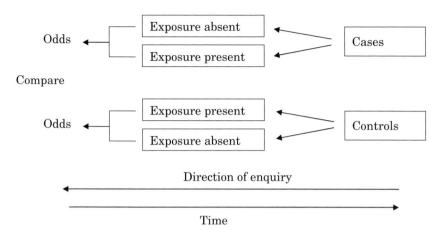

Fig. 2.6   A case–control study design.

Analytical studies

A better way to assess the strength of an association between a suspected risk factor and a disease is to perform a study which tries to analyse the effect of the proposed risk factor, while minimising interference from other variables such as age and sex, which might have an independent effect on the development of disease. Such variables are called confounding variables and are discussed in more detail later in this chapter. Analytical studies can be grouped into *observational* studies and *interventional* studies.

Observational studies are studies that describe the distribution of diseases in human populations and investigate possible aetiological factors to explain that distribution. The investigators have no control over who is or is not exposed to the factor under study. In interventional studies, the investigator decides who is exposed and who is not. Observational studies can be subdivided into *case–control* and *cohort* studies. Interventional studies can be subdivided into *clinical* trials and *community* trials.

Observational studies
(a) Case–Control studies

In this type of study people who have been identified as having the disease (the *cases*) are compared with people who do not have the disease (the *controls*) (Figure 2.6). Allocation to groups is on the basis of the presence or absence of disease. The investigator looks back (retrospectively) to discover if in the past the cases had more or less exposure to the proposed risk factor than the controls. Should this be the case then the investigator might conclude that there was, indeed, a relationship between exposure to the risk factor and development of disease (generally by calculating an Odds Ratio). It is important that the cases and the controls be as similar as possible (except for the presence of the disease) in order to reduce the effects of confounding variables. Failure to do this adequately leads to the introduction of *bias* into the results and may invalidate the study. Bias is discussed further later in the chapter.

A classic case–control study – oral contraceptives and pulmonary embolism[7]
In the late sixties, Vessey and Doll interviewed women who had been admitted to hospital with venous thrombosis or pulmonary embolism without medical causes (cases). The controls were women who had been admitted to the same hospital with other diseases and who were matched for age, marital status and parity. The investigators found that those who had pulmonary embolism were six times more likely to have used oral contraceptives compared to women who did not have the condition.

(b) Cohort studies
In a cohort study a comparison is made between subjects allocated to groups on the basis of their *exposure* to the proposed risk factor. The aim is to compare the development of the disease in an exposed group with that in an unexposed group. If the exposure occurred before the study started then the allocation to groups is done at the beginning of the trial and the exposed group compared with a selected, unexposed, control group. If, however, the exposure occurs during the study period then allocation is done at the end of the trial and those subjects who were not exposed act as the controls for those who were.

   All subjects are followed up to record the development of the disease and at the end of the trial the incidence of the disease in the exposed group is compared with the incidence in the unexposed group (usually calculated by a Relative Risk). Any difference between the two groups is likely to be due to the difference in their exposure to the risk factor provided that the groups are similar in regard to other factors such as age and sex. The evidence obtained from a cohort study is felt to be better than that from a case–control study because of the danger in the latter of introducing bias through inadequate selection of controls and the problems of reliable retrieval of historic information. Often a case–control study is followed by a cohort study when more evidence of an association is needed (Figure 2.7). However, cohort studies tend to be more time-consuming and expensive to perform.

A classic cohort study – the Whitehall study[8]   The Whitehall studies of civil servants study were set up in 1967 and included 18,000 men in the UK Civil Service. The first showed that men in the lowest employment grades were much more likely to die prematurely than men in the highest grades. The second Whitehall study that followed was set up to determine what underlies the social gradient in death and disease, and to include women. In 1985, all non-industrial civil

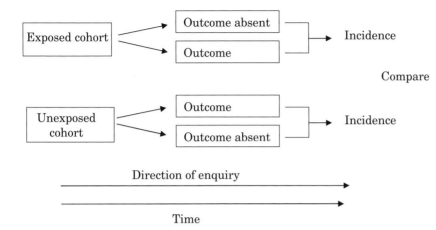

Fig. 2.7 A cohort study design.

servants aged between 35 and 55, in 20 departments in central London were invited to a cardiovascular medical examination at their workplace. The authors recruited 10,308 civil servants. This study found an inverse relationship between socio-economic position and the occurrence of coronary heart disease, diabetes and metabolic syndrome. A steep gradient in the incidence of coronary events with socio-economic status was observed in the study such that people of lowest socio-economic status were between two and three times more likely than the wealthiest to suffer coronary events.

Can you think of some of the possible reasons for the differences in health status observed among the civil servants?

Many differences between the civil servants could influence health status. These include their income and socio-economic status, access to and pattern of utilisation of health services, and lifestyle. For example, levels of smoking, obesity and physical activity could differ leading to increased risk of diabetes and heart disease.

Interventional studies

In interventional (sometimes called experimental) studies the investigators have control over who is and who is not exposed to the factor under investigation. Such intervention studies look at the effect of changing the exposure of the population to a factor. This is usually done by either removing a harmful factor or adding a beneficial or protective factor, and intervention studies provide information on prevention or treatment.

The whole population (termed the reference population) cannot be practically studied so two groups are chosen from the population to be representative. The reference group might be the whole population or those with a certain disease or condition. The desired intervention is administered to the intervention group while a placebo is administered to the control group.

Wherever possible it is important that the participants in the study have the same chance of being allocated to the intervention or control groups. The process of allocation is termed *randomisation*. A study where randomisation occurs between an intervention and control group is called a *randomised controlled trial* (RCT). It is regarded as the best form of evidence of association as the randomisation process should ensure that the two groups are similar except in terms of exposure to the intervention under study.

Both intervention and control groups are followed up and the development of disease in each group recorded. A significant difference in disease incidence between the groups may indicate that this was the result of the intervention and that the factor added or removed has a real effect on the development of the disease. Sometimes it is not possible to identify a control group and it may then be necessary to use the whole population before the intervention as an historical control against which the whole population after the intervention may be compared. These studies can be considered as cohort studies as they follow two groups of people over time to determine the outcome. The major difference is that the investigator has control over who is exposed and who is not. Intervention studies can be subdivided into clinical trials and community trials.

What measure of association do you expect to be used in intervention studies? Hint – remember these are similar to cohort studies
Relative risk.

(a) Clinical trials

These are studies of the effect of a specific treatment on patients who already have a particular disease, in comparison with another treatment (or a placebo) on a similar group of people, also with the disease (see Figure 2.8). These are normally only ethical when it is not known which of the treatments is more effective and the term used to denote this is *equipoise*.

Think through the following questions.
a. What do you understand by the term randomisation?
b. What do investigators attempt to achieve by randomisation?
c. What is the reference population?
d. Why are interventional studies regarded as providing better evidence?

a. The aim behind randomisation where study subjects are randomly allocated to the two groups (often termed as 'arms') in a trial is to produce comparable treatment and control groups.

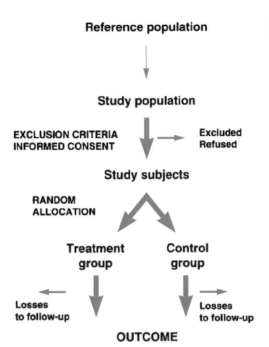

Fig. 2.8   Design of a clinical trial.

b. If it is effective, both known and unknown factors that could influence the outcome will be equally distributed between the two groups. This is the reason why the randomised controlled trial is such a powerful study design. Other epidemiological studies have to make statistical adjustments for known confounders.

c. The reference population is the population from which the study population is drawn and to which the results of the trial are to be extrapolated. If the study population is dissimilar to the reference population in some way (e.g. contains more people of one age group or sex or is generally sicker) then the results of the study may not be reliably applied to the rest of the population. This is called external validity a and discussed further later in the chapter.

d. Interventional studies are regarded as providing better evidence as they provide the best control for confounding factors so that we are able, with more certainty, to regard the results as truth.

A classic clinical trial – diabetes control [9]

In the Diabetes Control and Complications Trial (DCCT) a group of investigators from many centres tested whether intensive control of blood glucose in patients with insulin-dependent diabetes (IDDM) decreases long-term micro-vascular and neurological complications. Intensive control consisted of administration of insulin by external insulin pump or by three or more daily insulin injections and was guided by frequent blood-glucose monitoring. The control group received conventional therapy with one or two daily insulin injections. The researchers concluded that intensive therapy effectively delays the onset and slows the progression of diabetic retinopathy, nephropathy and neuropathy in patients with IDDM as the rate of neuropathy was around four times higher in the control group.

(b) Community trials

These trials are undertaken in community settings and the unit of intervention could be individuals, families or communities, or geographical areas.

A classical community trial – perinatal and maternal mortality in rural Pakistan[10]

This RCT involved randomising communities to the intervention and control groups. Seven subdistricts (talukas) of a rural district in Pakistan were randomised: three, were assigned to the intervention group where traditional birth attendants were trained and issued disposable delivery kits; female health workers linked traditional birth attendants with established services and documented processes and outcomes; and obstetric teams provided outreach clinics for antenatal care. Women in the four control talukas received usual care and there was no additional input from the research team. The authors concluded that training traditional birth attendants and integrating them into an improved health-care system were achievable and effective in reducing perinatal mortality as the Odds Ratio for perinatal death was 0.7 and that for maternal mortality was 0.74 in the study group.

Summary

Table 2.7 summarises the main features of the different types of epidemiological study.

Interpreting results of epidemiological studies

Before we conclude that the results of studies are valid (true), we need to consider the factors that might fully or partly explain the observed results. They include *chance* and *error* (random or systematic).

Chance

The observed results of a study could be due to chance. The effects of chance are quantified using statistical techniques and the two common measures employed are probability (*P value*) and *confidence interval* (CI). These are explained here but readers are advised to refer to statistical texts to expand further their knowledge in this area [11, 12].

Table 2.7. Main features of the different types of epidemiological study

Design	Descriptive/ Observational/ Interventional	Retrospective/ Prospective	Aim	Specific comparison group/No such group
Case-series (clinical and population)	Descriptive	Retrospective	Describes diseases in individuals	No
Cross-sectional	Descriptive	Retrospective	Describes disease or risk factors in populations	Usually not
Case-control	Observational	Retrospective	Examines causes of disease	Yes
Cohort (prospective and retrospective)	Observational	Prospective and retrospective	Examines causes of disease and/or outcomes due to exposure to risk factors	Usually, yes (though it may be integral to the study population)
Trial	Interventional	Prospective	Tests effectiveness of interventions to prevent or treat disease	Yes, with exceptions

The P value is the probability (ranging from zero to one) that the results observed in a study (or results more extreme) could have occurred by chance. Convention is that we accept a P value of 0.05 or below as being statistically significant and we call this the significance level. This means that when a P value of less than 0.05 is quoted it suggests that the association is real and not due just to chance. Because this means that 5% of the time (one time in 20) we would find an association purely by chance, when we are making many comparisons we often use a P value of 0.01, so that P values of 0.01 or below are deemed statistically significant and signify a real association.

The confidence interval (CI) quantifies the uncertainty in measurement. It is defined as 'a range of values for a variable of interest constructed so that this range has a specified probability of including the true value of the variable.' The range of values is called the confidence interval, and the end points of the confidence interval are called confidence limits. It is conventional to create confidence intervals at the 95% level – this means that 95% of the time properly constructed confidence intervals should contain the true variable of interest. One useful feature of confidence intervals is that one can easily tell whether or not statistical significance has been reached, just as when using the P value. If the confidence interval interval spans the value reflecting 'no effect' (e.g. the value 1 for a relative risk), this represents a difference that is not statistically significant. If the confidence interval does not enclose the value reflecting 'no effect' this represents a difference that is statistically significant. Apart from statistical inference, confidence intervals show the largest and smallest effects that are likely, given the observed data.

Error

Estimates of measures of associations such as Relative Risk and Odds Ratio may differ from their true value. This may be a result of random error or of systematic error. Random error results in an estimate being equally likely to be above or below the true value. Systematic error, which is caused by a consistent discrepancy in the measurement, results in an estimate being above or below the true value, depending on the direction of the discrepancy. For example, while measuring blood pressure random error could occur due to the time of measurement, the status of the person whose blood pressure is measured and random fluctuations. However, the causes of systematic error are different: for example, use of the wrong cuff size and deafness in the person making the measurement. In observational studies there is a greater potential for various biases to be introduced that need to be addressed.

Random error

The major cause of random error in epidemiological studies is *sampling error* caused simply by the random nature of the sample.

Random error means that we might conclude that there is no association when there is one. This is called a *type II* or beta error and is harmful as we do not become aware of risk factors for disease or effective treatments. A study must be designed with sufficient *power* to detect an association if one exists. Power is often increased by increasing the sample size in the study or by optimising the ratio of cases to controls, or exposed to unexposed.

Random error might also lead us to conclude that there is an association where none exists. This is potentially more harmful as we may decide to intervene in an ineffective way based on these results (e.g. to give an ineffective drug with potentially adverse effects). This is named *type I* or alpha error. Setting a significance level of 0.05 means that there will be a 5% chance of making an alpha error and, if the potential harms are great, we might set an alpha level (significant *P* value) of 0.01.

Sampling error cannot be eliminated, but one of the aims of good study design is to reduce it to an acceptable level within the constraints imposed by the availability of finite resources. Ways to reduce random error include taking multiple readings and training those taking measurements to ensure standardisation.

Systematic error

Systematic error may take one of three main forms, selection bias, information bias or confounding.

Selection bias   This is a major problem in case-control studies where it gives rise to non-comparability between cases and controls. It is found when cases (or controls) are chosen to be included in (or excluded from) a study by using criteria that are related to exposure to the risk factor under investigation.

Example. In a case control study of the aetiology of lung cancer, controls were selected from people who were suffering from non-malignant respiratory disease. Smoking is a cause of chronic bronchitis and thus the controls would have a higher prevalence of smoking than the population from which the people with lung cancer was drawn. As a consequence, the strength of the association between smoking and lung cancer would be underestimated. The controls should have been selected from the general population, which would have avoided this bias.

Much of the effort that goes into the design of good case-control studies is spent on the careful selection of controls in order to eliminate selection bias.

Information bias   This involves study subjects being misclassified either according to their disease status, their exposure status, or both. Differential misclassification occurs when errors in classification of disease status are dependent upon exposure status or vice versa. For example, in a case–control study, a case's recall of his or her past 'exposure' to risk factors may differ from the recall of a control because the process of having the disease will have caused the person to think much more about possible exposures than is the case for the controls.

Example. In a case–control study investigating the association between congenital defects in new-born babies and maternal exposure to X-rays, women with babies with congenital defects are more likely to recall their X-rays due to apparent association. The effect of this would be to over-estimate the strength of association, as the cases would appear to have a higher exposure to the risk factor.

Confounding   This occurs when an estimate of the association between an exposure and a disease is confused because another exposure, linked to both, has not been taken into account. For a variable to be a confounder, it must be associated with the exposure under study and it must also be independently associated with disease risk in its own right (see Figure 2.9). Both these criteria are met in the two examples below.

Example 1. Consider a study of the association between work in a particular occupation and the risk of lung cancer. A comparison of death rates due to lung cancer in the occupational group and in the general population may appear to show that the occupational group has an increased risk of lung cancer. If this still persists after taking into account the different age structures of the two groups, it is necessary to consider whether people in the occupational group smoke more (or less) heavily than people in the general population. If this is not taken into account, the inference is invalid.

Example 2. Age at menopause may confound estimates of the association between replacement oestrogens (taken for relief of menopausal symptoms) and breast-cancer risk. This is because an early age at menopause is associated with both a reduced risk of breast cancer and a greater use of replacement oestrogens.

Fig. 2.9   Confounding

- The relationship can be considered as triangular

- The spurious confounded association results from one of the causes of disease (confounding factor) being associated with the apparent risk factor

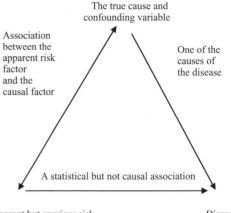

The true cause and confounding variable

Association between the apparent risk factor and the causal factor

One of the causes of the disease

A statistical but not causal association

Apparent but spurious risk factor for disease

Disease

Confounding may be avoided by appropriate study design, as could be achieved in Example 2 by only studying women who had their menopause at a particular range of ages. However, it may also be controlled for in the analysis, provided that the confounding factors have been identified and information on them has been collected. The control of confounding at analysis is a widely used strategy, much of the statistical methodology in epidemiology being concerned with this issue.

For each of the examples a–c consider the following questions:
- **What is the apparent association?**
- **What else might cause the outcome and could it also be related to the apparent cause?**
- **Therefore what is the confounded factor and what is the confounding (causal) factor?**
- **How can we check whether the possible confounder is having an effect?**
    a. **People who drink alcohol have a raised risk of lung cancer**
    b. **People living in an affluent seaside resort have a higher mortality rate than the country as a whole**
    c. **African Americans are heavier users of crack cocaine than 'white' Americans**

See Table 2.8.

As can be seen from the exercise above, we need to consider the potential confounders before we conclude that the association is causal. In case (b) although we observe higher mortality in coastal towns this is not due to the geographical area but the different age structure between resort towns and other areas of the

Table 2.8. Confounding questions answered

The confounded association	One possible explanation	The confounded factor	The confounding (causal) factor	To check the assumption
a. People who drink alcohol have a raised risk of lung cancer	Alcohol drinking and smoking are behaviours which go together	Alcohol which is a marker for, on average, smoking more cigarettes	Tobacco which is associated with both alcohol and with the disease	See if the alcohol–lung cancer relationship holds in people not exposed to tobacco: if it does, tobacco is not a confounder
b. People living in an affluent seaside resort have a higher mortality rate than the country as a whole	A holiday town attracts the elderly, so has a comparatively old population	Living in a resort is a marker for being, on average, older	Age which is associated with both living in a resort and with death	Look at each age group specifically, or use age standardisation to take into account age differences
c. African Americans are heavier users of crack cocaine than 'white' Americans	Poor people living in the American inner city are particularly likely to become dependent on illicit drugs	Belonging to the racial category 'African American'	Poverty and the pressures of inner-city living, including the easy availability of drugs	Use statistical techniques to adjust for the influence of a number of complex socio-economic factors

country. Resort towns tend to have a higher proportion of elderly as people tend to settle in these areas after retirement. Here age is a potential confounder because it is a surrogate for age-related causal factors. There are various ways of tackling confounders including advanced statistical techniques such as multivariate analysis.

Validity (truth)

Once we have established that the results from the epidemiological studies are not due to chance or error (including confounding) we need to determine if our results are *valid* and if any association seen is causal. Validity is the extent to which a variable or intervention measures what it is supposed to measure, or accomplishes what it is supposed to accomplish.

In the context of epidemiological studies validity has two components, internal and external validity. The *internal validity* of a study refers to the integrity of the experimental design and relates to inferences about the study population itself. The *external validity* of a study refers to the appropriateness by which its results can be applied to non-study patients or populations. This will depend upon the similarities or otherwise between study population and the population to which the results are extrapolated. This is often termed the generalisability of a study.

When we are assured that the results of a study are valid we can consider, where relevant, the issue of *causality*. Much of epidemiology seeks to relate causes to the effects they produce, that is, determine aetiology. Epidemiological evidence by itself is rarely sufficient to establish causality, but it can provide powerful circumstantial evidence. A statistical association between two or more events or other variables may be produced under various circumstances. The presence of an association does not necessarily imply a causal relationship.

To learn more about aetiology, associations between the disease and the hypothesised cause resulting from natural experiments must be observed. According to Hill, causality is more likely if the association can be shown [13] to be:

1. strong (e.g. is statistically significant and has a large relative risk)
2. dose-related (i.e. the greater the risk factor the greater the effects)
3. in the right time sequence (cohort studies show that exposure precedes outcome)
4. independent of recognised confounding factors
5. consistent between different studies (We are more likely to believe an association which has been demonstrated several times and we now look for systematic reviews and meta-analyses to increase our confidence in associations.)
6. plausible. However we need to be aware that this may not always be necessary because as medical science advances all the time and some of the biological mechanisms will evolve in future years. In the 1980s, HIV/AIDS research was in its earliest stages. A relationship was discovered between the incidence of AIDS-like symptoms in homosexual men (the largest portion of the population displaying these symptoms at the time), and the use of alkyl nitrites, more commonly called 'poppers'. As science stood at that time the biological agent had not been identified and various mechanisms were put forward including the 'poppers' hypothesis[14]'. However, with the discovery of the causative agent, all these theories disappeared and a biological mechanism was established.
7. Reversible (removing the exposure should remove the risk).

Two kinds of cause are sometimes distinguished. A necessary cause is one whose presence is required for the occurrence of the effect. A sufficient cause is one which can cause the effect alone. In practice most causal factors are neither necessary nor sufficient, but contributory.

In this chapter we have described the ways in which we measure the extent of health problems within and between populations and the scientific basis for conclusions we reach on disease causality, prevention and treatment. Without this knowledge we cannot know where best to concentrate our efforts to have the greatest effect on population health. We recommend the accompanying book in this series which provides a more detailed coverage of the field of epidemiology [15]. The next chapter continues this theme and looks at how we judge the strength of evidence on which we base health care decisions.

FURTHER READING

Huw T. O. Davies. What are confidence intervals? *Hayward Communications*, **3** (1), 1–8. (www.evidence-based-medicine.co.uk/ebmfiles/WhatareConfInter.pdf)

D. E. Lilienfeld and P. D. Stolley, *Foundations in Epidemiology*, New York, Oxford University Press, 1994.

J. Deeks, Swots corner: What is an odds ratio? *Bandolier*, **25**, March 1996. Available online at www.jr2.ox.ac.uk/Bandolier/band25/b25-6.html.

J. M. Last, *A Dictionary of Epidemiology*, 4th edn, New York, Oxford University Press, 2001.

REFERENCES

1. C. Hennekens and J. Burling *Epidemiology in Medicine*, Boston, MA, Little, Brown and Company, 1987.
2. Hippocrates. *The Genuine Works of Hippocrates*, transl. Frances Adams, Baltimore, MD, Williams & Wilkins, 1939.
3. *Genes, Behavior, and the Social Environment: Moving Beyond the Nature/Nurture Debate*. National Academic Press, Washington, DC, 2006.
4. G. Rose, Sick individuals and sick populations. *International Journal of Epidemiology*, **30** (3), 2001, 427–32.
5. R. Doll and A. B. Hill, The mortality of doctors in relation to their smoking habits; a preliminary report. *British Medical Journal*, **228**, 1954, 1451–5.
6. R. Doll, and R. Peto, Mortality in relation to smoking: 20 years' observations on male British doctors. *British Medical Journal*, **273**, 1976, 1525–36.
7. M. P. Vessey and R. Doll, Investigation of relation between use of oral contraceptives and thromboembolic disease. *British Medical Journal*, 1968, **2**, 199–205.
8. J. E. Ferrie, P. Martikainen, M. J. Shipley and M. G. Marmot, Self-reported economic difficulties and coronary events in men: evidence from the Whitehall II study. *International Journal of Epidemiology*, **34** (3), 2005, 640–8.
9. The Diabetes Control and Complications Trial Research Group. The effect of intensive treatment of diabetes on the development and progression of long-term complications in insulin-dependent diabetes mellitus. *New England Journal of Medicine*, **329** (14), 1993, 977–86.
10. A. H. Jokhio, H. R. Winter and K. K. Cheng, An intervention involving traditional birth attendants and perinatal and maternal mortality in Pakistan. *New England Journal of Medicine*, **352** (20), 2005, 2091–9.
11. D. G. Altman, *Practical Statistics for Medical Research*, London, Chapman & Hall/CRC, 1991.
12. B. R. Kirkwood and J. A. C. Sterne, *Essential Medical Statistics*, 2nd edn, Oxford, Blackwell Science, 2003.

13. A. B. Hill, The environment and disease: association or causation? *Proceedings of the Royal Society of Medicine*, **58**, 1965, 295–300. (online at www.edwardtufte.com/tufte/hill)

14. J. P. Vandenbroucke and V. P. Pardoel, An autopsy of epidemiologic methods: the case of "poppers" in the early epidemic of the acquired immunodeficiency syndrome (AIDS). *American Journal of Epidemiology*, **129** (3), 455–7.

15. P. Webb, C. Bain and S. Pirozzo, *Essential Epidemiology. An Introduction for Students and Health Professionals*, Cambridge, Cambridge University Press, 2005.

3

Evidence-based health care

Key points

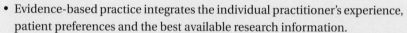

- Evidence-based practice integrates the individual practitioner's experience, patient preferences and the best available research information.
- Incorporating the best available research evidence in decision making involves five steps: *asking* answerable questions; *accessing* the best information; *appraising* the information for validity and relevance; *applying* the information to care of patients and populations; and *auditing* that same care for evidence of change.
- Although practitioners need basic skills in finding evidence, a health librarian is an invaluable asset.
- There are specific checklists available to appraise research papers critically, and every practitioner should possess the skills to appraise the published literature.
- The major barriers to implementing evidence-based practice include the impression by practitioners that their professional freedom is being taken away, lack of access to appropriate tools and resource constraints.
- Various incentives including financial ones are used to encourage evidence-based practice.

Introduction – what is evidence-based health care?

How much of what health and other professionals do is based soundly in science? Answers to the question 'is our practice evidence based?' depend on what we mean by practice and what we mean by evidence. Some studies have estimated that less than 20% of all health-care interventions are underpinned by robust research [1]. This varies from discipline to discipline. For example, studies

Essential Public Health, eds. Stephen Gillam, Jan Yates and Padmanabhan Badrinath.
Published by Cambridge University Press. © Cambridge University Press 2007.

examining clinical decisions in the field of internal medicine found that most primary therapeutic clinical decisions are based on evidence from randomised controlled trials [2].

Sackett [3] defined evidence-based medicine (EBM) as 'the conscientious, explicit, and judicious use of current best evidence in making decisions about the care of individual patients. The practice of evidence based medicine means integrating individual clinical expertise with the best available external clinical evidence from systematic research' [3]. The expansion of EBM has been a major influence on clinical practice over the last ten years. The demands of purchasers of health care keen to optimise value for money have been one driver. A growing awareness among health professionals and their patients of medicine's potential to cause harm has been another. Since the early nineties, EBM has steadily embraced other disciplines and public health is no exception. Public health practitioners with limited resources need to target resources efficiently. Public health interventions are often costly and policy makers need evidence to invest appropriately. In this chapter we examine the nature of what is nowadays more broadly referred to as evidence-based health care (EBHC) and discuss its limitations.

The tools necessary for EBHC

The tools needed to practice in an evidence-based way are common across disciplines. Doctors, public health practitioners, nurses and allied health professionals all need the skills to ensure that the work they do, whether with individual clients or patients, or in the development of programmes and policies, is based on sound knowledge of what is likely to work.

Of the following five essential steps, the first is probably the most important:
- convert information needs into answerable questions, i.e. by asking a focussed question
- track down best evidence
- appraise evidence critically
- change practice in the light of evidence
- evaluate your performance.

Step 1. Asking a focussed question

Before seeking the best evidence, you need to convert your information needs into a tightly focussed question. For example, it is not enough to ask 'Does aspirin help patients with myocardial infarction (heart attack)?' We need to convert this into an answerable question: 'Does treating patients who have had a heart attack with aspirin, as opposed to not treating with aspirin, reduce subsequent risk of death (mortality)?'

The PICO approach can be used as a framework to focus a question by considering the necessary elements. It contains four components (shown below with our aspirin question from above as an example):

Patient or the population (patients who have had a heart attack)

Intervention (aspirin)

Comparison intervention (no aspirin)

Outcome (mortality)

For example, suppose you want to find the evidence for the effectiveness of using steroids in adults with tuberculosis of the covering of the brain, i.e. TB meningitis. Form a focussed clinical question using the PICO format.

patient or the population – adults with TB meningitis

intervention – using steroids

comparison – not using steroids

outcome – mortality

This gives us the question 'How effective at reducing mortality is using steroids in adults with TB meningitis compared with not using steroids?'

Some practitioners add a fifth element to the question – time. It may be important to determine the timeframe, for example when using aspirin after a heart attack we may only be interested in mortality in the subsequent three months, but when considering the effectiveness of cancer treatment we might want to know about mortality rates after five years.

Step 2. Tracking down the evidence

The second step in the practice of evidence-based health care is to track down best evidence.

Doctors may all too easily assess outcomes in terms of surrogate pathological end points rather than commonplace changes in quality of life or the ability to perform routine activities ('the operation was a success but the patient died'). Traditionally, doctors making decisions about what works have attached much weight to personal experience or the views of respected colleagues. Over time, doctors' knowledge of up-to-date care diminishes [4] so there is a constant need for the latest evidence and simple ways to access and use it. A study of North American physicians has shown that up-to-date clinical information is needed twice for every three patients seen but they only receive 30% of this due to lack of time, dated textbooks and disorganised journals[5].

So, rather than rely on colleagues or textbooks, EBHC encourages the use of research evidence in a systematic way. Once a question has been formulated, the research base is then searched to find articles of relevance.

Table 3.1. Levels of evidence

I–1	A well done systematic review for two or more RCTs
I–2	An RCT
II–1	A cohort study
II–2	A case–control study
II–3	A dramatic uncontrolled experiment
III	Respected authorities, expert committees, etc . . .
IV	Someone once told me . . .

So what do we look for? What is evidence? Care needs to be taken in relying on published articles. Many reviews reflect the prejudices of their authors and are anything but systematic. Even mainstream journals have a propensity to accept papers yielding positive rather than negative findings, e.g. in assessing treatments (so-called 'publication bias' [6]). Most books date rapidly. Hence the prominence nowadays accorded properly conducted systematic reviews at the top of the hierarchy of evidence. A widely used ranking of the strength of evidence is shown in Table 3.1.

This list reminds us of the three main types of epidemiological study: descriptive, observational and interventional, which were considered in Chapter 2. When searching for evidence we should look for the highest level suitable to our question. A question relating to the effectiveness of an intervention will most appropriately be answered by a randomised controlled trial (RCT). The RCT is the gold standard as robust randomisation ensures that study and control groups differ only in terms of their exposure to the factor under study; the observed results are due only to the intervention and not to confounding variables. We can find answers to questions about the causes of a disease from case–control or cohort studies. However, questions beginning 'Why?' are often not answered by these kinds of study. Not all that is measurable is of value, and not all that is of value can be measured. What factors, after all, go to make a 'good nurse' or a 'good public health practitioner' and how easily are they measured? It is not possible to answer the question 'Why do women refuse an offer of breast screening?' with any of the study types mentioned so far. Another example would be: 'What leads to inappropriate use of medicines in elderly inpatients?' In these cases one looks for a qualitative study. Qualitative studies use methods such as interviews, diaries and direct observation to provide detailed information to describe the experiences of participants. Qualitative data are then analysed rigorously to lead to conclusions. Detailed coverage of qualitative methodology is beyond the scope of this book (see Pope and Mays' book [7] for an introduction to this topic) but it is important to remember that not every question can be answered using the classical hierarchy above. Qualitative methods can generate a wealth of knowledge to contextualise many of the decisions health professionals must make.

Evidence-based practitioners need to be aware of two key concepts in determining what is evidence: clinical effectiveness and cost-effectiveness. Clinical effectiveness can be pragmatically defined as the extent to which an intervention achieves the aims for which it is designed. This applies similarly to public health interventions. Cost-effectiveness is discussed in Chapter 9. However, what counts as effectiveness varies from the vantage point of patient and professional reflecting the different meanings they attach to the condition under treatment, the intervention and outcomes desired. The continuing debate over the proper place of complementary therapies in the NHS nicely illustrates these different vantage points.

Why do patients continue to use interventions, e.g. complementary therapies, which professionals consider to be ineffective?

Doctors are sceptical of their benefits on the basis of scientific evaluations which show either that most such therapies are not effective or that there is no evidence that they are [8]. The public continue to use them, presumably because they meet personal needs that conventional treatments do not. The professionals' view of complementary therapies is reflected in the campaign to restrict their use in the NHS[7].

Consider the questions below. What studies would be most appropriately conducted to answer them: RCT, cohort, case–control, cross-sectional, qualitative?

a. For what conditions do patients call their GP out of hours?

b. What are the barriers to handwashing in a hospital setting?

c. Does paternal exposure to ionising radiation before conception cause childhood leukaemia?

d. What is the most sensitive and specific method of screening for genital chlamydial infection in women attending general practice?

e. Does laparoscopic cholecystectomy cause less morbity and a swifter return to work than a small-incision cholecystectomy?

f. Do clinicians change their practice as a result of education?

g. For a given patient with asthma, does beclamethasone give better symptomatic control than fluticasone?

h. How do patients and carers view the service provided by a mental health team?

i. How does smoking cessation affect the risk of stroke in middle-aged men?

j. Is this new vaccine effective against bird flu?

k. Do cooking sessions and information provision improve people's diet in deprived community settings?

a. cross-sectional study
b. qualitative study
c. case–control study
d. cross-sectional study
e. randomised controlled trial
f. cohort study
g. randomised controlled trial
h. qualitative study
i. cohort study
j. randomised controlled trial
k. cohort study

There are various sources of evidence. These include primary and secondary sources of literature. Primary sources are the thousands of original papers published every year in research journals. However, to deal with the vast amount of information available, more and more people now turn to secondary sources of evidence and the single most important source of systematic reviews is the Cochrane Database (www.cochrane.org/). The Cochrane Collaboration (named after Archie Cochrane, an early pioneer of EBM) is an international endeavour to summarise high-quality evidence in all fields of medical practice. It has slowly transformed many areas of clinical practice. In the accompanying CD you will find more information about the Cochrane Library and relevant internet links.

So, it is important to have basic skills in searching the literature, although the help of expert librarians may be needed. Research papers are catalogued in a variety of databases searchable on the internet. For many medical or public health queries the database Medline is a good starting place. Other databases are available for specialist queries such as those in the fields of mental health and nursing. Using the PICO format here is helpful as it can be used to generate search terms with which to query the databases. Databases may have tools to support the user in this such as the 'Clinical Queries' tool in PubMed (which is a US National Library of Medicine's service to search the biomedical research literature; www.ncbi.nlm.nih.gov/entrez/query/static/clinical.shtml)

We can use our example question from earlier to demonstrate how a search might work. Our focussed question was 'How effective at reducing mortality is using steroids in adults with TB meningitis compared with not using steroids?'

What study type would be appropriate for answering this question?
Randomised controlled trials are possible, where participants with TB meningitis are randomised to receive steroid or a placebo, to give a measure of the relative effectiveness of steroid treatment.

Using the PICO format, list the keywords we need to use to search databases through a search function such as PubMed's Clinical Queries.

Adults, TB meningitis, steroids, mortality. In Clinical Queries, as we select an option to indicate our interest is in therapy (i.e. intervention studies) the term 'randomised controlled trial' is automatically added to the keywords. In other search systems or databases this may need to be added manually.

The journal articles found using this strategy are:

1. G. E. Thwaites, D. B. Nguyen, H. D. Nguyen *et al.,* Dexamethasone for the treatment of tuberculous meningitis in adolescents and adults. *New England Journal of Medicine,* **351**(17), 2004, 1741–51.

2. S. Kumarvelu, K. Prasad, A. Khosla *et al.,* Randomized controlled trial of dexamethasone in tuberculous meningitis. *Tubercular Lung Disease,* **75**(3), 1994, 203–7.

3. N. I. Girgis, Z. Farid, M. E. Kilpatrick *et al.,* Dexamethasone adjunctive treatment for tuberculous meningitis. *Pediatric Infectious Disease Journal,* **10**(3), 1991, 179–83.

Look at the result above. Are these articles relevant?

Yes. The chemical name for the steroid is dexamethasone. The first presents the results of a study published in the *New England Journal of Medicine.*

In the search for evidence it should be remembered that not every piece of information which might help us answer our question may be published. Studies may be in progress which could inform our action; negative studies, which could help tell us what NOT to do, may not have made it as far as a publication; many pharmaceutical companies have unpublished information; conference reports might provide helpful information. As we move down the hierarchy it becomes more difficult to find this kind of evidence (called 'grey' literature) from readily available sources but some databases and repositories are available. This is a good time to seek the help of an expert librarian!

Refer to the CD for more exercises to develop your skills in searching the literature to answer your questions.

Step 3. Appraising the evidence

To be able to determine whether we should act on the results of the studies found in the search we must be able critically to appraise a range of study types. It is important to have an understanding of the basic epidemiological concepts outlined in Chapter 2, to be able to understand the results presented and to have a systematic approach to the appraisal. In brief, we are looking to determine whether we believe the results sufficiently to act on them and change our practice. In order to do this we ask a series of question about the study which include:

- Did the research ask a clearly focussed question and carry out the right sort of study to answer it?
- Were the study methods robust?
- Do the conclusions made match the results of the study?
- Can we use these results in our practice? This might include an assessment of whether the results are 'big' enough to make a real difference and whether the same results are likely to occur in our own situation.

There are standard checklists available to support systematic appraisal of different types of study designs. We can use these to help determine how valid the findings of the study are, and whether the findings can be generalised to our own population.

Table 3.2 shows a checklist for appraising a randomised controlled trial, the most appropriate primary design to generate evidence of effective interventions. This checklist is taken from the critical appraisal skills programme (CASP) in Oxford (see www.phru.nhs.uk/learning/casp_rct_tool.pdf).

It is important to be able to analyse critically the results of all study types but, as the volume of scientific literature increases, it is perhaps most important to be able to use systematic reviews effectively to guide practice. It has been estimated that a general physician needs to read for 119 hours a week to keep up to date; medical students are alleged to spend 1–2 hours reading clinical material per week – and that's more than the doctors who teach them [9]. Also, a single study of insufficient sample size or of otherwise poor quality may yield misleading results. The right answer to a specific question is more likely to come from a systematic review. This is a review of all the literature on a particular topic, which has been methodically identified, appraised and presented. The statistical combination of all the results from included studies to provide a summary estimate or definitive result is called meta-analysis.

Antman's classic study of research into the effectiveness of thrombolysis demonstrates the importance of systematic review and meta-analysis for proponents of EBM [10]. The first study, showing that streptokinase reduced mortality following myocardial infarction, was published in 1960. The results of Antman's meta-analysis are shown in Figure 3.1. Whilst early RCTs showed a treatment effect (Odds Ratio below 1), the confidence intervals around these effect-size estimates were wide, showing imprecision, and went above 1, which indicates the possibility of no effect. The power of meta-analysis is clearly demonstrated by the narrowing of these confidence intervals as the number of RCTs increased. From around 1970 the beneficial effect of thrombolysis seems clearly apparent but some thirty years after the first RCT and nearly twenty years after meta-analysis might have decided the question, thrombolytics were still not being routinely recommended in clinical practice. Because reviews have not always used scientific methods, advice on some life-saving therapies has often been delayed. Other treatments have been recommended long after controlled trials have shown them to be harmful.

Table 3.2. The CASP critical appraisal tool for randomised controlled trials

Screening questions

1. Did the study ask a clearly focused question?

Yes / No / Can't tell

Consider if the question is 'focused' in terms of:

the population studied

the intervention given

the outcomes considered

2. Was this a randomised controlled trial (RCT) and was it appropriately so?

Yes / No / Can't tell

Consider:

why this study was carried out as an RCT

if this was the right research approach for the question being asked

Is it worth continuing?

Detailed questions

3. Were participants appropriately allocated to intervention and control groups?

Yes / No / Can't tell

Consider:

how participants were allocated to intervention and control groups. Was the process truly random?

whether the method of allocation was described. Was a method used to balance the randomisation, e.g. stratification?

how the randomisation schedule was generated and how a participant was allocated to a study group

if the groups were well balanced. Are any differences between the groups at entry to the trial reported?

if there were differences reported that might have explained any outcome(s) (confounding)

4. Were participants, staff and study personnel 'blind' to participants' study group?

Yes / No / Can't tell

Consider:

the fact that blinding is not always possible

if every effort was made to achieve blinding

if you think it matters in this study

the fact that we are looking for 'observer bias'

5. Were all of the participants who entered the trial accounted for at its conclusion?

Yes / No / Can't tell

Consider:

if any intervention-group participants got a control-group option or vice versa

if all participants were followed up in each study group (was there loss-to-follow-up?)

if all the participants' outcomes were analysed by the groups to which they were originally allocated (intention-to-treat analysis)

what additional information you would like to have seen to make you feel better about this

Table 3.2. (*cont.*)

6. Were the participants in all groups followed up and data collected in the same way?

Yes / No / Can't tell

Consider:

> *if, for example, they were reviewed at the same time intervals and if they received the same amount of attention from researchers and health workers. Any differences may introduce performance bias.*

7. Did the study have enough participants to minimise the play of chance?

Yes / No / Can't tell

Consider:

> *if there is a power calculation. This will estimate how many participants are needed to be reasonably sure of finding something important (if it really exists and for a given level of uncertainty about the final result).*

8. How are the results presented and what is the main result?

Consider:

> *if, for example, the results are presented as a proportion of people experiencing an outcome such as risks, or as a measurement, such as mean or median differences, or as survival curves and hazards*
>
> *how large this size of result is and how meaningful it is*
>
> *how you would sum up the bottom-line result of the trial in one sentence*

9. How precise are these results?

Consider:

> *if the result is precise enough to make a decision*
>
> *if a confidence interval were reported, would your decision about whether or not to use this intervention be the same at the upper confidence limit as at the lower confidence limit?*
>
> *if a p-value is reported where confidence intervals are unavailable*

10. Were all important outcomes considered so the results can be applied?

Yes / No / Can't tell

Consider whether:

> *the people included in the trial could be different from your population in ways that would produce different results*
>
> *your local setting differs much from that of the trial*
>
> *you can provide the same treatment in your setting*

Consider outcomes from the point of view of the:

> *individual*
>
> *policy maker and professionals*
>
> *family/carers*
>
> *wider community*

Consider whether:

> *any benefit reported outweighs any harm and/or cost. If this information is not reported can it be filled in from elsewhere?*
>
> *policy or practice should change as a result of the evidence contained in this trial*

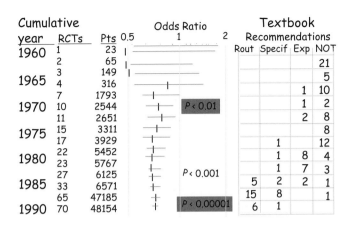

Fig. 3.1 Results of meta-analyses of thrombolysis for myocardial infarction (MI), according to when they could have been carried out, and the textbook recommendations at the time (Pts = patients): routine, in specified circumstances as experimental treatment or not recommended.

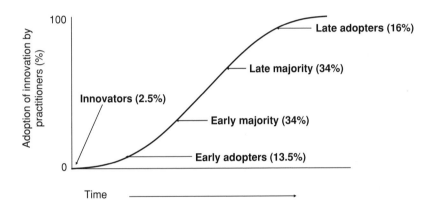

Fig. 3.2 Diffusion of innovation.

Step 4. Changing practice in light of evidence

Actually following through on the results of your appraisal of new evidence – implementation – is the most difficult of the five steps. Some change can be self-initiated; other circumstances require change in those around you. The implementation of effective public health interventions often requires change in others and public health practitioners often act as advocates for EBHC encouraging other professionals to act on results of an assessment of the evidence base. The management of people and an understanding of how they will react are invaluable. Everett Rogers' classic model [11] of how people take up innovations helps to understand different people's responses to change (Figure 3.2). It was based on observations on how farmers took up hybrid seed corn in Iowa. The model describes the differential rate of uptake of an innovation, in order to target promotion of the product, and labels people according to their place on the uptake curve. Rogers' original model described the 'late adopters' as 'laggards' but this seems a pejorative term when there may be good reasons not to take up the innovation. How soon after their introduction, for example, should nurses and doctors be prescribing new, usually more expensive, inhalers for asthma?

Individuals' 'change type' may depend on the particular change they are adopting. This depends on the perceived benefits, the perceived obstacles, and the motivation to make the change. People are more likely to adopt an innovation if it has the following attributes [12]:

- Relative advantage – the degree to which an innovation is perceived as better than the idea it supersedes. The higher the perceived relative advantage, the more likely the innovation will be adopted.
- Compatibility – the degree to which an innovation is perceived as consistent with the existing values, past experiences and needs of potential adopters. If the innovation is perceived as an extreme change, then it will not be compatible with past experiences and is less likely to be adopted.
- Complexity – the degree to which an innovation is perceived as relatively difficult to understand and use. Innovations that are perceived as complex are less likely to be adopted.
- Observability – the degree to which the results of an innovation are visible to others. If the observed effects are perceived to be small or non-existent, then the likelihood of adoption is reduced.
- 'Trialability' – the degree to which an innovation may be experimented with on a limited basis. This may include trying out parts of a program or having the opportunity to watch others using a new program. Trialability is positively related to the likelihood of adoption.

Pharmaceutical companies use this model in their approaches to nurses and doctors. Good local sales representatives know who in their area is an early adopter. Early adopters are often opinion leaders in a community. Early on in the process of promotion they will target those people with personal visits, whereas they may send the late adopters an information leaflet only, as the latter will not consider change until more than 80% of their colleagues have taken up the new product.

Anyone hoping to change people's behaviour is looking for the 'tipping point'[13]. This is the point or threshold at which an idea or behaviour takes off, moving from uncommon to common. You see it in many areas of life, new technologies like the uptake of mobile phones, fashion garments or footwear, books or television programmes. The change in behaviour is contagious like infectious-disease epidemics, a social epidemic. Using the model of diffusion, the tipping point comes at the point between the early adopters and the early majority. It applies equally to changing behaviour of professionals and the public.

This same technique can be used with staff going through a process of change. It is important to identify change types and opinion leaders. Knowing likely opponents is important because, if they can be persuaded to support the change, they

> ## Box 3.1 Evidence of effectiveness of interventions to change professional behaviour
>
> There is good evidence to support:
> - **Multifaceted interventions.** By targeting different barriers to change, these are more likely to be effective than single interventions.
> - **Educational outreach.** This is generally effective in changing prescribing behaviour in North American settings. On-going trials will provide rigorous evidence about the effectiveness of this approach in UK settings.
> - **Reminder systems.** These are generally effective for a range of behaviours.
>
> There are mixed effects in the following:
> - **Audit and feedback.** These need to be used selectively.
> - **Opinion leaders.** These need to be used selectively.
>
> There is little evidence to support:
> - **Passive dissemination of guidelines.** However, there is some evidence to support use of guidelines if tailored to local needs and associated with reminders.

are likely to become important advocates. Understanding people's psychological reaction to change is a key to helping overcome their resistance.

Changes to systems, structures and culture are underpinned by changes in the way people within the organisation behave. There are many approaches to securing change in the behaviour of health care professionals, including:
- guidelines dissemination, e.g. via Clinical Evidence, Map of Medicine
- local opinion leaders
- clinical audit and feedback
- educational outreach
- continuing professional development
- patient-mediated approaches
- patient-specific reminders / prompts
- financial levers / contracting.

The Cochrane Library review topic 'Effective practice and organisation of care' (see www.cochrane.org/reviews/en/topics/61.html) has several systematic reviews on what works in practice and organisational change. These are summarised in Box 3.1. Such reviews of effectiveness have reached the conclusion that there is no magic bullet (see Chapter 15). Most interventions are effective under some circumstances; none is effective under all circumstances. A diagnostic analysis of the individual and the context must be performed before selecting a method for altering individual practitioner behaviour. Interventions based on assessment of potential barriers are more likely to be effective.

Step 5. Evaluating the effects of changes in practice

Most commonly, this step will involve a clinical audit (see Chapter 8). Depending on how frequently the intervention or activity under scrutiny is performed, a review of behaviour will be undertaken some months after instigation of the change.

If we go back to the example of use of aspirin in the elderly after myocardial infarction, page 59, under step 1, how do we know that practice has changed?

There are various ways of ascertaining whether practice has changed. We could review notes of patients who have had a heart attack to determine how many of them have been prescribed aspirin. Once we identify professionals who are not prescribing aspirin we need to identify the barriers. These could include lack of knowledge or the possible fear of side effects and these could be addressed by training. Whitford and Southern [14] found that 85% of patients were prescribed aspirin at discharge from the hospital after a heart attack and this remained at 82% after a year in the community. However, for beta blockers (another drug that benefits patients after a heart attack) the results were less encouraging with under 50% being prescribed the drug. In recent years there have been moves to use financial incentives to improve quality of care in the NHS and the example of treating patients with coronary heart disease is one where setting treatment targets linked to payments is aimed at improving the uptake of effective care [15].

Evidence-based practice is not solely the province of the health sector. Here is an example of EBHC in the community setting.

Your community is concerned about the high rates of childhood obesity locally and local councillors have asked you for help. Keeping in mind the principles of EBHC list the steps you would take and how would you proceed?

1. You need to frame an answerable question. This might be 'What community-based interventions are successful at reducing obesity levels in children aged up to 16 years?'
2. Identify the evidence for the specific intervention. A simple search in Clinical Queries using the key words obesity, children and community, yields several studies including articles on exercise therapy, healthy nutrition, reducing television watching and interventions targeted at parents and ethnic minority populations.
3. Critically appraise the evidence. A closer look at the papers may show that some are not relevant to the local situation (e.g. as they do not consider obesity outcomes or are pilot studies only). There may be promising studies,

the results of which could be applied locally (e.g. establishing dance classes for ethnic-minority girls [16]).

4. Develop ways of implementing the evidence if found to be appropriate. One option might be to canvas local teachers to find an 'early adopter' willing to pilot the use of dance classes after school for local pupils.

5. Undertake an evaluation to determine if the intervention has produced the intended outcome. The introduction of a new intervention should always be accompanied by an explicit evaluation strategy which identifies the objectives of the intervention and plans to measure success in a robust way.

Limitations to EBHC

Evidence is only one influence on our practice. Education alone may not change deeply ingrained habits, e.g. patterns of prescribing. Knowledge does not necessarily change practice. Hence we need to consider employing other incentives to change. Financial incentives are used to promote interventions known to be effective (e.g. target payments to increase immunisation uptake). Recently in the NHS the Quality and Outcomes Framework (QOF) payment system has been introduced to improve the quality of clinical care and promote evidence-based practice [15]. Evidence suggests that financial incentives might improve provider performance in preventive interventions such as offering a smoking cessation service [17]. Chapter 16 looks in more detail at quality improvement in health care.

The most strident criticisms of EBHC have come from those physicians who resent intrusions into their clinical freedom. The use of evidence-based protocols has been demeaned [18] as 'cookbook medicine'. A more powerful philosophical argument is mounted by those arguing that a rigid fixation on randomised controlled trials risks ignoring important qualitative sources of evidence [17].

In addition, there may be times when high-quality evidence from the upper echelons of the hierarchy simply does not exist. This should not prevent action! The lack of RCTs does not mean an intervention is ineffective, it means that there is no evidence that it is effective, a clear distinction. In these cases one looks further down the hierarchy and uses the best level of evidence available. When no research evidence exists there is nothing wrong with asking colleagues for their opinions, the practice of EBHC simply means we should at least carry out the search.

In conclusion, the terms 'evidence-based medicine' and 'evidence-based health care' were developed to encourage practitioners and patients to pay due respect – no more, no less – to current evidence in making decisions. Evidence should enhance health care decision-making not rigidly dictate it[19]. Public health practitioners need to consider their population's health and social care needs and what effective interventions are available to meet them. The choice of interventions needs to be tempered by research evidence. Finally, the practitioner must consider society's and individuals' preferences. The art of EBHC lies in bringing all these considerations together.

REFERENCES

1. R. Smith, Where is the wisdom . . .? *British Medical Journal*, **303**, 1991, 798–9.
2. G. Michaud, J. L. McGowan, R. van der Jagt, G. Wells and P. Tugwell, Are therapeutic decisions supported by evidence from health care research? *Archives of Internal Medicine*, **158**(15), 1998, 1665–8.
3. D. L. Sackett, W. M. Rosenberg, J. A. Gray, R. B. Haynes and W. S. Richardson, Evidence based medicine: what it is and what it isn't. *British Medical Journal*, **312**, 1996, 71–2.
4. P. G. Ramsey, J. D. Carline, T. S. Inui *et al.*, Changes over time in the knowledge base of practicing internists. *Journal of the American Medical Association*, **266**, 1991, 1103–7.
5. D. G. Covell, G. C. Uman and P. R. Manning, Information needs in office practice: Are they being met? *Annals of Internal Medicine*, **103**, 1985, 596–9.
6. K. Dickersin, The existence of publication bias and risk factors for its occurrence. *Journal of the American Medical Association*, **263**, 1990, 1385–9.
7. C. Pope and N. Mays (eds.), *Qualitative Research in Health Care*, 2nd edn, UK, BMJ Books, 2000.
8. E. Ernst, A systematic review of systematic reviews of homeopathy. *British Journal of Clinical Pharmacology*, **54**, 2000, 577–82.
9. D. L. Sackett, W. S. Richardson, W. Rosenberg, and R. B. Haynes, Evidence-based medicine: how to practise and teach EBM. Edinburgh, Churchill Livingstone, 1997, pp. 8–9.
10. E. M. Antman, J. Lau, B. Kupelnick, F. Mosteller and T. C. Chalmers, A comparison of results of meta-analyses of randomized control trials and recommendations of clinical experts. *Journal of the American Medical Association*, **268**, 1992, 240–8.
11. E. M. Rogers, New product adoption and diffusion. *Journal of Consumer Research*, **2**, 1976, 290–301.
12. E. M. Rogers, *Diffusion of Innovations*, 4th edn, New York, Free Press, 1995.
13. M. Gladwell, *The Tipping Point: How Little Things can Make a Big Difference*, Boston, MA, Little, Brown and Company, 2000.
14. D. L. Whitford, and A. J. Southern, Audit of secondary prophylaxis after myocardial infarction. *British Medical Journal*, **309**, 1994, 1268–9.
15. T. Doran, C. Fullwood, H. Gravelle, *et al.*, Pay-for-performance programs in family practices in the United Kingdom. *New England Journal of Medicine*, **355**(4), 2006, 375–84.

16. T. N. Robinson, J. D. Killen H. C. Kraemer *et al.*, Dance and reducing television viewing to prevent weight gain in African-American girls: the Stanford GEMS pilot study. *Ethnicity and Disease*, **13**(1 Suppl. 1), 2003, S65–77.
17. J. Roski, R. Jeddeloh, L. An *et al.*, The impact of financial incentives and a patient registry on preventive care quality: increasing provider adherence to evidence-based smoking cessation practice guidelines. *Preventative Medicine*, **36**(3), 2003, 291–9.
18. B. G. Charlton and A. Miles, The rise and fall of EBM. *Quarterly Journal of Medicine*, **12**, 1998, 371–4.
19. S. E. Straus, and F. A. McAlister, Evidence-based medicine: a commentary on common criticisms. *Canadian Medical Association Journal*, **163**, 2000, 837–41.

4

Improving population health

Key points

- Health promotion focuses on the social, economic and environmental determinants of health and aims to help people increase control over their own health.
- Many different groups and organisations are involved in health promotion within and without the NHS for it encompasses health policy, education, legislative action and community development.
- Disease prevention at the level of the high-risk individual is increasingly effective but population-wide approaches have greater potential to improve population health.
- Psychological models of behaviour change suggest ways of intervening in support of both individuals and organisations managing change.

Disease prevention

Cervical cancer is twenty times more common in Columbia than in Israel. In Nepal, 20% of children die before the age of five, compared with 1% of children in the UK. Ischaemic heart disease death rates vary by a factor of two in different wards in Luton. In other words, diseases that are common in one place will usually prove to be rare somewhere else. Such variations suggest that common diseases – with their roots in lifestyle, social factors and the environment – are preventable. However, there are several misconceptions about prevention.

Prevention and cure are not alternative ways of dealing with illness. Much that we consider 'cure' in the classical medical sense is, in reality, prevention. (Consider, for example, the treatment of high blood pressure or hypothyroidism).

Essential Public Health, eds. Stephen Gillam, Jan Yates and Padmanabhan Badrinath.
Published by Cambridge University Press. © Cambridge University Press 2007.

Although some treatments do effect a permanent 'cure', most merely prevent or retard the development of pain, handicap or more serious consequences.

It is often held that 'prevention is cheaper than cure'. Successful reduction of incidence rates of common diseases ought in theory to reduce health-care costs. In practice, this hope has been frustrated and the costs of health services have generally risen in inverse proportion to disease rates (consider how cardiology services have expanded as death rates from heart disease have declined). Preventive medicine such as screening can be very expensive. For example, according to the UK National Screening Committee, the annual cost of the NHS cervical screening programme is approximately 157 million – but it saves around 4500 lives each year (www.nsc.nhs.uk, as accessed in November 2006).

Preventive medicine is but one small part of the wider field of health promotion. In the introduction page 4, we listed three main approaches to improving the population's health. How health care can be made more effective is examined in Chapter 16, but most of the activities that promote health occur beyond the world of clinical medicine. How we change unhealthy behaviours and alter social determinants of health is the subject of this chapter.

Natural history of disease

We need to begin by looking at the progression of disease in the community. This is represented simply in Figure 4.1. The first stage in the development of a disease is exposure to risk. A risk factor is an aspect of personal behaviour or lifestyle, an environmental exposure or an inherited characteristic, which is known to be associated with a particular health-related outcome (see Chapter 2).

What behavioural and other risk factors do you associate with the onset of cardiovascular disease?
Your list might include: tobacco smoking, high-fat diet and abnormal lipid profiles, raised blood pressure, diabetes mellitus and raised blood glucose, lack of exercise and haemostatic factors: e.g. raised fibrinogen, inflammatory markers such as C reactive protein, homocysteine and stress (though the evidence is highly contested!).

The next step is to consider factors and processes that determine whether or not a disease is manifest. Pathological processes may ensure a disease progresses to be symptomatic but many other factors will determine whether or not a person with symptomatic disease seeks or gains access to health services. These include increasing awareness of the meaning of symptoms (influenced by education and cultural factors) or whether or not appropriate care is available. A further set of factors determine the outcome of any episode of care. Outcomes can broadly be classified into three: death, disability and recovery.

Fig. 4.1   Natural history of
disease in the community.

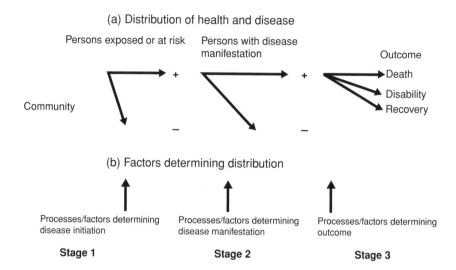

(a) Distribution of health and disease

Persons exposed or at risk   Persons with disease
                               manifestation
                                                          Outcome
                                                          Death
                               +   +   Disability
Community   Recovery

                            −   −

(b) Factors determining distribution

Processes/factors determining   Processes/factors determining   Processes/factors determining
disease initiation   disease manifestation   outcome

      Stage 1   **Stage 2**   **Stage 3**

**What processes or factors might determine the outcomes for someone
diagnosed with diabetes mellitus?**

Age, severity of disease, level of education or health awareness which might
influence adherence to dietary and treatment regimes, socio-economic status
which may have a bearing on dietary and other relevant lifestyle choices (e.g.
exercising to reduce obesity), ethnicity if written material to assist self-care is
inappropriate, quality of care in general practice, access to specialist hospital
care or services in the community (e.g. retinal screening), availability of funding
to provide optimal drug therapy, level of support from carer or others.

At any one time, all three stages of a disease exist in the community (see Figure
4.1). The processes and factors working at each stage may overlap. Medical care,
however, has tended to concentrate on treating outcomes but this is the end stage
of a complex process. To reduce the burden of disease at stage 3, we need to tackle
stages 1 and 2 as well. The community's health needs are the totality of what is
required to interrupt the natural history at all three stages.

Levels of prevention

Preventive activities are commonly categorised at one of three levels:
• Primary prevention – these are actions designed to prevent the occurrence of
  the problem, e.g.
      health education
      genetic counselling
      immunisation
      protection from carcinogens.

- Secondary prevention – these are actions designed to detect and treat the occurrence of a problem before symptoms have developed, e.g.
  - screening
  - early diagnosis.
- Tertiary prevention – these are actions designed to limit disability once a condition is manifest, e.g.
  - limitation of disability
  - rehabilitation
  - prevention of relapse.

Illustrate the different levels of prevention by considering ischaemic heart disease.

Primary prevention	=	Encourage healthy life styles: not smoking, healthy diet, exercise.
Secondary prevention	=	Detection of risk factors, e.g. high blood pressure, raised cholesterol levels, hyperglycaemia . . . and action to reduce these.
Tertiary prevention	=	Cardiac rehabilitation and patient education after ischaemic events such as myocardial infarction to reduce risk factors.

The stages of the natural history can be seen to correspond to the three levels of prevention. Simplistically, the aim of public health practice can be described as shifting the problem to the left in terms of its natural history and shifting the problem upwards in terms of the level of prevention.

Strategies for prevention

The epidemiologist Geoffrey Rose described two broad approaches to prevention (Figure 4.2):
- The high-risk strategy aims to protect those individuals at the high end of the risk distribution. They are usually a small proportion of that distribution.
- The population strategy aims to reduce the underlying causes. It is concerned with factors that affect the whole population [1].

The high-risk strategy avoids interference with those who are not at special risk. Interventions are appropriate to the individuals targeted and this strategy is regularly accommodated within the ethos and organisation of medical care. Appropriate targeting improves its cost effectiveness. However, the high-risk strategy has a limited impact on the behaviour of populations and has hitherto been limited by our ability to predict individuals' futures. Population strategies, on the other hand, by tackling behaviours and other risk factors en masse offer large benefits for populations. Taking strokes as an example, a 5 mm lowering of blood pressure across the population might achieve a 33% reduction

Fig. 4.2   High-risk individual
and population-based strategies
for prevention.

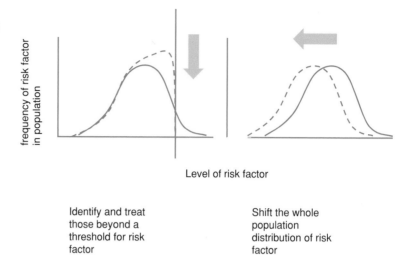

Identify and treat
those beyond a
threshold for risk
factor

Shift the whole
population
distribution of risk
factor

in strokes (approximately 75,000 in the UK each year). This compares with a 15% reduction in the number of strokes, if all cases of hypertension (defined as those people with blood pressure higher than a set threshold) were detected and treated.

However, with a population strategy, the benefits to the individuals may be small and both subjects and health professionals may be poorly motivated to implement mass strategies. This is the so-called *prevention paradox*: where preventive measures bringing large benefits to the community offer little to each participating individual. However, recent evidence affirms that countries able to implement strategies targeted at individuals on the basis of baseline risks will also see major health gains [2]. In other words, Rose's famous dichotomy is less clear cut. Thus, preventive medicine must embrace both approaches but – at least in low-to-middle-income countries yet to introduce simple policy changes aimed at smoking and dietary change – the power resides with the population strategy.

It is important in passing to distinguish two kinds of preventive measures. The first consists of removing or reducing an unnatural exposure, e.g. stopping smoking, reducing dietary intake of saturated fat and salts. The second type of mass preventive measure consists of adding some unnatural factor in the hope of conferring protection (e.g. folic acid to prevent neural tube defects, fluoridation of water supplies to prevent dental caries, even statins to reduce blood lipid levels and prevent excess risk of heart disease). For such measures there can be no prior presumption of safety and the required evidence of benefit must be stringent.

The public health approach to screening presents a further ethical dilemma with its focus on maximising participation in screening rather than on informed participation. For example, current recommendations for the primary prevention of coronary heart disease in groups at high risk depend on screening through primary care and provision of risk-related advice or treatment. However, we lack evidence for the cost effectiveness of multiple-risk-factor interventions delivered through primary care [3]. Presenting the uncertainties associated with the assessment and reduction of cardiovascular risk to individuals may actually be more cost effective than screening conducted in a traditional, public health paradigm if it results in participants who are more motivated to reduce their risks [4].

Prevention in clinical practice

A sharp distinction between health and disease is a medical artefact for which nature provides no support. Not so long ago, this proposal was regarded as revolutionary. A spectrum of disease is now seen to be the norm rather than the exception; even infectious diseases come in all sizes from obvious clinical cases to symptomless infections.

Physiological variables such as blood pressure, serum cholesterol, body mass index, and bone mineral density are important in the aetiology of common diseases. They are not direct causes of disease, like smoking, but are intermediates between those external factors and disease itself. Risk can be reduced by lowering high levels of these variables by drug treatment or lifestyle change. However, there is a view that changing the average values of these physiological variables is not worthwhile, a view that implies the presence of thresholds in the dose–response relations between the level of the variable and the risk of disease. This view is reinforced by terminology that regards extreme values as indicating a disease state (such as hypertension, hypercholesterolaemia, osteoporosis and obesity) and average values as being 'normal' (normotensive, normocholesterolaemia). Clinical guidelines specify risk-factor thresholds; these have been set at successively lower levels over time and redefined as 'action levels' but they still deny treatment below specified values.

The notion that we intervene only when an individual risk factor reaches a threshold is misguided. Meta-analyses of cohort studies have been used to plot the relationships between risk factors and diseases [5]. Far from demonstrating risk-factor thresholds, these plots yield reasonably straight lines, and this is so whether the level of the risk-factor on the horizontal axis is plotted using an arithmetical or proportional scale (Figure 4.3). In other words, there is a constant proportional change in risk for a given change in the risk factor from any starting level. These continuous dose–response relationships have a crucially important implication: anyone at high risk should be 'treated'.

For example, blood-pressure-lowering drugs should not be limited to people with high blood pressure, nor cholesterol-lowering drugs to people with high serum cholesterol concentrations. The constant proportional relations indicate that the absolute reduction in risk from changing the risk factor will be large in

Fig. 4.3 Incidence of ischaemic heart disease (with 95% confidence intervals) according to diastolic blood pressure, serum cholesterol and body mass index – data from cohort studies [5].

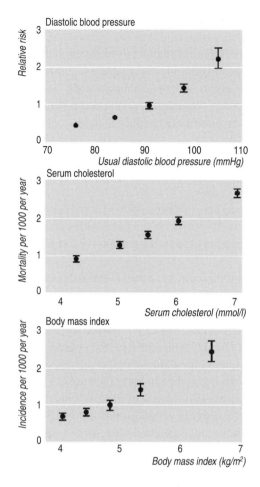

people who are at high risk for any reason (existing disease, smoking status or older age, for example), regardless of the starting value of the risk factor.

The major determinant of risk is existing disease. Without preventive treatment, mortality from heart disease in people who have had a myocardial infarction in the past is about 5% per year for the rest of their life. Mortality from stroke in people who have had a stroke is similar. Both rates are much higher than in people with no history of cardiovascular disease; coronary mortality is 0.3% per year in men aged 60, for example, or about 0.5% per year in men with high cholesterol or blood pressure [6]. Anyone with existing disease (a previous myocardial infarction or stroke for example) should be treated, irrespective of the level of the risk factors being modified.

Another problem with the notion of intervening only above a threshold level is illustrated in the case of cardiovascular disease and age. In people without known cardiovascular disease, age is the most important determinant of risk. Mortality from ischaemic heart disease and from stroke doubles with about every eight years of increasing age [5]. In England and Wales 95% of deaths from heart disease occur in the quartile of the population at oldest age (men ≥ 55 and women ≥ 60). Offering preventive treatment only to people with relatively high values of a variable means that only a small proportion of those destined to have disease events will be targeted. People of a given age with relatively high values of the physiological variables are at similar risk as people a few years older with average levels; it is illogical to offer preventive treatment to the former but not the latter. In people without cardiovascular disease, intervention to change risk factors should be introduced when a person's risk of a disease event over the next few years exceeds a specified value. Because there is substantial benefit from lowering these physiological variables from any starting value in persons at high risk, all the reversible risk factors should be changed, not just those judged 'abnormal.' Reducing only variables with high values loses most of the potential benefit.

Behaviour change

Some public health programmes can impose benefits on people without them having to change their own behaviour (e.g. the provision of clean water). However, many preventive projects require some behaviour change on the part of the public/patient. Unless frontline health professionals have the skills to assist in that behaviour change, the goals of the programme may be thwarted. This section looks at ways of changing behaviour.

Much of human disease is due in whole or in part to the attitudes and behaviour of individuals. Cholera, typhoid, poliomyelitis and infectious hepatitis are all transmitted faeco-orally, so their spread depends upon personal habits, as well as policies for public sanitation, and the way food is prepared. The most important single cause of lung cancer is the habit of smoking cigarettes; the causes of coronary heart disease include a diet high in fat and salt and low in fruit and vegetables, physical inactivity and the use of tobacco. Cleanliness, smoking, diet and physical activity are all personal matters. However, the behaviour underlying each is, to a large extent, determined by the values of society and resultant attitudes. By changing knowledge and attitudes, one hopes to change behaviour, prevent many of these diseases and thus promote health. In reality, the link between these three is less straightforward [7].

Knowledge does not always lead to 'correct' behaviour. For example, many drivers who do not wear seat belts know what happens to an unrestrained driver in an accident. Knowledge and behaviour can be out of step for many reasons (Table 4.1).

Simply telling people what is good for them is not an effective health change strategy. Four pre-conditions are necessary for behaviour change to take place.

Table 4.1. Why behaviours may persist

- No perception of personal threat from the behaviour
- Rewards of present behaviour
- Benefits of change too long-term
- Social pressure
- Belief that change will have no effect or that there is no value or benefit in the outcome of the change
- Belief that 'I cannot change'

You must

1. want to change
2. believe you can change
3. believe change will have the desired effect
4. know how to change.

Self-efficacy is the belief in your own ability to effect change. Patients with low self-efficacy will find it hard to make changes because they lack confidence in their capacity to determine what happens to them. Self-efficacy is closely related to self-confidence and self-esteem. Where patients have low self-efficacy, it may be raised in various ways, for example, helping the patient remember or recognise someone else who made the change ('If they did it, then so can I'). Action efficacy is the belief that the change will remove the threat caused by the original behaviour. Achieving early successes breeds confidence thus reinforcing both self- and action efficacy. It is particularly important that a person with low self-efficacy does not have further experiences that will reinforce his/her poor self-image. Setting realistic, measurable goals is more likely to ensure successful practice. Physical feedback that tells you that you are doing something right increases self-efficacy (e.g. the 'feel good' factor in exercise which fuels the desire for more exercise).

Stages of behavioural change

Prochaska and DiClemente [8] have provided a well-known model of behaviour change (Figure 4.4). The stages can be illustrated by the example of someone giving up smoking.

- Pre contemplation – At this stage, the smoker does not perceive that he/she has a problem. Others, though, might be pointing out a problem.
- Contemplation – The smoker begins to recognise that he/she has a behaviour which is a problem for them. He/she thinks about the problem – is it bad enough to need action? What action might I take? Who could help? At this stage, the smoker might discuss his/her problems with others, including those who have previously been smokers.

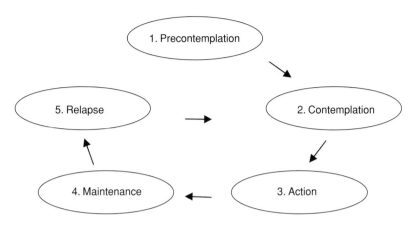

Fig. 4.4   Stages in behaviour change.

- Action – This is when the attempt to change behaviour takes place. It can include seeking advice; joining a support group; using a nicotine patch; keeping charts of progress.
- Maintenance – Once the smoker has reached the desired level of performance (say, abstinence), he/she has to keep to that level. This may involve special strategies for recognising a high-risk situation (e.g. 'When I go to the pub with the bowls team, there's always a lot of smoking') and designing strategies for dealing with them (e.g. 'When the game is finished, I will remind the team that they must not let me have a cigarette even if I ask for one in the pub').
- Relapse – Despite a patient's best efforts, relapses occur and patients need to be warned that this can happen. The commonest triggers of relapse are events that trigger a low emotional state, e.g. accidents, job loss, relationship difficulties or social pressure, especially when the pressure catches the patient unawares. The role of the health professional is to accept the relapse as normal and not as an indication of weakness on the patient's part; to talk the relapse through and see what the patient can learn from it; and help the patient re-establish short-term targets.

Health promotion

Health has a wide variety of meanings ranging from an ideal state to the absence of medically defined disease. The former was encapsulated in the famous World Health Organisation definition of health as 'a state of complete mental, physical and social well-being and not merely the absence of disease or infirmity.' Unfortunately, health of this sort is more aspirational than obtainable. In the 1980s, the WHO promoted a more realistic definition of health in terms of the ability to function 'normally' in one's own society. Of more practical use is a definition of health which states the means by which its foundations can be achieved. These

---

Box 4.1 Tobacco control as a health promotion programme

The links between tobacco use and adverse health events such as heart disease, lung cancer and chronic obstructive airways disease are well documented. Efforts to control the risks of tobacco illustrate well the four routes for health promotion.

- **Health education.** This is central and takes the form of major education campaigns such as television adverts and posters as well as interventions used to support those wanting to quit. Smoking cessation interventions have been funded and made widely available across the UK and several high-profile media campaigns have worked to increase the awareness of the public. Quit rates increase during times of these campaigns [12].

- **Legislation.** The increase in tax on tobacco products, age restrictions, smoking bans in public places and advertising restrictions have worked in several developed countries to bring the smoking rates down. Restrictions on smoking in public places have the knock-on effect of reducing smoking in homes [13]. Unfortunately, the tobacco companies have increased marketing in less developed countries where the resources available for effective control are limited.

- **Community development.** This includes, for example, educational initiatives within schools, local policy development, working to understand and bridge cultural barriers to cessation, and work with teenage mothers on smoking in pregnancy.

- **Healthy public policy.** This is distinct from legislative action as it is often non-mandatory policy. The banning of smoking and provision of cessation advice in workplaces are policy initiatives which provide supportive environments for those wanting to quit and triggers to those who may be at the precontemplation or contemplation stage.

---

foundations include basic requirements such as adequate food, safe water, shelter, safety and security as well as education and information. The chosen definition of health itself has important implications for policy as it determines whether the emphasis is on multi-sectoral approaches or on technological solutions to tackling particular diseases.

Health promotion is identified [9] as 'the process of enabling people to exert control over and to improve their health'. Health promotion is not something that is done *on* or *to* people, it is done *with* people either as individuals or as groups. The purpose of this activity is to strengthen the skills and capabilities of individuals to take action, and the capacity of groups or communities to act collectively *to exert control* over determinants of their health. There are four main routes for health promotion (these are illustrated in the example in Box 4.1).

1. Health education – These are activities which are intended to lead to health-related learning. Typically health education consists of interventions directed at individuals and led by professionals (for example, a community nurse or midwife encouraging a pregnant woman to stop smoking). Client-led interventions encourage individuals to make their own choices (for example, helping young people identify their own concerns and working with them to develop their own confidence and skills). Using a personal counselling approach to support behaviour change is preferable to crude 'health persuasion' ("You know, you really should eat less chips, Mrs Jones") which can appear authoritarian and may reinforce power differentials between 'professional' and 'patient'.

2. Legislative action – Interventions are led by professionals or experts but are intended to protect the health of the community (for example, lobbying for legislation for compulsory fluoridation by water companies). This approach also includes multi-agency working and can include health protection issues such as compulsory notification of diseases (see Chapter 10).

3. Community development – Interventions take place within a defined community to identify local health issues and work with local people to take action on those concerns (for example, residents on a housing estate setting up a food cooperative). A community empowerment model is often used which aims to support members of communities to develop personally, form mutual support groups to tackle health-related issues identified by communities themselves and engage in collective political and social action to bring about change.

4. Healthy public policy – Tones and Tilford [10] have defined health promotion as:

Health education × Healthy public policy   (4.1)

Healthy public policy focuses on the underlying determinants of good health and well-being. These can be summarised by the prerequisites of health as defined in the 1986 Ottawa Charter [11] – food, shelter, stable ecosystems, sustainable resources, peace, education, equity, income, social justice. In many cases individuals can have little impact on their 'share' of these prerequisites. In a time of war your ability to obtain the peace, shelter, food, indeed any of the prerequisites, is likely to be limited and beyond your control. If your income is low and you have no transport you may be unable to access cheaper, healthier food choices. Thus healthy public policy covers the ways in which states can impact on the social, political, cultural and economic contexts in which we live and from there our ability to obtain the resources which promote health. Policies which ensure fair taxation, reduce national debts, impose restrictions on sales and marketing such as tobacco licensing and advertising legislation, and healthy building policies would all come under the heading of healthy public policy.

The WHO's Bangkok Charter of 2005 [14] affirms that the promotion of health:
- is central to the global development agenda
- is a core responsibility for all of government
- is a key focus of communities and civil society
- is a requirement for good corporate practice.

The charter recognises the need to work in partnership with the corporate sector – hitherto demonised multinationals – to create healthier environments in which individuals can make choices. The values underpinning the charter are those of social justice, equity, human dignity, peace and security. The need to find constructive ways of working with the private sector is reflected in the World Health Organisation Framework Convention for Tobacco Control [15] which includes an article helping tobacco growers to find economically viable alternative activities.

Who is responsible for health promotion?

The wide variety of influences on health means that health promotion is not the sole province of one professional group or organisation. The challenge for those working in the field and particularly for health promotion specialists has always been to develop the skills and capacity of others so that they can then promote health as an integral part of their work.

National-level organisations have a part to play. In the UK organisations such as the Health Education Authority and then the Health Development Agency (HDA) have worked to help people to make sustainable improvements in health and are working to reduce health inequalities. This function now forms part of the National Institute for Health and Clinical Excellence (NICE) which draws together evidence for public health interventions. National departments for health take various forms and provide the strategic framework for health care but other government departments are also crucial in creating change at a national level. Hence, the importance of the Labour government's appointment of a Minister for Public Health in 1997 to work across government departments.

Local health-care organisations are often expected to take the lead on local action to promote health through partnerships in which local government has a crucial role to play. Within local authorities, health promotion may be traditionally associated with environmental health officers, but departments of transport, housing, planning, leisure, education and social services are also taking a more active role with the increasing recognition of the wider determinants of health.

Health promotion specialists are core members of the multi-disciplinary and multi-organisational public health team. They are usually employed within health care or local government with responsibility for developing strategy and stimulating and co-ordinating activities to promote health. They work in settings such as hospitals, schools and workplaces.

Health professionals and others who make up the primary health-care team have an essential role to play in health promotion. Moreover, health promotion is a core function for professional groups such as practice nurses, health visitors and school nurses. The relationships they establish with local people and communities mean they are all well placed to provide one-to-one support and advice.

Finally, the voluntary, non-governmental sector has an important part to play in health promotion. Voluntary organisations are often commissioned to provide outreach services to community groups and set up community-based projects. Voluntary organisations can advocate on behalf of local people and are important partners in community development work.

Making health promotion effective

In tackling determinants, health promotion will include actions directed towards changing both those things within the more immediate control of individuals, such as individual health behaviours, and those outside the immediate control of individuals, such as social, economic and environmental conditions, which influence health. Effective interventions have the following characteristics [16]:

1. They are planned on the basis of a thorough analysis of the problem that indicates reasonable linkages between the short-term impact of interventions and subsequent changes in the determinants of health and in health outcomes.
2. They are informed by established theory and evidence relevant to the type of intervention planned.
3. There is sufficient public and political awareness of the issue and the need for action.
4. Resources are available to implement and sustain a programme.
5. They are of sufficient size, duration and sophistication to be detectable above the 'background noise' of more general changes in society.
6. Programmes which combine different intervention methods, rather than relying on a single methodology, are most likely to be successful.

There are five distinct phases in developing a health promotion intervention:
a. problem definition
b. solution generation
c. capacity building
d. implementation
e. process, impact and outcome evaluation.

A case study relating to HIV/AIDS prevention (Box 4.2) briefly illustrates these phases.

Box 4.2 Case study: HIV

Context: A post-industrial town with a population of 200,000, 10% of whom are from ethnic minorities. A recent influx of people from Zimbabwe has coincided with a five-fold increase in HIV seroprevalence and the incidence of AIDS. Of people newly identified with HIV 90% are from sub-Saharan Africa. Local epidemiological analysis has identified this community, and men who have sex with men, as key target groups. Additional research into the views of the local African population has revealed variable levels of understanding concerning the virus, the screening process and how to prevent infection with HIV. A community-based voluntary organisation working with this community is newly established. The local genito-urinary medicine (GUM) department is struggling to meet national access targets.

In the light of the national strategy for sexual health and HIV [17], a multi-agency group (including representation from the Primary Care Trust, the Strategic Health Authority, relevant hospital departments, local-authority departments and a range of voluntary organisations representing users) met to **define the problem** and **generate solutions**.

The first and overriding prerequisite for progress was to **build capacity** in various areas addressing, for example:

- Low levels of HIV awareness in key target groups.
- A lack of HIV counsellors able to promote and undertake screening.
- Lack of knowledge among key health personnel, e.g. general practitioners and practice nurses in the prevention and management of HIV.
- Comparable knowledge deficits in the education sector, e.g. among school nurses, teachers.
- Staff shortages in the local GUM department.
- Limited understanding in the general population.
- Lack of resources for community-based organisations seeking to create links in the community, e.g. in churches, schools and clubs.

The district HIV Strategy included several health-promoting aims which, in turn, were converted into concrete objectives. For example:

1. To increase access to HIV/STI (sexually transmitted infection) testing within the local population thereby reducing the risk of onward transmission. Key actions included:

   expansion of community-based services for testing and management of HIV in general practice

   setting up outreach clinics in collaboration with the local GUM department

   training key personnel in primary and secondary care on pre-test counselling

2. To reduce vertical transmission from mother to child by developing a programme of preventive work targeting high-risk groups on the basis of local epidemiology. Key actions included:

> targeting African and Caribbean communities via awareness-raising work in schools, training community-based volunteers (e.g. from faith groups, colleges, voluntary organisations), building community partnerships.
>
> continued work with voluntary organisations serving men who have sex with men
>
> increasing the provision of needle exchange schemes.

3. To improve public awareness of HIV, reducing stigma and discrimination through:

> local campaigns on World Aids Day
>
> awareness raising events within the African community
>
> service reviews with voluntary organisations
>
> educational initiatives within health and social care
>
> increasing uptake of training in key settings, e.g. education, social services
>
> developing and implementing a user-involvement strategy.

Implementation of the new strategy has inevitably required new money, some of which has come from dedicated central funding via the Department of Health, some of which has been pared from existing local budgets. The steering group is overseeing a programme of **evaluation** that monitors, for example, the changing incidence of HIV infection, numbers of staff trained in different sectors, uptake of screening tests, the deployment of new staff, waiting times in the GUM department, public attitudes and levels of satisfaction through consumer surveys.

Conclusion

All health promoters at national and local level can work to influence personal behaviour and use policy-making and enactment to secure change. A commonly cited example of successful health-promotion legislation at national level is seat-belt legislation; seat-belt use appears to reduce motor-vehicle fatalities and serious injuries by at least 40% [18]. In developed countries, increasing attention is being paid to the design and provision of environments which encourage healthy behaviours such as physical activity. In developing countries health promotion still focuses on crucial interventions such as condom use, clean water and basic hygiene. Population strategies place heavy emphasis on health education but early enthusiasm for risk-factor interventions was tempered by the lack of evidence for their effectiveness. Furthermore, health inequalities by social class have persisted and even widened. Though politicians are inclined to retreat in the face of criticisms of the so-called nanny state, there is plenty of evidence that the electorate want governments to take a lead in developing healthy public policies [19]. New approaches to promoting health such as social marketing, which uses techniques developed in the commercial sector, place a greater emphasis on individual choice [20]. The primary determinants of disease remain economic and social. Therefore its remedies must in part be economic and social. These are considered further in Chapters 14 and 17.

REFERENCES

1. G. Rose, *The Strategy of Preventive Medicine*. Oxford, Oxford University Press, 1992.
2. R. Jackson, J. Lynch, and S. Harper, Preventing coronary heart disease. *British Medical Journal*, **332**, 2006, 617–8.
3. S. Ebrahim and G. Davey Smith, Multiple risk factor interventions for primary prevention of coronary heart disease (Cochrane Review). *The Cochrane Library*, Issue 1, 2001.
4. A.-L. Kinmonth and T. Marteau, Screening for cardiovascular risk: public health imperative or matter for individual informed choice? *British Medical Journal*, **325**, 2002, 78–80.
5. M. R. Law and N. J. Wald, Risk factor thresholds: their existence under scrutiny. *British Medical Journal*, **324**, 2002, 1520–6.
6. J. D. Neaton Wentworth, Serum cholesterol, blood pressure, cigarette smoking, and death from coronary heart disease. *Archives of Internal Medicine*, **152**, 1992, 56–64.
7. S. Rollnick, P. Mason, and C. Butler, *Health Behaviour Change. A Guide for Practitioners*. Edinburgh, Churchill Livingstone, 2005.
8. J. Prochaska and C. DiClemente, Stages and processes of self-change of smoking: towards an integrated model of change. *Journal of Consulting and Clinical Psychology*, **51**, 1983, 390–5.
9. M. Lalonde, A new perspective on the health of Canadians. Ottawa, Government of Canada, 1974.
10. K. Tones and S. Tilford, *Health Promotion: Effectiveness, Efficiency and Equity*, 3rd edn, Cheltenham, Nelson Thornes, 2001.
11. World Health Organisation, *Ottawa Charter for Health Promotion*. Geneva, WHO, 1986.
12. D. McVey and J. Stapleton, Can anti-smoking television advertising affect smoking behaviour? Controlled trial of the Health Education Authority for England's anti-smoking TV campaign. *Tobacco Control*, **9**, 2000, 273–82.
13. R. Borland, H.-H. Yong, K. M. Cummings *et al*. Determinants and consequences of smoke-free homes: findings from the International Tobacco Control (ITC) Four Country Survey. *Tobacco Control*, **15**, 2006, 43–50. (suppl_3):

14. World Health Organisation. Bangkok Charter for Health Promotion in a Globalised World. Bangkok. WHO, 2005.

15. World Health Organisation. Framework Convention for Tobacco Control, Geneva, WHO, 2005.

16. D. Nutbeam, Effective health promotion programmes. In *Oxford Handbook of Public Health Practice*, 1st edn, D. Pencheon, C. Guest, D. Melzer, and J. A. Muir Gray (eds.), Oxford, Oxford University Press, 2001, ch. 4.2.

17. Department of Health. Better prevention, better services, better sexual health – the national strategy for sexual health and HIV. London, Department of Health, 2001.

18. M. Mackay, Seat belt use under voluntary and mandatory conditions and its effect on casualties. In *Human Behaviour and Traffic Safety*, L. Evans and R. Schwing (eds.), New York, Plenum Press, 1985.

19. King's Fund. *Public Attitudes to Public Health Policy*. London, King's Fund, 2004.

20. *National Social Marketing Centre for Excellence. Social Marketing Pocket Guide.* London: Department of Health, 2005.

5

Screening

Key points

- Screening is a tool to identify people at increased risk of a condition so that preventative action can be taken.
- Established criteria are used to judge when a screening programme should be introduced. These take account of the importance of the condition, the test, the treatment and the effectiveness of the programme as a whole.
- The performance of a screening test can be evaluated using calculations of sensitivity, specificity, predictive values and likelihood ratios. Knowing when to use each of these measures is an important public health skill.
- Screening will always identify so-called false negatives and false positives.
- Screening programmes are evaluated in the short and long term and potential sources of bias are considered in determining their effectiveness.
- Screening can incur harm and raises ethical questions. Health professionals and the public need to be aware of both the costs and benefits to society and individuals from screening as a public health activity.

Introduction

Screening is one of the most important preventive public health activities. This chapter provides some examples of effective screening programmes, considers what criteria are needed to demonstrate the effectiveness of a programme, how screening tests can be used to guide action and how screening programmes can be evaluated.

The UK National Screening Committee (see www.nsc.nhs.uk) defines screening as:

Essential Public Health, eds. Stephen Gillam, Jan Yates and Padmanabhan Badrinath.
Published by Cambridge University Press. © Cambridge University Press 2007.

a public health service in which members of a defined population, who do not necessarily perceive they are at risk of, or are already affected by a disease or its complications, are asked a question or offered a test, to identify those individuals who are more likely to be helped than harmed by further tests or treatment to reduce the risk of a disease or its complications.

It is different from a diagnostic test in that it identifies those at increased risk rather than those having a disorder. Screening can be termed 'mass' screening when it is applied to the whole population or targeted screening when it is aimed at specific parts of the population. 'Opportunistic' screening (or case finding) is applied to those who seek medical attention for another, perhaps unrelated, condition.

Should we establish a new screening programme?

Screening incurs harms as well as benefits. Screening tests may wrongly identify disease (false positives) or detect disease which would never have had any harmful clinical implications. This results in unnecessary diagnostic tests which may have harmful physical effects as well as cause worry and concern for individuals. Those who are detected as having a disease early may feel labelled by that condition. This can also lead to psychological harm; however, the overall psychological impact of screening is not easy to determine as, for example, a false positive may be reassuring for some and extremely worrying for others. In addition, there are opportunity costs to be paid during the screen, diagnosis and treatment. These come primarily in the form of time and money for an attendance, which may prove to have been unnecessary for the individual. Policy is shifting towards informed choice so that patients have the potential risks and benefits of the screen explained clearly to them through good-quality information to ensure the resulting choice reflects the decision-maker's values. The effects of informed choice may be to reduce emotional distress and increase motivation to change behaviours. However, it may also decrease uptake, but not consistently across the population (as not everyone will have the skills to access or interpret information), and so could increase inequity [1].

This potential for harm leads to ethical debates when a population of people, who believe themselves healthy, are offered an intervention which may determine that they are in fact at higher risk of disease. As relatively high coverage is needed to produce health gains this leads to target setting for coverage rates and incentives to encourage screening. Those offered screening may find it difficult to make an informed decision about participation. This is because it is not easy to weigh the harms and benefits that accrue over a long period and it is difficult for individuals to understand health outcomes which have a low probability of occurrence. Explaining screening is not always easy for health professionals.

Thus it is important to weigh up the benefits and harms of a potential screening programme before implementing it and to evaluate the effects carefully. There are established criteria for doing this, initially outlined by Wilson and Jungner in 1968 [2] and updated variously since to take account of the more rigorous standards of evidence required and an increased awareness of the potential for harm. The criteria used for evaluating the viability, effectiveness and appropriateness of a screening programme can be split into four categories relating to: the condition, the test, the treatment and the programme itself. Breast and cervical cancer are used as examples throughout this section to show how these criteria might be met.

The condition

The condition screened for should be an important problem. A population-wide intervention such as screening will only be effective if it can prevent significant disease. For rare conditions without major health effects screening would not be worthwhile.

Breast cancer comprises a heterogeneous group of diseases and is the most common cancer in women (around 22% of all cancer cases). There are over a million cases worldwide per year (over 40,000 in the UK) and incidence is around four times higher in more-developed countries than less-developed ones. There are around half a million cases of cervical cancer worldwide per year (around 3,000 in the UK) and mortality is nearly three times higher in less-developed regions compared to more-developed regions. Thus, both breast and cervical cancer give rise to a high burden of disease (see Figure 5.1) although the incidence of cervical cancer is lower than many other cancers and may become too low to be considered an important problem in the UK.

From the charts in Figure 5.1, which three cancers would you suggest should be considered for screening programmes in women in the UK based solely on the burden of disease?
The three cancers with the highest incidence and highest death rates for women are breast, lung and colorectal.

In men, prostate cancer has the highest incidence followed by lung and colorectal. Lung cancer, followed by prostate and colorectal, has the highest death rate.

The natural history of the condition sought should be adequately understood and there should be a recognisable latent or early symptomatic stage. To make gains in morbidity or mortality it must be possible to identify an early stage of disease so that early intervention can prevent progression. For example, in cervical cancer

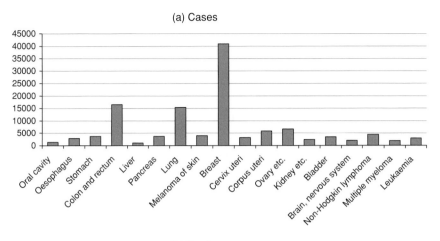

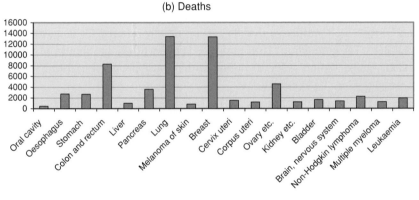

Fig. 5.1 Estimated number of female cases (a) and deaths (b) from selected cancers in 2002 from GLOBOCAN 2002.

the presence of abnormal cells provides a pre-cancerous stage which is detectable and the likelihood of these abnormalities progressing to cancer is known.

All practicable, cost-effective primary prevention measures should have been implemented. It is better to prevent the onset of disease rather than have to detect it early and then treat. Thus screening programmes are generally only established for conditions where preventive measures have not led to significant reductions in disease prevalence or incidence, such as cancers.

The risk factors associated with an increased risk of breast cancer are: increasing age, late childbearing (first child after the age of 30), having no children, early menarche, late menopause, family history (first-degree relative, particularly premenopausal) and carriage of a particular genetic mutation. In more developed countries cultural shifts are towards late childbearing and fewer or no children, so that preventing these risk factors poses problems. Other potential risk factors such as diet, alcohol, prolonged use of hormone replacement therapy and stress are still being investigated and may also play a part. The main risk factor for the development of cervical cancer is infection with certain strains of human papilloma virus (HPV) which is sexually transmitted. Increased risk is also associated with sexual intercourse at an early age, smoking, multiple sexual partners, long-term oral contraceptive use, low socio-economic status, immunosuppressive therapy and some nutrient deficiencies. This criterion raises questions about the future relevance of cervical screening programmes which were established before a link to HPV was discovered. There is now increasing interest in preventing cervical cancer through interventions aimed at reducing the incidence and prevalence of sexually transmitted infections such as vaccination.

The test

There should be a suitable test available which is simple, safe, precise and validated. As screening only identifies those at increased risk it is necessary to have a clearly valid test for the condition so that those who do not need further investigation can be reassured and those that do can be rapidly referred for diagnosis and treatment. The population distribution of screening test values should be known and an agreed 'cut-off' value identified so that those people warranting further investigation can be identified.

The test or examination should be acceptable to both the public and to professionals. Screening programmes depend, for their effectiveness, on high proportions of the target population complying with screening offers. If the screening or diagnostic test is not acceptable this will reduce the effectiveness of the programme as many will not attend.

There should be an agreed policy on further diagnostic investigation. Those who receive a positive screen result must be informed of the choices available to them and access to diagnostic services should be available equitably for the whole screened population.

Cervical cancer develops from altered cells in the cervix and microscopy can be used to detect abnormal cells (dysplasia) at early stages. A screen for cervical abnormalities involves a scrape (smear) or brush of the cervix and examination of the removed cells under a microscope. The standard test is a smear (Papanikolaou or Pap test) and a more recent innovation is liquid based cytology (LBC). The sensitivity of the smear test for cervical cancer is expected to improve with a move to LBC where samples are taken using a brush and suspended in a liquid medium. Women with abnormalities are then investigated further using colposcopy (examination of the cervix using a lighted microscope) and any areas of abnormal cervix can be biopsied (sampled) or removed.

Screening via mammography (breast X-ray) detects abnormalities in the breast tissue. Any abnormal areas seen under X-ray can be investigated further by other types of imaging such as ultrasound or by collecting cells for further microscopy by biopsy. Not all abnormalities will be due to or progress to invasive disease, but the mammogram provides information which may identify cancers that are too small to be felt, and further investigations are required to conform the nature of the abnormality.

Thus, for breast and cervical cancer the screening and diagnostic tests are considered unpleasant by some but have been shown over time to be acceptable. However, there are still concerns about whether this is consistent across all parts of the population, for example cultural differences occur when women are not comfortable with intimate examinations and the percentage of people invited who attend screening may be lower in some populations than others for this reason.

The treatment

There should be an accepted and effective treatment for patients with recognised disease, facilities for treatment should be available and such treatment optimised by all health-care providers. Implementing a screening programme which raises hopes and uncovers demand for treatment services that do not exist or do not have a firm evidence base would be unethical and an uneconomical use of resources.

There should be an agreed policy on whom to treat as patients, including management of borderline disease. Treatment policies for cancers are, in the main, in place well before screening is established. Treatments may, however, be invasive and unpleasant and this must be explained clearly before screening is undertaken. In some screening programmes the treatment becomes more of an issue, for example screening for Down's syndrome during pregnancy. There is a simple blood test that will tell a mother-to-be that she may be at increased risk of her foetus having Down's syndrome. A diagnostic test to confirm this involves invasive sampling of the amniotic fluid or placenta and this carries a small risk of miscarriage. The only treatment to prevent a known Down's baby is to have the pregnancy terminated. Thus, the diagnosis and treatment may not be acceptable to pregnant women, and the attitudes of health-care staff to treatment options has an impact on the woman's decision whether or not to accept screening.

The programme

There should be robust evidence that the screening programme is effective in reducing mortality or morbidity. Evidence from randomised controlled trials of screening programmes should be considered before initiating a screening programme. Much screening activity, for example in childhood, is no longer undertaken for lack of evidence that it is effective [3].

There should be evidence that the programme is acceptable to the public and professionals and that the benefits outweigh the harms. All elements of the screening programme from invitations through to treatment should be considered and be acceptable. The outcomes of the programme in terms of morbidity and mortality should outweigh the physical and psychological harms caused by the test, diagnostic procedures and treatment.

The cost of early diagnosis and treatment should be economically balanced in relation to the total expenditure on health care. Within a limited health-care budget all health and health-care costs must be justified in terms of cost effectiveness. Implementation of a screening programme must be demonstrated to be an efficient use of health-care funds in comparison to other interventions possible for specific conditions.

The programme must be adequately resourced. As well as all the staffing and other resource implications of the testing, diagnosis and treatment, screening programmes require significant money for management and monitoring, quality assurance and long-term evaluation. All these resource implications must be determined before the programme is established.

Following successful trials in Sweden the UK introduced breast-cancer screening in 1990 and the programme covered the whole UK population by the mid 1990s. Women aged 50–70 are invited for a mammogram and two X-ray views are taken to maximise the chance of detecting abnormalities. Women are recalled every three years. Mammographic screening has been shown to reduce mortality in women aged 50–69 years by an estimated 35%. Among women screened regularly over a ten-year period between the ages of 50 and 70, it is estimated that cumulative mortality from breast cancer is reduced from 8.0 to 5.2 per 1000. It is estimated that this screening programme saves around 1400 lives each year in England [4]. In younger women (40–49) screening is of less benefit and screening more frequently than every three years is not predicted statistically to improve mortality [5].

In the UK, cervical screening was carried out ad hoc from the mid 1960s until 1988 when a co-ordinated programme was established. There have been no controlled trials of cervical screening but observational studies show that mortality has decreased after the introduction of screening programmes [6, 7]. In the UK it has been estimated that the introduction of cervical screening reversed an upward trend in cervical cancer mortality and will result in fewer deaths per year (estimates vary from several hundred lives saved to several thousand depending upon the data and model used [8, 9]). The time between successive screens (called the screening interval) is determined by establishing the additional number of cervical cancer cases which can be detected at different intervals and opting for the most cost-effective programme. In the UK women are screened three yearly from

25 to 49 and five yearly from 50 to 64. Above and below these ages the balance of harm to benefit of screening is less certain. Women over 65 are no longer offered screening unless they have not been screened since aged 50 or have had recent abnormalities. The three-year interval for breast cancer was determined in the same way.

In the UK the National Screening Committee oversee the introduction of new screening programmes and robust evidence for all of the criteria is needed for a new screening programme to be agreed.

Thinking back to our question earlier about screening for the major cancers in the UK, we can consider why some of these screening programmes have not been introduced in the light of the criteria outlined above.

Many of the criteria for assessing the need for a population programme have not been met for prostate cancer. In particular, there is a lack of knowledge about the epidemiology and natural history of the disease, a poor level of accuracy in the screening tests, and a lack of good-quality evidence concerning the effectiveness and cost-effectiveness of treatments for localised prostate cancer. In addition the evidence suggests that a screening programme would not reduce deaths [10] There is little evidence for the effectiveness for screening for lung cancer in those at risk (cigarette smokers).

Examples of effective screening programmes

Screening can be targeted at various stages of the life course. Some examples of screening programmes established in the UK at each life stage are given in Table 5.1.

Old age

There are currently no screening programmes in the UK which are targeted at older people. Two conditions which could, theoretically, be screened for are osteoporosis and Altzheimer's disease but there is insufficient evidence that such programme would be cost effective. The UK National Screening Committee determines UK screening policy and is continually reviewing its policy on screening in old age. The committee is also currently discussing the utility of screening in men aged over 65 for abdominal aortic aneurysm which can be fatal.

Immigration screening

Screening of all ages on immigration may also occur. In the UK, immigrants and those wishing to stay in the UK for longer than six months are screened for tuberculosis and immigrants and refugees to the US are screened for a range

Table 5.1. Screening programmes in the UK, 2006

Life stage	Population offered screening	Diseases screened for
Antenatal	All pregnant women (some programmes are being phased in)	Anaemia
		Bacteriuria
		Blood group
		Rhesus status
		HIV
		Hepatitis B
		Down's syndrome
		Spina bifida
		Other foetal anomalies
		Tay Sachs disease
		Thalassaemia
Newborn	All newborn babies	Congenital hypothyroidism
		Phenylketonuria (PKU)
		Cystic fibrosis
		Haemoglobinopathies
		General physical examination with particular emphasis on the eyes, heart and hips
		Automated hearing screen
Children	All children	Growth abnormalities (height and weight at school entry)
		Visual impairment (between 4th and 5th birthdays)
Adults	Women of certain ages	Breast cancer
		Cervical cancer
	All older people	Colorectal cancer
	Men and women aged 16–24	Chlamydia
	Diabetics	Sight-threatening retinopathy

Source: National Screening Committee, www.nsc.nhs.uk.

of infectious diseases including HIV, TB, gonorrhoea, syphilis and leprosy. Whilst this detects disease in the individuals it is termed screening as it intends to protect the resident population from the effects of communicable diseases.

Evaluating screening programmes

Screening test performance

No screening test can be 100% perfect. It only picks up those people thought to be at increased risk of disease and some of these may not in fact develop the condition. It is important in population terms to be able to predict the numbers of false results (either false negatives or false positives), to be able to judge the best screening test for a particular condition. It is also important on an individual basis to be able to predict how likely a test result is to reflect the true status of the patient.

Two measures used are *sensitivity* and *specificity*. Sensitivity is the proportion of truly diseased persons, as measured by the gold standard, who are identified as diseased by the test under study; specificity is the proportion of truly non-diseased persons as measured by the gold standard, who are identified as non-diseased by the test under study. A sensitive test will identify all (or almost all) the true positives, but in doing so will wrongly identify some truly negative cases as positive ('false positives'). A specific test will only identify positives if it is certain (or almost certain) that they are truly positive, but in doing so will wrongly identify some truly positive cases as negative ('false negatives'). A sensitive test keeps the false negative rate low, and a specific test keeps the false positive rate low. In the design of tests, as the tests are made more specific, they become less sensitive, and vice-versa. A balance is needed and the calculated sensitivities and specificities are used to determine the best screening test for each condition.

Calculating sensitivity and specificity

In calculating these measures one needs to know the numbers screened and the numbers deemed later to have the disease by a 'gold-standard' diagnostic test. These people are termed 'test' and 'true' positives and negatives.

The 2×2 in Table 5.2 illustrates this: a is the number of people who truly have the disease who have a positive test result (true positives); b is the number of people who truly do not have the disease who have a positive test result (false positives); c is the number of people who truly have the disease who have a negative test result (false negatives); and d is the number of people who truly do not have the disease who have a negative test result (true negatives).

Table 5.2. Generic 2×2 table showing the possible outcomes of a screening test and used to calculate its validity

		('True')		
		Positive	Negative	
	Positive	a	b	a + b
('Test')				
	Negative	c	d	c + d
		a + c	b + d	a + b + c + d (Total)

Table 5.3. A 2×2 table for a urine glucose test as a screen for diabetes

Result of urine test for glucose (screening 'test')	Result of glucose tolerance test (gold-standard diagnostic 'true')		
	Positive	Negative	
Positive	6	7	13
Negative	21	966	987
	27	973	1000

Using terms from the 2×2 table sensitivity, specificity and false test rates can be calculated:

Sensitivity $= a/(a + c)$ (5.1)

False positive rate $= b/(a + b + c + d)$ (5.2)

Specificity $= d/(b + d)$ (5.3)

False negative rate $= c/(a + b + c + d)$ (5.4)

For example, urine analysis can be used to screen for the likelihood of diabetes. The validity of this test has been considered [11] – see Table 5.3.

Use the formulae to calculate the sensitivity and specificity for this test.
Sensitivity $= 6/27 = 22\%$
Specificity $= 966/973 = 99\%$
This test is very specific but not very sensitive. This means that, at a population level, it is not very effective at picking up positive cases of diabetes but is quite good at identifying people who do not have diabetes. It is unlikely that a test with such a low sensitivity would be used as a widespread screening tool without further information being available for the clinician to inform decision-making on the best course of action following the test. More information is needed and can be provided by calculating the predictive values and a likelihood ratio for the test.

Returning to our examples of breast and cervical screening we can examine the reported validity of these tests. The sensitivity of mammography in women aged over 50 ranges from 68% to over 90%, with most trials and programmes achieving sensitivities of around 85%. In women aged 40–49 the sensitivity has been reported to be lower, with estimates between 62% and 76%. The specificity of breast screening by mammography ranges between 82% and 97% [12]. For fluid-based cervical screening, the sensitivity has been reported as 90% and the specificity 85%. For the conventional Pap test, the sensitivity was found to be 79% and the specificity was 89% [13].

Table 5.4. A 2×2 table for a urine glucose test as a screen for diabetes in high (15%) prevalence population

	Result of glucose tolerance test (gold-standard diagnostic)		
	Positive	Negative	
Positive	33	8	41
Result of urine test for glucose (screening)			
Negative	117	842	959
	150	850	1000

Predictive values and likelihood ratios

The sensitivity and specificity of a test does not depend on the prevalence of the disease in question. In other words they are the same, no matter which population you screen. However, screening tests can vary considerably in their ability to predict the true disease state of an individual. This is termed the predictive value and depends on how prevalent is the disease. Take the diabetes test again as an example.

The prevalence of the condition in the example in Table 5.3 is 2.7% (27 true positives in a population of 1,000). In this case the predictive values can be calculated:

Positive predictive value $= a/(a + b) = 6/13 = 46.2\%$

Negative predictive value $= d/(c + d) = 966/973 = 97.8\%$

This can be interpreted to mean that a patient with a positive urine test result has a 46.2% chance of really having diabetes but a patient with a negative result has a 97.8% chance of NOT having diabetes. In this case the test is good at ruling out diabetes but not so good at ruling it in!

What difference does it make to this prediction if the prevalence of the condition is higher? Table 5.4 shows the same sensitivity and specificity but in a population where the prevalence of diabetes is 15% (150 cases out of 1,000).

Use Table 5.4 to calculate the positive and negative predictive values of the test in this population.

Positive predictive value $= 33/41 = 80\%$
Negative predictive value $= 842/959 = 88\%$

This demonstrates that when there is already a greater likelihood of the disease being present (a prevalence of 15% compared to 2.7%) the test is a better predictor, both of true negatives and true positives. This begs a question. What if we already suspected the patient may have diabetes from other information? We might be testing an elderly patient who has come to clinic complaining of increased urination, tiredness and excess thirst. An individual clinician might then be more likely to have a higher index of suspicion and trust a positive result more. Because this is the way people really think in real situations, sensitivities and specificities (and even predictive values) are not always useful tools on a patient-by-patient basis.

Estimates of positive predictive value in the UK Breast Screening Programme range from 6% to 8% for prevalent screening, meaning that 6% to 8% of women recalled for further tests after their first screening have cancer. The positive predictive value is higher for incident screens (women who are having their second or subsequent mammogram) and has been estimated at between 12% and 14% [14]. Assuming a sensitivity of 90% and specificity of 85% for cervical cancer, because the prevalence of the disease is so low (less than 3,000 cases per year in the UK), the positive predictive value is very low and the negative predictive value very high (almost 100%).

Here *likelihood ratios* can be useful. We start before the test with a probability that the patient has the condition we are interested in. This is called the pre-test probability. A positive likelihood ratio tells us how much more likely it is that a condition is present when the test result is positive. A negative likelihood ratio tells us how much more likely the patient is not to have the condition after a negative test result.

For example, say we thought our elderly patient already had a 50% chance of having diabetes from his symptoms (a probability of 0.5 or 50:50 odds, ie odds of 1:1 – this is called the pre-test odds). The post-test odds is the pre-test odds multiplied by the likelihood ratio and the likelihood ratios from the test can be calculated using:

Negative test:

Negative likelihood ratio = (1-Sensitivity)/Specificity　　　　　　　　　　(5.5)

Positive test:

Positive likelihood ratio = Sensitivity/(1-Specificity)　　　　　　　　　　(5.6)

Using the sensitivity and specificity of the urine analysis test from earlier we can calculate:

$$\text{Negative likelihood ratio} = (1 - 0.22)/10.99$$
$$= 0.78 - 0.99$$
$$= 0.79$$

$$\text{Positive likelihood ratio} = 0.22/(1 - 0.99)$$
$$= 22$$

 If the test came in negative we could alter our first estimate of the odds (1), by the negative likelihood ratio (0.79):

Post-test odds $=$ Pre-test odds $\times$ Likelihood ratio

$$= 1 \times 0.79$$

$$= 0.79$$

The probability of the patient having diabetes can be calculated from this using:

Post-test probability $=$ Post-test odds$/$(Post-test odds $+ 1$)   (5.7)

So:

Post-test probability $= 0.79/(0.79 + 1) = 0.44(44\%)$

In this case, even though the test was negative, there is still a 44% chance that the patient has diabetes. This value is lower than our initial pre-test probability of 50%, but a negative test result here is unlikely to deter further diagnostic tests.

The positive likelihood ratio of 22 is so high that with a positive result we would be pretty certain our patient had diabetes and would be likely to initiate treatment.

To summarise, sensitivities and specificities tell us how good the test is and are used to determine which is the best test for any condition. Predictive values tell us how the test utility varies across populations and likelihood ratios are useful to interpret test results for individual patients where we have additional information on the likelihood of a disease being present before we do the test.

Monitoring screening programmes

Criteria based on those of Wilson and Jungner summarised above are generally used to determine whether to put a screening programme in place but they do not guarantee that a screening programme will work in practice. The programme must be evaluated to ensure that it is safe and acceptable in the short term and meets its aims of morbidity or mortality reduction in the long term. In the UK all new screening programmes are established with quality assurance programmes that consider a range of short-term outcomes (see Box 5.1).

As well as determining a test's validity, it is necessary to consider potential sources of bias and health-related long-term outcomes.

Sources of bias in screening

Selection bias

We hope that screening programmes attract the population we intended to screen but there is the potential for those who respond to our invitations to be

Box 5.1 Monitoring screening programmes

The following information can be used to judge the effectiveness of a screening programme:

- clinical or laboratory expertise of those responsible for screening tests
- coverage achieved
- number of referrals
- number referred who attend for specialist diagnosis
- number of test positives who are confirmed as true positives
- number of false positives
- number of true cases missed
- number of cases effectively treated
- the impact of the screening programme on other related services
- the delays between different steps of the programme and resulting anxiety
- the quality, accuracy and readability of the information provided to patients about the programme
- the extent of the benefit accruing to those effectively treated
- the cost of the programme, the cost per case detected and the value of the benefits obtained

systematically different from the target population in some way. For example, there is some evidence that South Asian women are less likely to be offered and take up prenatal screening [15] and the UK National Screening Programme statistics show that uptake is also lower in women aged over 60 years. Such studies and statistics demonstrate to those running the screening programme that efforts are needed to minimise the biases we have in the types of women who are screened.

Lead time bias

Lead time bias occurs when detection by screening seems to increase disease-free survival but this is only because disease has been detected earlier and not because screening is delaying death or disease. Figure 5.2 shows how this works: person A and B develop disease, then die at the same time; however, it appears that A lives longer than B because she found out about her disease earlier through screening. This is one reason why it is important to evaluate a programme using mortality as an outcome and to compare screened and unscreened populations. Where there is a lead time bias no improvements in mortality will be demonstrated.

Length time bias

Length time bias occurs if the screening programme is better at picking up milder forms of the disease. Figure 5.3 shows this. Length time bias means that people who develop disease that progresses more quickly or is more likely to be fatal

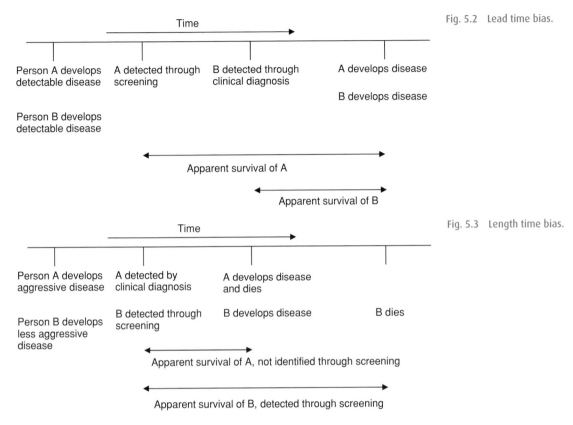

Fig. 5.2   Lead time bias.

Fig. 5.3   Length time bias.

(person A) are less likely to be picked up by screening and their outcomes may not be included in evaluations of the programme. Thus the programme looks to be more effective than it is. The programme evaluation must compare the type of disease which is picked up through screening with that picked up by routine diagnosis. Where length time bias occurs the screening programme will systematically identify disease which has a better prognosis.

Conclusion

Screening is an important public health intervention which has been demonstrated to have had a major impact on mortality for certain conditions. However, screening carries risks to individuals and is a good example of an area of public health where the needs of individuals and the needs of populations may conflict. Professionals working in screening, whether counselling individuals on screening choices or supporting screening at a population level, need to be aware that their beliefs colour the way they communicate with people. There are links to further resources and educational and training materials on the CD.

REFERENCES

1. T. M. Marteau and A. L. Kinmonth, Screening for cardiovascular risk: public health imperative or matter for individual informed choice? *British Medical Journal*, **325**, 2002, 78–80.

2. J. M. Wilson and G. Jungner, Principles and practice of screening for disease. Geneva, World Health Organization, 1968 (Public Health Paper Number 34).

3. D. M. B. Hall, *Report of the Joint Working Party on Child Health Surveillance: Health for All Children*, 3rd edn, Oxford, Oxford University Press.

4. Advisory Committee on Breast Cancer Screening, Screening for breast cancer in England: past and future. *NHSBSP Publication No 61*, 2006.

5. The Breast Screening Frequency Trial Group. The frequency of breast cancer screening: results from the UKCCCR Randomised Trial. *European Journal of Cancer*, **38**, 2002, 1458–64.

6. International Agency for Research on Cancer (IARC) Working Group on the Evaluation of Cervical Cancer Screening Programmes. Screening for squamous cervical cancer: duration of low risk after negative results of cervical cytology and its implication for screening policies. *British Medical Journal*, **293**, 1986, 659–64.

7. P. D. Sasieni, J. Cuzick and E. Lynch-Farmery, Estimating the efficacy of screening by auditing smear histories of women with and without cervical cancer. The National Co-ordinating Network for Cervical Screening Working Group. *British Journal of Cancer*, **73**(8), 1996, 1001–5.

8. M. Quinn, P. Babb, J. Jones and E. Allen, on behalf of the United Kingdom Association of Cancer Registries, Effect of screening on incidence of and mortality from cancer of cervix in England: evaluation based on routinely collected statistics. *British Medical Journal*, **318**, 1999, 904.

9. J. Peto, C. Gilham, F. E. Matthews and O. Fletcher, The cervical cancer epidemic that screening has prevented in the UK. *The Lancet*, **364**, 2004, 249–56.

10. S. Selley, D. Gillatt, J. Coast, A. Faulkner and J. Donovan, Diagnosis, management and screening of early localised prostate cancer. *Health Technology Assessment*, **1**(2), 1997.

11. D. K. G. Andersson, E. Lundblad and K. Svardsudd, A model for early diagnosis of type 2 diabetes mellitus in primary health care. *Diabetic Medicine*, **10**, 1993, 167–73.

12. F. Bianchini and H. Vainio, *Breast Cancer Screening Techniques*. International Agency for Research on Cancer (IARC) Handbooks of Cancer Prevention, vol. 7, Lyon, IARC Press, 2002.

13. S. M. Sulik, K. Kroeger, J. K. Schultz *et al.*, Are fluid-based cytologies superior to the conventional Papanicolaou test: a systematic review. *Journal of Family Practice*, **50**(12), 2001, 1040–4046.

14. R. G. Blanks, S. M. Moss and J. Patnick, Results from the UK NHS breast screening programme 1994–1999. *Journal of Medical Screening*, **7**(4), 2000, 195–8.

15. R. E. Rowe and L. L. Davidson, Social and ethnic inequalities in the offer and uptake of prenatal screening and diagnosis in the UK: a systematic review. *Public Health*, **118**(3), 2004, 177–89.

6

Health needs assessment

Key points

- Health needs should be distinguished from the need for health care which is nowadays defined in terms of ability to benefit.
- Health care needs assessment is central to the planning process.
- There are three commonly contrasted approaches to needs assessment: corporate, comparative and epidemiological.
- Many toolkits and other resources have been developed to assist those undertaking health-care needs assessments.

Theoretical perspectives

Health professionals spend much time learning to assess the needs of individuals; many know less about defining the needs of a population. The need for health underlies but does not wholly determine the need for health care. Health-care needs are often measured in terms of demand, but demand is to a great extent 'supply-induced' (see Chapter 14). For example, variations in general-practice referral or consultation rates have less to do with the health status of the populations served than with differences between doctors, such as their skills or referral thresholds [1].

There is no generally accepted definition of 'need'. Last's notion of the 'clinical iceberg' of disease [2] (see Chapter 1) has been supported by various community studies indicating much illness is unknown to health professionals. Needs can be classified in terms of diseases, priority groups, geographical areas, services or using a life-cycle approach (children/teenagers/adults/elderly). Bradshaw's often-quoted taxonomy highlighted four types of need [3]:

Essential Public Health, eds. Stephen Gillam, Jan Yates and Padmanabhan Badrinath.
Published by Cambridge University Press. © Cambridge University Press 2007.

- expressed needs (needs expressed by action, for instance visiting a doctor)
- normative needs (defined by experts)
- comparative needs (comparing one group of people with another)
- felt needs (those needs people say they have).

Health or health care?

Health is famously difficult to define. As we saw in Chapter 4, the World Health Organisation's definition of health embraces the physical, social, and emotional well being of an individual, group, or community and emphasises health as a positive resource of life, not just the absence of disease [4]. Health needs accordingly encompass education, social services, housing, the environment and social policy.

The need for health care is the population's ability to benefit from health care, which is in turn the sum of many individuals' ability to benefit [4]. As well as treatment, health care includes prevention, diagnosis, continuing care, rehabilitation and palliative care. The ability to benefit does not mean that all outcomes will be favourable but implies outcomes that will, on average, be effective. Some benefits may be manifested in changes of clinical status; others, such as the benefits of reassurance or the support of carers, are difficult to measure. Diagnosis and reassurance form an important part of primary care when many people may require no more than a negative diagnosis. Health care needs assessment thus requires knowledge of the incidence of the health problem (risk factor, disease, disability), its prevalence, and the effectiveness of services to address it.

Individual or population?

Clinicians focus on the individual and need is defined in terms of what can be done for the patients they see. However, this may neglect the health needs of people not receiving care, e.g. attending surgery or outpatients departments. Traditionally, the clinical view enshrined in such notions as 'clinical freedom' has taken little account of treatment cost. Services of doubtful efficacy are provided if they may be even remotely beneficial to patients. In contrast, the public health view seeks to prioritise within finite budgets. Individual clinical decisions may be made without considering the opportunity costs of treatment, while at a population level such opportunity costs must be minimised if the health of the population is to be maximised.

The ethical conflicts raised are not easily resolved. Health professionals will only reluctantly withhold interventions of minor benefit for the greater good of potential patients. Tension between what is best for the individual and what may be best for society will always present a dilemma for clinicians. In reality, a complex range of considerations, of which cost-effectiveness is but one, will always determine both clinical and strategic decision-making (see Chapter 9).

Need, supply or demand?

Health care is never organised as a 'pure' market. Its products are heavily sub-sidised and regulated in all countries. The main reason for this is asymmetry of information whereby patients lack knowledge of their own treatment needs and depend on providers to make appropriate decisions. The clinician acts as the patient's 'agent' to translate demands into needs. However, the literature on variation in referrals, prescribing and other activity rates reveals that this agency relationship is complex.

Professional perceptions of need may differ from those of consumers [5]. The latter are more likely to be influenced by external factors such as media coverage and the opinions of relatives and friends. Consumers' priorities vary with age, health status and previous experience of health service use.

The health problems considered to constitute need may change over time. Much universal screening activity, for example in the field of child health surveil-lance, is no longer supported by research evidence. New needs accrue with the development of new technology. There is usually a time lag before lay demand (for health) reflects scientific evidence of need (for health care). Unfortunately, an even longer time lag distorts the provision of health services. Their supply is affected by historical factors, and by public and political pressures. The closure of hospital beds is ever politically charged. Health services tend to be regarded as untouchable even when their usefulness has been outlived, while medical inno-vations are generally implemented before they have been fully evaluated.

The relationship between need, demand and supply is illustrated in Figure 6.1. It shows seven fields of services divided into those for which there is a need but no demand or supply (1), those for which there is a demand but no need or supply (2), those for which there is a supply but no need or demand (3), and various other degrees of overlap. Any intervention can be fitted into one of these fields. Rehabilitation after myocardial infarction may be needed but not supplied or demanded. Antibiotics for upper-respiratory-tract infec-tion may be demanded but not needed or supplied, and so on. Much effort is required on behalf of patients, providers and purchasers to make the three cycles more confluent. Something is known about how to change professional behaviour through financial incentives, protocols, education, audit and even con-tracts (see Chapter 16); the factors influencing patient preferences are less well understood.

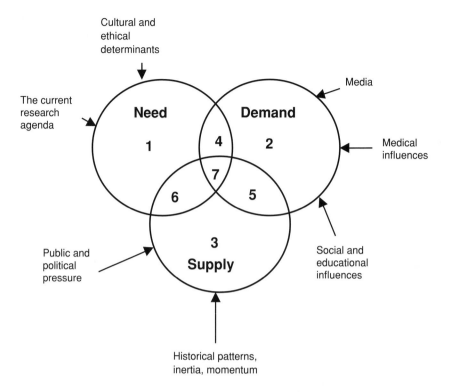

Fig. 6.1   Need, demand and supply.

 From Figure 6.1, seven types of service can be identified. See if you can provide examples of services in each segment. For example, preventive or health-promoting interventions such as the fortification of flour with folic acid come into the category of interventions that are needed and supplied (in some countries) but not necessarily demanded (segment 6).

1. Services where there is a need but no demand or supply – Family-planning and contraceptive services are needed in many parts of the developing world to improve women's reproductive health. They are frequently neither *demanded* nor *supplied*.

2. Services for which there is a demand but no need or supply – Patients may ask for (*demand*) expectorants for coughs and colds. However, cough mixtures are ineffective and should be seldom prescribed (no *need* or *supply*).

3. Services for which there is a supply but no need or demand – The provision of routine health checks in people over 75 years. Most people do not request these (no *demand*), but in some practices they are provided (*supply*). Research suggests that the benefits of such checks do not outweigh the costs (no *need*).

4. Services for which there is a need and demand but no supply – Substance misuse is a common and dangerous affliction. Methadone maintenance

programmes can reduce the physical risks of heroin addiction and may increase the chances of drug misusers giving up (*need*), but it is not always available (no *supply*).

5. Services for which there is a demand and supply but no need – People may request (*demand*) and be prescribed (*supply*) long-acting benzodiazepines for insomnia. In the long term this is not effective (no *need*).

6. Services for which there is a need and supply but no demand – Even when it is offered, not all health-care staff take up the opportunity of Hepatitis B immunisation (*supply* but no *demand*). Yet they are at risk of Hepatitis B infection and immunisation is effective at preventing it (*need*).

7. Services for which there is a need, demand and supply – People with insulin-dependent diabetes ask for (*demand*) insulin, it is effective at maintaining their health (*need*) and the UK National Health Service, unlike many others, can afford to provide it (*supply*).

Health needs assessment (HNA) in practice

In the UK, after the so-called 'internal market' between health-care purchasers and providers was introduced in the early 1990s, purchasing decisions based on the needs of the population to achieve 'health gain' came into focus. Health Authorities and subsequently primary care trusts have been required to assess the needs of their population and to use these needs to set priorities and improve health. Public health practitioners, with their training and origins in epidemiology, disease control and health promotion, developed a number of techniques to assess population needs. At the same time, there was greater interest in involving the general public in shaping services, and a number of techniques have been developed to assess health needs from the user's perspective.

The aim of a health needs assessment is to describe health problems in a population and detect differences within and between different groups in order to determine health priorities and unmet need. It should identify where people are able to benefit either from health service care or from wider social and environmental change, and balance any potential change against clinical, ethical and economic considerations; that is, what should be done, what can be done and what can be afforded [6]– See Box 6.1.

Health needs assessment is thus a method that:
- is objective, valid and takes a systematic approach
- involves a number of professionals and the general public
- involves using different sources and methods of collecting and analysing information (including epidemiological, qualitative and comparative methods)
- seeks to identify needs and recommends changes to optimise the delivery of health services.

> **Box 6.1 Five objectives of a health care needs assessment [7]**
>
> 1. **Planning**. This is the central objective of needs assessment: to help decide what services are required; for how many people; the effectiveness of these services; the benefits that will be expected; and at what cost.
> 2. **Intelligence.** Gathering information to get an overview and an increased understanding of the existing health care service, the population it serves and the population's health needs, i.e. what is the base-line?
> 3. **Equity.** Improving the allocation of resources between and within different groups.
> 4. **Target efficiency.** Having assessed needs, measuring whether or not resources have been appropriately directed: i.e. Do those who need a service get it? Do those who get a service need it? This is related to audit.
> 5. **Involvement of stakeholders**. Carrying out a health care needs assessment can stimulate the involvement and ownership of the various players in the process.

Assessing needs and priorities

Assessing needs and priorities is important because the NHS and health systems across the world face similar pressures. These include the rising cost of health care due to continuing scientific advances, increasing life expectancy and rising public expectations. At the same time, most countries face similar dilemmas: health service resources are limited and people face inequitable access to existing care. People whose health needs are greatest are least likely to have access to health care (the 'inverse care law' referred to several times throughout this book). Finally, there are concerns about the appropriateness, effectiveness and quality of that care. The challenge is to make decisions that maximise the benefit for the population, taking into account the resources available. Needs assessment helps this decision-making and involves at least three steps:

Step 1. Identifying health priorities by defining the population under scrutiny and collecting and analysing routine data – comparative needs assessment

Routine data indicate what it is that people are dying from and why they consult general practices, hospitals and social services. This will help to prioritise topics for local discussion (Step 2) with a range of other local agencies and professionals. These data allow comparisons to be drawn between local services and those available in other geographical areas. It is also possible to compare these data with previously set standards. For example, one might compare rates of heart operations with standards set in the National Service Framework for coronary heart disease.

Many data are already available and provide information to 'start the ball rolling'. Chapter 7 gives an indication of routinely available information, which may be accessed from health care organisations. Such information can be reproduced in packs and used in meetings. Discussions about the data will help lead to a consensus on what areas are priorities. They can also be a starting point to involve the public.

There are some disadvantages. The data may be quite old (it often takes up to two years for routine data to become available), diseases may have been misdiagnosed or not reported and hospital data may reflect different admission policies for the same condition. Nevertheless, it does help to start the process and is a means to approaching others who have a contribution to make.

Step 2. Agreeing local priorities by involving other agencies, users and the public – corporate needs assessment

There are a confusing number of terms for this process including community appraisals, rapid appraisals and community surveys. Many of the techniques have been pioneered in developing countries by researchers using qualitative methods [8] – unstructured or semi-structured interviews, for example. These approaches to understanding behaviours and beliefs may reduce the distorting effect of measuring needs through the eyes of health professionals.

Professionals from other agencies, including local government and the voluntary sector, may have differing ideas from health professionals, and it is important to take these ideas into account. It is also important to consider the ideas of users and carers about what improves their health. These factors may include having a job, adequate housing, better choice of food or a bus route. It is important to be aware of the limitations of professional knowledge. There are a number of ways of getting the public involved including:

- Citizens' juries – representatives of the public or local opinion leaders are selected. Experts give evidence and jurors have an opportunity to ask questions and debate.
- User consultation panels – local people are selected as representatives of the locality. Typically, members are rotated to include a broad range of views. Topics are considered in advance and members are presented with relevant information. A moderator facilitates the meeting.
- Focus groups – semi-structured discussion groups of six to eight people led by a moderator.
- Questionnaire surveys – these can be postal or distributed by hand. This is often most appropriate when the issues behind questions are well known.

- Panels – these are large, sociologically representative samples (around 100) of a population in a health authority, which are surveyed at intervals.
- Interviews – for example, with patients after a clinic visit on the quality of care, or with health workers on what they know of people's perceptions of local needs.
- Rapid appraisal – involves the public directly in the assessment and definition of local needs through a series of face-to-face interviews with local informants who have a knowledge of the community. From these interviews, and from appraisal of local documents about the neighbourhood or community, a list of priorities is drawn up. This is then assessed collectively by means of a public meeting. Working groups develop action plans. The approach is 'bottom up' and the key philosophy is not only of public involvement but of a collective response to health needs.

Step 3. Undertaking an epidemiological needs assessment

This stage involves examining specific priorities in more detail. It looks carefully at matters such as the size of the problem, what is currently being provided and what interventions may help. Recommendations can then be made on what changes are needed. Priorities for the purposes of HNA may comprise:

- a whole speciality such as mental health
- a disease such as coronary heart disease
- a client group such as substance misusers
- groups waiting for interventions such as those waiting for hip operations
- vulnerable groups such as ethnic minorities
- socially deprived groups such as tenants of particular housing estates.
  An epidemiological approach to assessing health needs measures:
1. The size of the problem. It looks at how much illness or ill health there is in the community by assessing the incidence and prevalence.
2. The current services that exist to meet this burden. It examines how local provision compares with other areas, whether the services meet the needs or whether they are over- or under-provided.
3. Whether the services are effective. If new services are required to meet unmet need it looks at what is known about what works or will make a difference.

Resources for health care are always finite so the purpose of this type of needs assessment is to identify health improvements which can be achieved by reallocating resources to remedy over-provision (sometimes) and unmet need.

Policy, planning and strategy development

The planning cycle should originate in an assessment of needs: where are we now and where do we want to get to? The rest of the cycle is mostly concerned with how to get there (Figure 6.2). Comprehensive needs assessment will generate a

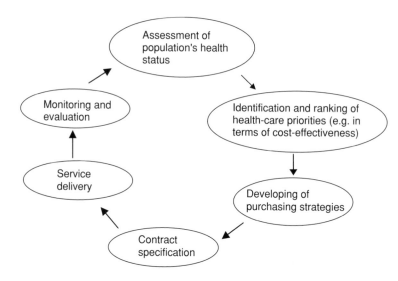

Fig. 6.2   The planning cycle.

bewildering array of possible needs. There are many ways of identifying priorities and this issue is discussed in Chapter 9.

At whatever level in the system priorities are being agreed, the process should involve as many of the people who will be affected by the choice as reasonably possible. Teams need to take careful stock of their current work when making a decision. In many important areas work may already be ongoing (for example, heart disease prevention). Few health professionals are not already overloaded. There is little point in setting grandiose objectives that cannot realistically be attained.

Audit and evaluation (to see whether we have got to where we want to go) is therefore integrally related to needs assessment (Chapter 8). Indeed the selection of audit topics should be framed by systematic assessment of priority needs. It can too often be governed by ad hoc medical choices.

A description of the planning process may falsely imply an orderly sequence. Few practitioners with experience of planning and policy-making will subscribe to this myth of rational planning (Chapter 15). In real life, it is rarely possible to maintain forward progress around the cycle for long. The process is iterative rather than cyclical. The commonest causes of disruption, other than shortage of finance, are vague objectives, lack of information and changing circumstances, people and politics. An understanding of the contingent nature of much planning is important in effecting change.

However, consideration of both the planning process and policy-making process as a cycle is helpful when working at a local level within the NHS or partner organisations such as local authorities or voluntary-sector organisations. The policy cycle is often portrayed in a similar way to the planning cycle (see Figure 6.3).

Table 6.1. An example of local policy and planning – obesity

Step in the policy process	Step in the planning process	What might happen locally
Assessment of health status		Local obesity levels 25% in adults and 20% in children
Problem identification		Stakeholders identify the following problems: poor school menus, little school sport, poor access to cheap leisure centres
Identification of policy options		Options include: amend education authority policies, work with local authority to increase leisure facilities
Choice of policy		A consensus is reached on the priority area: work on childhood obesity with the education authority
Policy implementation	Assessment of population's health status	Obesity levels in primary school children are identified as particularly high
	Identification and ranking of health care priorities (e.g. in terms of cost-effectiveness)	Creating healthier diets is ranked locally as more important than increasing school sport
	Development of purchasing strategies	Local purchasing is arranged through local suppliers to reduce food miles
	Contract specification	The quantity and quality of food is specified and the menus agreed
	Service delivery	Food is delivered and prepared to new menus in local schools
	Monitoring and evaluation	Menus and uptake are monitored
Policy evaluation		Height and weight is monitored on school exit

Fig. 6.3   Generic policy-making cycle.

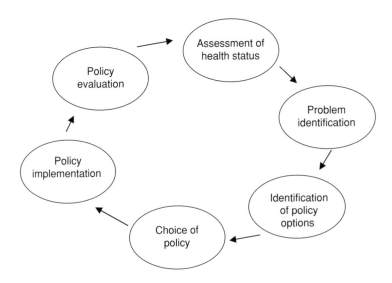

You have been asked to undertake an assessment of health care needs in a local prison. What steps are likely to be involved and what questions would you be seeking to answer?

See Figure 6.4. For further details, explore the toolkit developed for health care needs assessment in prisons [9], a good example of the resources available.

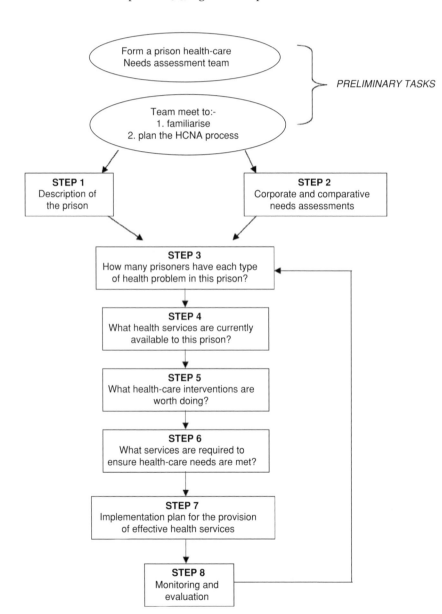

Fig. 6.4   Assessment of needs in a local prison.

As an example, consider the development of a local obesity strategy to meet the stated government-policy aims of 'halting the year-on-year rise in obesity among children aged under 11 by 2010 in the context of a broader strategy to tackle obesity in the population as a whole' (Department of Health Public Service Agreement Target). The aim of developing a local strategy to achieve this would reflect a rational approach; an attempt to set out the logical steps needed to reach the goal. With an understanding that the process is cyclical, the actions needed form a logical sequence. How this might work is summarised in Table 6.1.

Context is as important for strategy development and implementation as it is for policy-making. Some of the contextual elements which would be relevant to the development of an obesity strategy are: local obesity levels, the availability of healthy food, views of local health professionals, views of local schools, the availability of exercise opportunities, local political imperatives, local commercial interests, and the views of the public locally.

Which of the contextual elements listed above would have to be considered in planning to improve school meals? Are there other factors which would need to be taken into consideration when implementing this plan?

All the contextual elements would be relevant in this example. Other factors to consider include the costs of the plan and ensuring that changes are sustainable.

Conclusion

The policy-making process is often summarised as a cycle (See Figure 6.4). The nature of policy-making and recent national health policy are considered in more detail in Chapter 15.

FURTHER READING

1. S. Gillam and S. Murray, *Needs Assessment in General Practice*. Occasional Paper 73, London, Royal College of General Practitioners, 1996.
2. J. Hooper and P. Longworth, *Health Needs Assessment Workbook*. London, Health Development Agency, 2002.
3. J. Wright, *Health Needs Assessment in Practice*, London, BMJ Books, 1998.
4. A. Stevens and J. Raftery (eds), *Health Care Needs Assessment. The Epidemiologically Based Needs Assessment Reviews*, Oxford, Radcliffe Medical Press, Series 1 and 2, 1997.

REFERENCES

1. M. Roland and A. Coulter, *Hospital Referrals*. Oxford, Oxford University Press, 1993.
2. J. M. Last, The iceberg: completing the clinical picture in general practice. *Lancet* **2**, 1963, 28–31.

3. J. S. Bradshaw, A taxonomy of social need. In G. McLachlan (ed.), *Problems and Progress in Medical Care: Essays on Current Research*, 7th series, London, Oxford University Press, 1972.

4. A. Stevens and J. Raftery, *Health Care Needs Assessment*. The Epidemiologically Based Needs Assessment Reviews. Oxford, Radcliffe Medical Press, vols. 1 and 2, 1994.

5. A. Bowling, Health care rationing: the public's debate. *British Medical Journal*, **312**, 1996, 670–4.

6. J. Wright and D. Kyle, Assessing health needs. In *Oxford Handbook of Public Health Practice*, 2nd edn, D. Pencheon, C. Guest, D. Melzer and J. A. Muir Gray (eds.), Oxford, Oxford University Press, 2006, ch. 1.3, pp. 20–31.

7. A. Stevens and J. Gabbay. Needs assessment, needs assessment. . . *Health Trends*, **23**, 1993, 20–3.

8. H. Annett and S. Rifkin, Guidelines for rapid participatory appraisal to assess community health needs: a focus on health improvements for low income urban and rural areas. Geneva, World Health Organisation, 1995.

9. T. Marshall, S. Simpson and A. Stevens, Toolkit for health care needs assessment in prisons. Department of Public Health and Epidemiology, University of Birmingham, 2000.

7

The health status of the population

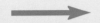

Key points

- Determining the health status of a population is essential before planning effective interventions to improve health and to prevent disease.
- Health measures used to compile such a health profile include:
  mortality (for example, all deaths, deaths from specific causes, in specific subsets of the population standardised to account for different population structures, deaths in and around childbirth, years of life lost)
  objectively measured morbidity (for example, infectious disease rates, hospital activity, primary care data, registered diseases)
  self-reported health and risk status (for example, from surveys)
  assorted data on road accidents, occupational diseases, vital statistics, determinants of health.
- Data may be collated at regional or national level by statistical organisations or public health observatories.

Introduction

Public health practitioners are frequently called upon to determine the health status of a population. This is central to understanding the health experiences of the people within the population and to planning effective interventions to improve their health. Over time, this use of data becomes public health surveillance enabling the use of routine data and collection of specific data to provide the information necessary for public health decision-making.

It is important to consider both health and disease, to consider what contributes to well-being as well as what conditions we must address. Both qualitative and quantitative measures are important as not every outcome can be measured or counted easily. We can count deaths, numbers of operations or measure blood

Essential Public Health, eds. Stephen Gillam, Jan Yates and Padmanabhan Badrinath.
Published by Cambridge University Press. © Cambridge University Press 2007.

> **Box 7.1 Finagle's law**
>
> The information you have is not the information you want. The information you want is not the information you need. The information you need is not what you can get or is not known. The information that is known can't be found in time.

pressure, but people's perceptions of their care or feelings of well-being can only be measured qualitatively. In addition it is important to consider both self-reported (subjective) and measured (objectively verified) elements so that care can be carefully planned and monitored and shown to meet the needs of patients and the public. As well as absolute counts it is useful to have information on disease trends to help predict the need for interventions in the future. Lastly, the information must be related to knowledge of health service structure (e.g. numbers of doctors), processes (e.g. admission rates) and outcomes (e.g. death) so that action can be taken. This chapter outlines some of the key indicators of health status which are typically included within a health profile. Therefore this chapter links to many of the other public health tools – it is integral to the understanding of needs (Chapter 6), it requires skills in epidemiology (Chapter 2), it is necessary to evaluate services (Chapter 8) and it informs prioritisation decisions (Chapter 9). We see once more that public health skills are not used in isolation but must be integrated in practice.

Note that the data described in this chapter come with a 'health warning' (Box 7.1). Data are not without flaws and should never be used without first considering their completeness, accuracy and relevance. Data can be difficult to collect, collate and analyse and it is worth considering carefully the use to which the data will be put and whether they are fit for purpose (Box 7.2).

Measuring mortality

One of the most commonly used epidemiological measurements is the incidence of death. It is generally the starting point for a health profile but does not describe the extent of ill health within a population. Many countries require physicians to record cause of death and these mandatory reports form the basis of mortality files. Although many countries have vital registration systems it is important to remember reasons why these may not be completely accurate, such as limited recording of multiple pathologies in old age or non-statutory birth and death registration systems (see Chapter 1).

For comparative purposes, it is usual to express the number of deaths as a rate:

Box 7.2 Is the data you have fit for purpose?

You should ask the following questions of any data obtained:

1. Are the data related clearly to specific ages and sexes? If the disease you are interested in varies by age or sex you may need to standardise rates of death or morbidity or use age specific rates to allow comparisons.
2. Are the data clearly related to a specific time period? Time trends are helpful in supporting the planning of health care or other public health interventions. It often takes time to collate data and it is important to use the most up-to-date information available.
3. Are the data clearly related to specific geographical locations? You need to ensure that the data you have are related to your population and take care in extrapolating information from other populations to your own.
4. Are the data complete? Are there any population groups missing? Will whoever inputs the data have included every case? Some causes of death may be more easily identified and recorded more frequently than others and some may carry stigma (for example, HIV) and be less well recorded. Is the same data collected across geographical areas? – data coverage in rural areas may be less complete than urban ones.
5. Are the data accurate? What do the definitions of data fields mean? For example, what clinical indications would a field called 'coronary heart disease (CHD)' include? Has it been transcribed from original data allowing the introduction of errors? Are the data coded and are the codes used in the same way by everyone? Have the definitions changed over time if you are looking at time trends?
6. Are the data relevant to the question you have? It is often tempting to use readily available routine data without real thought as to whether they are right for the job!

The crude death rate is the average number of deaths in a given population time period, usually expressed per hundred thousand population over one year,

2,100 deaths occurred in an area of 250,000 population in 2006. What is the crude death rate?

2,100 deaths per 250,000 people means (2,100 / 250,000) × 1,000 = 8.4 deaths per 1,000 population.

200 of these were deaths due to cancer. What is the cancer death rate?

200 deaths per 250,000 people means (200 / 250,000) × 1,000 = 0.8 deaths per 1,000 population.

Differences in the age structure of populations affect crude rates and for most epidemiological purposes it is usual for them to be refined. This enables us to compare the mortality of our population with other similar populations. One way is to compare age- and sex-specific death rates. These are routinely published in the UK by National Statistics, for five- and ten-year age groups. In order to have a single summary figure which allows for different age or sex distributions, standardised death rates are used. These make use of a standard (or reference) population, e.g. the population of England and Wales in 2004.

The directly standardised death rate (DSR) is the death rate that would have occurred in the reference population if it had had the age- and sex-specific death rate of the population being studied (the study population). However, the age-specific death rates of every group must be known, making calculations tedious if more than one population is being studied, and age-specific death rates may not be available.

Indirect standardisation leads to a standardised mortality ratio (SMR), which is the ratio of the deaths observed in the study population to the number of deaths that would have occurred if it had the age- and sex-specific death rates of the reference population, multiplied by 100. This is the most common type of standardisation in the UK and is used to compare populations differentiated by such variables as geographical region, time and social class. The appropriate reference population varies, e.g. with occupation or social class it is the national population aged 15–64 years. The SMR can also be used to show trends, but in this case the reference population is the study population at one particular point in time. Standardised mortality ratios can be misleading if the populations being studied differ widely, from each other or from the reference population, in age and sex structure.

The crude death rates for two towns, A and B, are 10.4 per 1,000 and 20.1 per 1,000, respectively. The DSRs are 14.5 per 1,000 for A and 15.7 for B. What does this mean?

More people die in town B per year but, after accounting for age and sex, the two towns have roughly similar death rates. This may indicate that the age and/or sex structure of the two towns differs. It may be that town B has larger numbers of older people and a higher death rate would be expected. When the standardised death rates are compared this age structure difference is accounted for and the death rates look more similar. This demonstrates that differences in crude rates generally need more investigation.

The coronary heart disease SMR for your population is 130. What does this mean?

An SMR of 130 means that there are 30% more deaths from coronary heart disease in this population than would be expected if the age and sex structure were the same as the reference population. An SMR of 100 is the baseline, higher SMRs indicate worse health and SMRs lower than 100 indicate better health than expected. An SMR this high would suggest that interventions to prevent CHD are needed for this population and that more services for CHD will be needed by this population than the average.

Sometimes it is helpful to demonstrate the proportion of the overall mortality that may be ascribed to a specific cause and emphasise the importance of a particular cause of death. Here we use proportional mortality (also known as the attributable mortality rate). The definition is:

$$\frac{\text{Deaths assigned to the disease in a year}}{\text{Total deaths in the same population in the same year}} \times 100 \qquad (7.1)$$

What is the proportional mortality for cancer in the example in the questions on page 125.
Cancer deaths = 200, total deaths = 2,100. Proportional mortality = (210/2,100) × 100 = 9.5%

Since the 1850s there have been attempts to aid epidemiological analysis and health planning by standardising the classification of death statistics. This allows comparisons between countries and supports international collaboration by providing a common language. The international classification has been overseen by the World Health Organisation since 1948 and is called the International Classification of Diseases (10th revision) or ICD-10. Since 1948 the classification has also included causes of morbidity (see below).

Deaths around the time of childbirth or in infancy are helpful indicators in many countries of the scale of infectious disease or malnutrition and point to the need for public health interventions such as childhood vaccination programmes or improved breast feeding. Indicators used here are perinatal mortality, neonatal mortality, post-neonatal mortality, maternal mortality, stillbirth and infant mortality rates (actually ratios). The definitions of these are:
- perinatal mortality rate: stillbirths + deaths in the first week per 1,000 total births
- neonatal mortality rate: deaths in the first 28 days per 1,000 live births (early neonatal death – first week; late neonatal death – subsequent three weeks)
- post-neonatal mortality rate: post 28 days to first-year deaths per 1,000 live births
- maternal mortality rate: deaths from puerperal causes during pregnancy or within 42 days per 1,000 live births
- stillbirth rate (synonym, foetal death rate): stillbirths per 1,000 total births
- infant mortality rate: deaths at <1 year per 1,000 live births.

Table 7.1. Rates for different indicators

Indicator	Numerator	Denominator	Rate
Perinatal mortality	Stillbirths + first-week deaths = 41	Total births = 3,500	11.7 per 1,000 total births
Neonatal mortality	Deaths in 28 days = 22	Live births = 3,469	6.3 per 1,000 live births
Early neonatal mortality	Deaths in first week = 10	Live births = 3,469	2.9 per 1,000 live births
Late neonatal mortality	Deaths in subsequent 3 weeks = 12	Live births = 3,469	3.5 per 1,000 live births
Post-neonatal mortality	Post 28 days to first-year deaths = 5	Live births = 3,469	1.4 per 1,000 live births
Maternal mortality	Deaths from puerperal causes during pregnancy or within 42 days = 14	Live births = 3,469	4.0 per 1,000 live births
Foetal death rate	Stillbirths = 31	Total births = 3,500	8.9 per 1,000 total births
Infant mortality	Deaths at <1 year = 27	Live births = 3,469	7.8 per 1,000 live births

A population has 3,500 births in a year. Of these 31 are stillborn, 10 babies die within one week, another 12 die before 28 days and a further 5 die before they are a year old. For this year 8 mothers die in pregnancy and 6 women die within a month of giving birth. For this population calculate each of the indicators above. All rates should be given per 1,000.
See Table 7.1.

There are many causes of perinatal death, including congenital abnormalities, immaturity and low birth weight, maternal diseases in pregnancy and obstetric problems. Factors associated with increasing perinatal death are higher maternal age, higher parity, lower socio-economic class and ethnicity.

High rates of perinatal mortality are observed in UK-born Pakistani babies. What might be the reasons for this?

The reasons include the higher proportion of consanguineous marriages (inbreeding) resulting in congenital malformed babies and the lower economic status of these communities [1]. There is lower mortality in second-generation compared to first-generation Pakistani mothers [2] (perinatal mortality for second-generation mothers approaches that for the indigenous white population). It has been suggested that this may be due in part to a reduction in the stillbirth rate which may be due to factors such as longer gestational age.

Interventions to improve perinatal mortality include both those aimed at specific causes of death and those aimed at broader lifestyle factors. To prevent certain particular causes of perinatal mortality, rubella vaccination, antenatal screening for spina bifida and Down's syndrome and the use of anti-D in Rhesus haemolytic disease may be recommended. Given the strong associations between general aspects of lifestyle and perinatal mortality, there is a case for prevention on a broader front:

- economic: income and housing
- educational: health, parenthood education and sex education
- cultural: age of child bearing, diet, the use of tobacco, drugs and consumption of alcohol in excess
- medical: assessment of the value of antenatal care and the place of technology as a use of scarce resources
- research: to obviate our inadequate knowledge of the causes of antepartum haemorrhage, prematurity or the effects of stress during birth.

Another indicator of child health is the under-five mortality rate: the number of deaths of children less than five years old divided by the number of live births in a year multiplied by 1,000. This indicator measures child survival. It also reflects the social, economic and environmental conditions in which children (and others in society) live, including their health care. Data from UNICEF show that in the mid 1990s the under-five mortality rate varied from 5 per 1,000 in Sweden to 320 per 1,000 in Niger (see www.unicef.org/sowc96/swc96t9x.html).

In the UK the infant mortality rate has fallen from 25% of all deaths in 1901 to 4% in 2004. Deaths in adults are a more useful indicator for a UK public health practitioner and guide the planning of preventive measures and health-care services. Data from National Statistics for the UK shows that over 500,000 deaths were recorded in 2004. Of these, 14% were for cancer, 37% for circulatory diseases and 14% for respiratory causes. This explains the increased focus in the NHS on the management of these long-term conditions.

Life expectancy and years of life lost (YLL)

Mortality rates alone give only a partial picture of the public health impact of diseases. The significance of common causes of death (e.g. pneumonia at the end of life) may eclipse rarer but devastating causes of death earlier in life (e.g. road traffic fatalities). Life expectancy provides an estimate of the average expected lifespan of a population based on current patterns of mortality. Years of potential life relate to the average age at which deaths occur and the expected life span of the population, so provide a measure of the relative importance of conditions in causing mortality.

Years of life lost (YLL) are calculated for each person who died before the age of 75. For example, a person who died at the age of 30 would contribute 45 potential years of life lost. (Deaths in individuals aged 75 or older are not included in the calculation.) Years of life lost are the sum of the YLL contributed for each individual. They can be expressed as a rate, where the total years of life lost

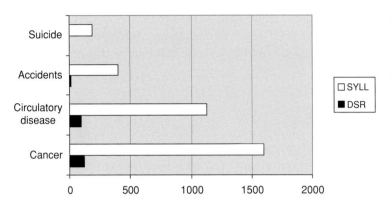

Fig. 7.1 Directly standardised death rates (DSRs) and standardised years of life lost (SYLL) (2002–2004) for selected causes, England. Data source www.nchod.nhs.uk.

by the total population less than 75 years of age are divided by the population count.

United Kingdom figures relating to YLL are published regularly by the National Centre for Health Outcomes Development as part of the Clinical and Health Outcomes Database (www.nchod.nhs.uk/)

Figure 7.1 illustrates that using YLL (in this case standardised to account for population differences) shows a much higher burden of disease than mortality (here directly standardised – DSR – to allow comparison).

Measuring morbidity

Morbidity is defined [3] as 'any departure, subjective or objective, from a state of physiological or psychological wellbeing. In this sense sickness, illness and disease are similarly defined and synonymous' (4). Morbidity statistics will be described (with the UK as an example) under the following headings:
1. Infectious diseases
2. Hospital data
3. Primary care data
4. Disease registers.

1. Infectious diseases

In the UK and many other countries certain communicable diseases are notifiable by law. This system provides a rich source of information on one aspect of the health of a population. A list of UK notifiable diseases is included on the CD. Other data are available from alternative surveillance systems (see Chapter 10) and are helpful in determining public health policy such as vaccination requirements, sexual health service needs and likely sources of communicable disease outbreaks in a population.

However, these notification and reporting systems may be incomplete. Despite this they have been shown to provide valid information that is relatively consistent and can be used as a crude indicator of change in prevalence in the community.

2. Hospital data

The origins of concern for recording hospital activity can be traced to the eighteenth century and an early proponent in the UK was Florence Nightingale. However, it was not until after the founding of the NHS in 1948 that a system for collecting these data was introduced. Today, hospital episode statistics (HES) data are collected on patient administration systems (PAS) and diagnostic/operation coding is added at hospital trust level. The following data are recorded:
1. demographic, e.g. age, sex, marital status, residence, ethnic codes
2. administrative, e.g., length of stay, waiting times and source of admission
3. clinical, e.g. speciality, main condition and operation details.
Hospital activity data are only a proxy measure of morbidity and represent process data on those treated by the hospital system. However, data about utilisation by speciality, principal diagnosis and operation can provide indices of morbidity. Accident and emergency and out-patient data are also available. Coding of the clinical elements of HES allows linkage to ICD-10 coding and international comparisons are possible.

3. Primary care data

The main focus for medical care outside hospitals in the UK is general medical practice. Some 90% of illness episodes are dealt with in the context of primary care. The most recent of the decennial National GP Morbidity Surveys was undertaken in 1998–99. Information was collected over a year and included individual consultation data such as date of birth of patient, diagnostic category, date of consultation and any hospital admission. General practitioners maintain disease registers to support the management of chronic conditions (e.g. coronary heart disease, diabetes, epilepsy). This source of data is useful as, although not always complete, it is available at very small population levels and can be used effectively to engage local clinicians in health improvement or health care quality initiatives. For example, an audit of statin prescribing to those people identified in a practice register as having coronary heart disease might be used to encourage greater rates of prescribing in women (which tend to be lower). Incentive systems may operate to encourage general practitioners to increase the amount of data collected which can be used for audit and monitoring as well as for one-to-one patient care during consultations.

4. Disease registers

It is possible to establish special data collection systems for some diseases. They provide richer sources of information than routine data but are costly to establish and maintain. A good example of a disease register is that for cancer. Cancer registration is established in many countries including the UK, many European countries and the USA. In the UK in 1923 the Ministry of Health set up a system through the Radium Commission to follow up patients treated with radium. This was the origin of the regional Cancer Registries which collect details of age, sex, place of birth, occupation, site of primary tumour, type of tumour and date of initial diagnosis. Information about survival and incidence is obtained through linkage to the national death registration system. As with the other systems there are concerns about completeness of registration, accuracy and effectiveness of follow-up. However, the system has proved an invaluable source of cancer morbidity and survival data.

Self-reported health status

Not all ill health is reported and details of the behavioural determinants of health, such as diet, smoking, housing and physical activity levels cannot be collected solely through health-sector systems. Thus we need to consider other data sources when aiming for a complete profile of the health of our population.

Population surveys

Many countries administer regular health surveys. Typically they sample a population and ask a standard series of questions repeatedly over time, for example annually or decennially. Whilst these surveys tend to cover a range of topics such as employment, housing tenure and family nature they often have a health component. In the UK in 1971 the General Household Survey was developed as an instrument to examine the interaction between different education, employment, social security and health departmental policies. The sampling frame is obtained through the electoral registers from which households are identified. Approximately 12,000 households are approached annually to undertake a detailed interview questionnaire, which results in a response rate of about 70%.

The health section in this survey includes data about how activity is limited by acute or chronic illness, contacts with health and social services, consultations with GPs, hospital outpatients or admissions, smoking and alcohol consumption and other specific topics such as sight or hearing. The time period for recall varies from two weeks for acute illness and GP consultation to one year for in-patient care. One advantage of this system is the ability to cross-tabulate health data with other social variables such as housing, employment, income, etc. In the UK, National Statistics publishes the findings annually.

In addition, the Health Survey for England is administered annually and produces data on health status and related activities (e.g. smoking, obesity, diet, mental health, physical activity).

Some health information may be available from full population censuses. These are also carried out in many countries, often less frequently than smaller, sampled surveys. In the 2001 UK census information was collected on long-term limiting illness, provision of unpaid care, sickness and disability and general health. This showed that 1 in 10 people provide unpaid care (21% of these for over 50 hours per week), 18% of people say they have a long-term illness, disability or health problem, and 9% of people report their health as 'not good'. Data from the UK census is available at a local level and can help define the self-reported health of small populations. However, as the census takes place only every 10 years, the data become increasingly inaccurate as the next census approaches.

Local health surveys

It is also possible to carry out local health surveys to obtain a picture of the population's perception of important health issues. These are time-consuming and must be carried out with rigorous methodology to be valid but can provide information not obtainable in any other way.

Other sources of data

The following sources can provide useful information in building up a picture of morbidity and health risk in the community:

a. National Statistics – monitors, for example, births, migration, adoptions. Publications report on specific topics such as:

population trends published quarterly with demographic data

social trends reported annually

abortions

congenital malformations (the increased incidence of congenital malformations born to women taking thalidomide for morning sickness prompted the establishment of a national notification scheme in 1964)

longitudinal studies following a cohort identified in the 1971 census.

b. Social-security statistics include data on sickness and injury benefit payments and absences from work resulting from illness.

c. Registers such as disabled, blind and partially sighted registers held by local government authorities or organisations.

d. Notifiable occupational diseases (for example, occupational dermatitis, pneumoconioses, asthma or cancer; communicable diseases acquired through work such as legionella).

e. Accident reports for road accidents and Consumer Safety Unit of the Department of Trade and Industry for accidents at home.

f. School health reports including dental surveys.

g. National food surveys which collect data on food consumption and expenditure.

h. Indices of deprivation. These combine different deprivation-related domains and produce measures with which to compare different geographical areas. An example in the UK is the Index of Multiple Deprivation 2004 which incorporates domains relating to health and disability, employment, income, education and skills, crime, living environment and barriers to housing and services.

Collecting health-status information

It is often time-consuming and difficult to collate all the information described above. Public health observatories were established in 2000 to promote better use of health-related information. Their roles are to support local bodies by:

- monitoring health and disease trends and highlighting areas for action
- identifying gaps in health information
- advising on methods for health and health inequality impact assessment
- drawing together information from different sources in new ways to improve health
- carrying out projects to highlight particular health issues
- evaluating progress by local agencies on improving health and cutting inequality
- looking ahead to give early warning of future public health problems.

Summary exercise

Use the information in this chapter, your own knowledge and some additional research if necessary to complete Table 7.2

See Table 7.3 for the answers.

Table 7.2. Complete the advantages and disadvantages in health profiling

Type of data	Advantages in health profiling	Disadvantages in health profiling
Mortality statistics		
Notifiable infectious disease rates		
Hospital-episode data		
General practice (primary care) data		
National surveys		
Disease registers		

Table 7.3. Answer to Table 7.2

Type of data	Advantages in health profiling	Disadvantages in health profiling
Mortality statistics	Provides an indicator of a clear outcome Is generally easy to count Is often available at small population levels	Cause of death may be inaccurately recorded May be incomplete if no mandatory death registration system Does not give an indicator of the burden of long-term health conditions or of loss of potential life
Notifiable infectious disease rates	Good population coverage Mandatory Regularly updated Clinician and laboratory based, so local Provides trends over time	Not all infectious diseases are notifiable Time-consuming to collect and analyse so timeliness may be an issue
Hospital-episode data	Contain a patient identifier so can be linked to other person-based datasets Coded by disease categories Collected by hospital so local Covers the majority of major diseases Relatively complete	Process (rather than outcome) based There may be inconsistencies in coding across areas or over time Data is recorded twice (by clinicians and then entered onto a database by coders) and errors may be introduced
General practice (primary care) data	Local Provides a source of data that cannot be obtained elsewhere (for example, prevalence of heart failure)	May not be very complete There may be inconsistencies in coding across areas or over time There are usually incentives for completion which may skew what is collected It is time-consuming to collect, collate and analyse
National surveys	Random sampling should ensure the results are applicable to the whole population Can provide information not obtainable elsewhere (for example, subjective health status) Generally they have a core set of questions which can be used to determine trends over time	Those which do not have complete population coverage need care with extrapolation to a local population Response rates may be low (some groups tend to respond less well than others, for example young men) May not be very frequent so data become out of date Does not necessarily cover all population groups such as travellers and migrant workers
Disease registers	Rich source of disease-specific data which can be linked to other data sources Provides trends over time Local	Not all diseases are recorded in this way Time-consuming and expensive to maintain

Measuring the health status of the population extends beyond an assessment of traditional health-status indicators like death, disease and disability. A population health approach establishes indicators related to mental and social well being, quality of life, life satisfaction, income, employment and working conditions, education and other factors known to influence health. Many of the principles and tools discussed in Chapter 2 on epidemiology would help in this exercise.

Conclusion

As public health practitioners we must be familiar with the indicators that are established to monitor the health status of our communities. These indicators also help us to understand and evaluate the effects of current interventions and programs. In some cases, this information is available and just needs to be made more accessible. National and regional bodies such as National Statistics and public health observatories play a crucial role in this. For some indicators new research will be required to generate the information needed and we have a role in generating this information wherever feasible and appropriate.

Further reading and sources of data

Details on the major sources of data for health profiling (and the data sources used within this chapter) are given on the CD but the key sources are:

The World Health Organisation: www.who.int/en/

ICD-10 www.who.int/classifications/icd/en/

Clinical Health Outcomes Knowledge Base: www.nchod.nhs.uk/

Public Health Observatories: www.apho.org.uk/apho/

National Statistics: www.statistics.gov.uk/

Health protection information: www.hpa.org.uk/

REFERENCES

1. S. Bundey, H. Alam, A. Kaur, S. Mir and R. Lancashire, Why do UK-born Pakistani babies have high perinatal and neonatal mortality rates? *Paediatric and Perinatal Epidemiology*, **5**(1), 1991, 101–14
2. A. Hobbiss, Are perinatal and infant mortality rates improved for second generation Pakistani mothers? *Research Findings Register*, H1060R, 2002
3. J. M. Last, *A Dictionary of Epidemiology*, 4th edn, Oxford, Oxford University Press, 2004.

8

Health care evaluation

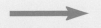

Key points

- Quality in health care is multidimensional but measurable.
- Evaluation of an intervention attempts to determine objectively whether the activity in question is meeting its objectives.
- Assessing the impact of public health interventions in the short term can present particular challenges.
- Clinical governance refers to the systems through which NHS organisations and staff are accountable for the quality of patient care.

Introduction

The last part of the planning cycle to which you were introduced on page 118 concerns evaluation. How can public health specialists know whether their interventions are having the desired effect? Clinicians can monitor the impact of their treatments on an individual patient basis but how do we examine the impact of a new service? In the first part of this chapter, we will look at what we mean by quality of care and consider one well-known framework for its evaluation. In the second half we will consider how quality of care is promoted across the NHS as a whole and the changing nature of the health professional's accountability.

Quality of care and its evaluation

Quality in health care means doing the right thing, at the right time, in the right way, to the right person – and having the best possible results. A more formal framework is provided by Maxwell who described six dimensions to quality [1]:

Essential Public Health, eds. Stephen Gillam, Jan Yates and Padmanabhan Badrinath.
Published by Cambridge University Press. © Cambridge University Press 2007.

> **Box 8.1 Issues important to patients**
>
> - Equality in access to services
> - Comprehensive information about services
> - Being listened to and treated confidentially
> - Quality of treatment, correct diagnoses
> - Care in an appropriate place
> - Staff consistency and familiarity with their case
> - Quick access to primary care, flexible GP hours
> - Shorter waits for outpatients and accident and emergency
> - Fewer cancelled operations
> - Choice of consultant, GP, alternative practitioners
> - Gender of doctor, treatment in single sex wards
>
> Adapted from: Christine Farrell, Ros Levenson and Dawn Snape, *The Patient's Charter: Past and Future* London, King's Fund, 1997.

- effectiveness (achieves intended benefit)
- acceptability (satisfies reasonable expectations)
- efficiency (making the best use of available resources)
- accessibility (those who need services will receive them)
- equity (resources are fairly shared)
- relevance (treatments are appropriate to their particular target groups).

Of course, it is not only health professionals who are interested in the quality of care they provide – as media interest in medical mishaps reminds us. Managers in hospitals and health authorities are charged to monitor quality as part of clinical governance (see below). Whether as users or voters, the general population have great interest in quality of health care and patients' priorities may differ from those who provide it. They may place clear information, caring communication and outcomes that improve activities of daily living higher up their list than technical aspects of care; such priorities may be difficult to assess (Box 8.1).

Evaluation has been defined as 'a process that attempts to determine as systematically and objectively as possible the relevance, effectiveness and impact of activities in the light of their objectives.' Where do we start when thinking about evaluation of a delivery system in the NHS? Avedis Donabedian, a guru in quality improvement circles, distinguished four elements [2]:

- structure (buildings, staff, equipments)
- process (all that is done to patients)
- outputs (immediate results of medical intervention)
- outcomes (gains in health status).

Thus, for example, early evaluation of the new national screening programme for colonic cancer may consider

- the volume and costs of new equipment (colonoscopic, radiographic, histopathological), staff and buildings (structure)
- the numbers of patients screened, coverage rates within a defined age range, numbers of true and false positives (process)
- number of cancers identified, operations performed (outputs)
- complication rates, colonic cancer incidence, prevalence and mortality rates (outcomes).

This distinction is helpful because for many interventions it may be difficult to obtain robust data on health outcomes unless large numbers are scrutinised over long periods. For example, evaluating the quality of hypertension management within a general practice, you may be reliant on process measures (the proportion of the appropriate population screened, treated and adequately controlled) as a proxy for good outcomes. The assumption here is that evidence from larger-scale studies showing that control of hypertension reduces subsequent death rates from heart disease will be reflected in your own practice population's health experience. Thinking about the care provided for people with a particular disease, evaluation – like resource allocation – can also be considered in terms of different elements of their care: prevention, diagnosis, treatment and rehabilitation.

Use a structure, process, output, outcome model to consider what measures might be relevant to the evaluation of the following services:
- **smoking cessation service**
- **immunisation programmes**
- **breast screening programme**
- **cardiac rehabilitation services**
- **hip replacement for osteoarthritis**
- **chronic-disease management (e.g. diabetes in general practice)**
- **provision of free fruit and vegetables to school children**
- **national programmes to Roll Back Malaria.**

See Table 8.1.

One of the biggest problems in evaluating large-scale public health interventions is the confounding effect of the many different factors influencing outcomes: background 'noise'. For example, assessing the impact of mass media campaigns against smoking might be complicated by the impact of new laws to prevent smoking in public places, changes to the national curriculum, increased taxation on cigarettes or background decline in the population prevalence of smoking. Similarly, it is difficult to measure the contribution of fruit and vegetable provision to, for example, reduction in bowel cancer rates, due to the multifactorial nature of the determinants of bowel cancer. Thus, measures of outcome may be limited. Remember that readily available measures of quality are not

Table 8.1. Examples of measures that might be relevant for evaluation

Service	Measures to be evaluated
Smoking cessation service	Number of smokers seen and counselled
	Prescriptions for nicotine replacement therapy dispensed
	Quit rates
	Costs (of material/staff etc.)
	Trends in smoking prevalence
	Death rates from smoking related diseases
Immunisation programmes	Numbers of vaccines administered
	Proportion of target population covered
	Costs (of vaccines distributed, maintaining cold chain, other disposables, staff deployed etc.)
	Disease incidence rates over time
Breast screening programme	Numbers of mammograms carried out
	Abnormality detection rates
	False positives at lumpectomy
	Proportion of target population covered
	Breast-cancer incidence (falling or rising?)
	Long-term mortality trends
	Costs (Staff, mammographic equipment, etc.)
Cardiac rehabilitation services	Numbers passing through programme
	Numbers as a proportion of all patients admitted with diagnosis of Myocardial infarction (MI), and as a proportion of all of those meeting appropriate referral criteria
	Percentages of patients in programme receiving recommended interventions post MI (aspirin, beta blockers, statins if not contraindicated)
	Impact on patients' quality of life
	Costs (Staff, materials accommodation, etc.)
	Long term re-infarction rates
	Mortality rates post MI
Hip replacement for osteoarthritis	Numbers of operations performed
	Lengths of stay
	Infection or other complication rates
	Readmission rates
	Proportion of patients requiring surgical revision
	Costs (prostheses, hospital stay and rehabilitation)
	Numbers on waiting lists
	Length of waiting
	Prevalence of unmet need for hip replacement within local community
	Patient-satisfaction surveys
	Impact on quality of life/activities of daily living

Table 8.1. (*cont.*)

Service	Measures to be evaluated
Chronic disease management (e.g. diabetes at general practice level)	Numbers on disease register
	Proportion receiving annual check (e.g. retinal screening)
	Proportion meeting appropriate standards for criteria of good care (e.g. blood pressure below 140/85, HbA1c haemoglobin levels less than 7, etc.)
	Proportion of patients with management plan
	Costs
	Rates of disease-related complications
Provision of free fruit and vegetables to school children	Number of supply contracts negotiated to provide seasonal fruit and vegetables
	Numbers of pieces of fruit or vegetable delivered
	Numbers of pieces of fruit or vegetable consumed by children
	Satisfaction ratings for children, parents and teachers
	Attitude surveys of children and parents to the consumption of fruit and vegetables
National programmes to Roll Back Malaria	Numbers of people treated with artemesinin-based medications
	Measures of distribution of insecticide-treated bednets
	Numbers/level of staff trained
	Spending on malaria-related activities in health and education sectors
	Outcomes – morbidity and mortality rates (especially in high-risk groups such as mothers and children)

necessarily the most important, and the most important elements of quality may not be easily measurable. For example, with their interest in equity of provision, public health specialists need to consider the accessibility of services, particularly to disadvantaged groups.

Can you think of other factors that might complicate the evaluation of public health interventions?

The complexity of the determinants of disease and of interventions designed to prevent them; the long time lag between some interventions and their expected effect (e.g. efforts to improve food labelling will not swiftly affect obesity levels).

Clinical governance

A common criticism of much of what health professionals do to try and improve the quality of their care is that it is piecemeal and poorly co-ordinated. Variable quality of care, particularly in the poorest, least healthy and least well-resourced parts of the country have long been a fact of NHS life. A landmark white paper called 'A first class service' was published by the Labour Government in 1998 [3]. It contained a blueprint for improving quality encapsulated in Figure 8.1

Table 8.2. Components of clinical governance

Processes for quality improvement	1. Patient and public involvement
	2. Risk management
	3. Clinical audit
	4. Clinical effectiveness programmes
	5. Staffing and staff management
Staff focus	6. Education, training and continuing personal and professional development
Information	7. Use of information to support clinical governance and health care delivery

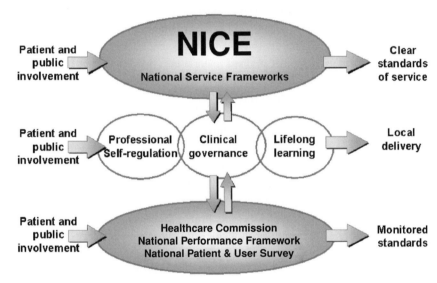

Fig. 8.1 Standards for the NHS.

While structures may change (the Commission for Health Improvement has been replaced by the Healthcare Commission; the National Institute for Clinical Excellence (NICE) has added public health to their remit to become the National Institute for Health and Clinical Excellence; the patient survey programme has been expanded; and performance indicators monitored by the Department of Health change from year to year) the importance of nationally set standards, individual responsibility for governance and robust monitoring remains high.

The term 'clinical governance' (borrowing on notions of corporate governance from the private sector) refers to the framework through which NHS organisations and their staff are accountable for the quality of patient care. It covers the organisations, systems and processes for monitoring and improving services. The different components of clinical governance are listed in Table 8.2.

Fig. 8.2   Audit cycle.

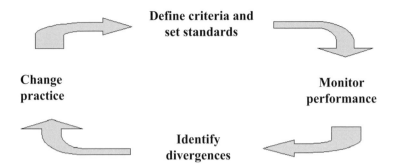

An element of clinical governance that has the potential to have a rapid impact on patient care is clinical audit. The clinical audit cycle (Figure 8.2) refers to the monitoring of performance against pre-defined standards. The example in Box 8.2 concerns the management of hypertension in general practice. Measurement of one's performance against defined criteria can be demanding but the real challenge is to make necessary adjustments and re-evaluate your performance – in other words to complete the cycle.

While there is scope for clinical audit within public health (for example, one might wish to audit the use of carbon monoxide measurement to monitor smoking status in smoking cessation clinics), a variation on clinical audit is often used for public health purposes. Health equity audit has been developed to identify how fairly services or other resources are distributed in relation to the health needs of different population groups or geographical areas (see Figure 8.3). The assessment of need against supply is called an equity profile. However, as with clinical audit, the intention of health equity audit is not only to measure baseline differences between different population groups but also to act before measuring again, i.e. to complete the cycle. Like clinical audit it is therefore a tool for making change happen. The purpose of health equity audit is to help services narrow health inequalities by using evidence on inequalities to inform decisions on investment, service planning, commissioning and delivery, and to review the impact of action on inequalities. In England, equity audit is mandatory for primary care trusts.

Examples of ways a primary health care team might identify and address inequities in access to their services include the following:

• Ethnic monitoring in large, heterogeneous practice populations to answer questions such as whether the patients on our diabetes register are representative of the practice population. Alternatively, are we failing to detect early cases in, for example, south Asian groups?

• Identifying a service lead for people with learning difficulties, a priority group that has repeatedly been found to receive sub-standard primary care.

Box 8.2 A routine example of clinical audit from frontline general practice

Hypertension audit – example

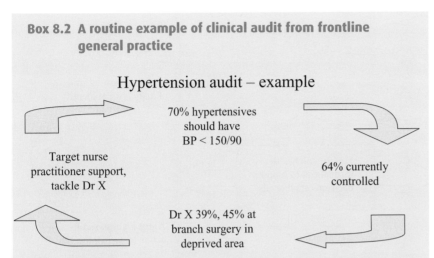

70% hypertensives should have BP < 150/90

64% currently controlled

Target nurse practitioner support, tackle Dr X

Dr X 39%, 45% at branch surgery in deprived area

One criterion used to assess the quality of care provided for people with hypertension is the proportion of patients whose blood pressures (BPs) lie below 150/90 (140/85 for people with diabetes). Under their new contract general-practice teams are rewarded for achieving a target of 70% of people with hypertension thus controlled (the standard). In this instance, the practice was surprised to find that they were only achieving 64% coverage. On closer examination of data, it transpired that coverage among hypertensive patients attending one branch surgery sited on a deprived estate was only 45%. Furthermore, only 39% of the patients in the care of Doctor X, who works predominantly from this site, were adequately controlled.

Various interventions were made to tackle these divergences. The clinical audit lead decided to monitor performance more closely. Patients whose blood pressure remained elevated and who had not been seen in the last six months were contacted by letter and asked to attend surgery. Doctor X was provided with a copy of the practice hypertension protocol (based on the British Society of Hypertension's guidelines) and asked to dedicate more time to this area of his clinical practice. The records of patients in the target group were tagged electronically so as to ease their identification at opportunistic consultation. More nurse time was channelled to supporting the branch surgery.

Regular monthly monitoring and sharing of the results across the team over the next half year revealed gratifying improvements. Six months later coverage rates were 62% among Doctor X's patients and 66% under the branch surgery; across the practice as a whole the 70% target was achieved.

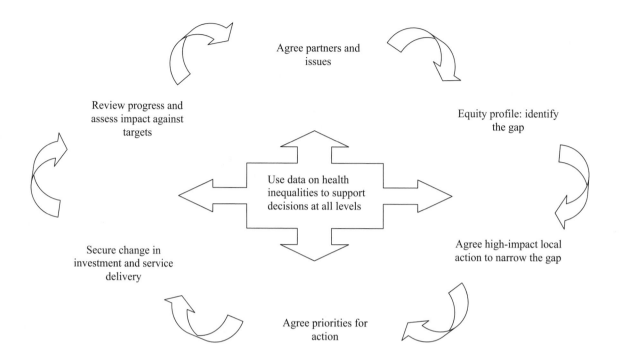

Agree partners and issues

Review progress and assess impact against targets

Equity profile: identify the gap

Use data on health inequalities to support decisions at all levels

Secure change in investment and service delivery

Agree high-impact local action to narrow the gap

Agree priorities for action

Fig. 8.3   The health equity audit cycle [4].

- Co-ordinated case management with local community mental health teams for care of the severely mentally ill.
- The 'basics' – appropriate use of interpreters, signage, translated leaflets – for patients who do not speak English.
- Using information technology intelligently to 'flag' to practitioners when they should consider certain treatment options (for example, cholesterol-lowering drugs if these have been found to be more often prescribed to men with coronary heart disease than women.)

Risk management

About 850,000 'adverse events' occur in the NHS each year involving 10% of admissions and costing an estimated two billion pounds per year. Four hundred people die or are seriously injured in events involving medical devices. Nearly 10,000 people are reported to experience serious adverse reaction to drugs. In an increasingly litigious environment, the numbers of written complaints about health care are increasing. The NHS pays out about 400 million pounds a year to settle clinical-negligence claims. Hospital-acquired infections, of which Methicillin Resistant *Staphylococcus aureus* (MRSA) is only the most graphic example, are estimated to cost the NHS nearly one billion pounds [5].

The first rule of quality assurance based on experience in private production systems and public services across the world is: when things go wrong and mistakes are made the problem arises more often from faulty systems than from faulty individuals ('bad apples'). In the report 'An organisation with a memory', the Department of Health laid down its approach to risk management in the NHS borrowing on experience in the airline industry [5]. It declared the need for:

- unified mechanisms for reporting and analysis when things go wrong
- mechanisms for ensuring that, where lessons are identified, the necessary changes are put into practice
- much wider appreciation of the value of the systems approach in preventing, analysing and learning from errors
- a more open culture in which errors or service failures can be reported and discussed.

The National Patient Safety Agency (NPSA) is a Special Health Authority created to co-ordinate the efforts of all those involved in health care, and, more importantly, to learn from patient safety incidents occurring in the NHS. As well as making sure that incidents are reported in the first place, the NPSA promotes an open culture across the health service, encouraging doctors and other staff to report incidents and 'near misses', when things almost go wrong. A key aim is to encourage staff to report incidents without fear of personal reprimand, and know that by sharing their experiences others will be able to learn lessons and improve patient safety. The NPSA also supports local organisations in addressing their concerns about the performance of individual doctors and dentists, through its responsibility for the National Clinical Assessment Service (NCAS).

In your experience, how 'open' is the culture of health care? How does increasing litigation affect the way in which doctors practice medicine and their willingness to share adverse events?

Accountability

To whom do you feel accountable in your work? Your peers? Your teachers? Your managers? Most health professionals would probably place patients at the top of a long list and, increasingly, the public have the means to ask critical questions about performance. In practice, a powerful driver of their behaviour is the respect and continuing support of work colleagues.

A range of professional bodies including the Royal Colleges set standards for postgraduate training and professional development. The General Medical Council (GMC) regulates the training and practice of doctors and may hold them to account in cases of medical malpractice. The Nursing and Midwifery Council works similarly on behalf of nurses. The GMC has been under stringent criticism since the Harold Shipman case for failing to protect patients' interests and is currently undergoing further reform. For the first time, procedures are being introduced for the appraisal and revalidation of medical practitioners. These are likely to be toughened to include assessments of knowledge, skills and attitudes as well as ensuring relevant systems are in place to improve quality of care. Other public health professionals may have professional bodies who oversee elements of practice such as the Chartered Institute of Environmental Health who set standards for environmental-health officers.

Dr Harold Shipman murdered at least 215 of his own patients between 1977 and 1988. The Baker report investigating these events subsequently recommended routine monitoring of general-practice mortality rates [6]. Why do you think this has proved difficult to implement?
Despite some encouraging pilot studies, no practical method of mortality monitoring has yet been agreed. Unusual mortality rates are mostly the result of unmeasured case mix factors (demography and deprivation) affecting practice populations [7]. The cost of exploring all potential outliers may be considerable. There is lack of support: many practitioners have yet to be convinced that the Shipman case exposed systemic flaws. They view him as an insane extreme, a 'one-off'.

In summary, health professionals are going to be increasingly accountable for their performance in future with greater control exercised through guidelines, protocols and monitoring systems. The trend is towards greater patient involvement in these processes. It is to be hoped that the current panoply of different agencies with often overlapping roles in this area will be rationalised through the formation of a Council for Healthcare Regulatory Excellence, which promotes best practice and consistency in the regulation of health-care professionals.

How the quality of health care is measured and improved in practice is considered further in Chapter 16.

REFERENCES

1. R. Maxwell, Quality assessment in health. *British Medical Journal*, **288**, 1984, 1470–2.
2. A. Donabedian, The definition of quality and approaches to its assessment. Ann Arbor, Michigan, Health Administration Press.
3. A first class service: quality in the new NHS. London, Department of Health, 1998.
4. Health equity audit: a guide for the NHS. London, Department of Health, 2003.
5. An organisation with a memory. London, Department of Health, 2002.
6. The Shipman Inquiry. Safeguarding patients: lessons from the past, proposals for the future. London, The Stationery Office, 2004.
7. M. Mohammed, K. Booth, D. Marshall *et al.*, A practical method for monitoring general practice mortality in the UK: findings from a pilot study in a health board of Northern Ireland. *British Journal of General Practice*, **518**, 2005, 676.

9

Decision-making in the health care sector – the role of public health

Key points

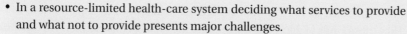

- In a resource-limited health-care system deciding what services to provide and what not to provide presents major challenges.
- In the UK funding decisions are made at three main levels: centrally at the Department of Health; locally within primary care trusts and practice collaboratives; and at the front line between clinicians and patients in hospitals and general practices.
- In order to make funding decisions it is necessary to determine the priority status of different options and to make decisions between them.
- Priority setting should be a transparent process based on a clear set of criteria, for example:

    Is there a need for the service?

    Is there an intervention or service which is proven to be effective and which will meet this need?

    Is the intervention acceptable and appropriate for the health-care system?

    Is the service cost effective?

    Is the service ethically justified?
- Priority setting needs to take place within a clear ethical framework.

Introduction

Health care systems are resource limited – budgets are finite and not every service one would like to provide can be funded. In publicly funded health systems, those responsible for procuring health care need to be able to explain how taxpayers' money has been spent. Decisions are made at both an individual patient and a population level. At an individual level the decision might be: should this patient

Essential Public Health, eds. Stephen Gillam, Jan Yates and Padmanabhan Badrinath.
Published by Cambridge University Press. © Cambridge University Press 2007.

get a prescription for a statin to lower her blood cholesterol and, if so, which statin should it be? At a population level the decision might be: will a primary care organisation employ a heart-failure specialist nurse or run an additional sexual health clinic? In the UK funding decisions are made at various levels. Individual clinicians, managers within primary care organisations and hospitals, managers in strategic health authorities and civil servants in the Department of Health all make decisions which affect what public health and treatment services are available to populations. Some decisions are more appropriately made by individuals at a local level but the need for some specialised services may be very low for small populations. For example, less than 20 liver transplants are needed for every million people and decisions over funding liver-transplant services are taken at larger population levels by specially configured service commissioning groups. In the UK a National Specialist Commissioning Advisory Group decides on very specialist services for rare conditions such as liver transplantation.

How these kinds of decisions are made is the focus of this chapter. We will look briefly at a framework for priority setting and consider what factors should be taken into account when comparing options. This will include an examination of basic health economic concepts. While this chapter primarily takes examples from health care, the same principles can be applied to decision-making in other areas relevant to the public's health such as the use of green spaces and parkland.

A framework for setting priorities

In order to plan services which are effective and can be adequately resourced it is important to consider the need for each service within a clear public health framework. A series of questions should be answered before a service is funded and these are shown in Figure 9.1. Each question is described in more detail below using as an example a decision on whether or not to make available services to help people stop smoking.

1. Is there a need for the service?

The assessment of needs is discussed in detail in Chapter 6. In health economics need is often defined as the capacity to benefit, so the use of needs assessment is crucial to determining which interventions for which health and health-care issues are likely to benefit the population most and so become priorities. Populations vary according to age, sex, ethnicity and many other determinants of health, and the need for health services will vary accordingly. Public health specialists' role here is to ensure that services are targeted to those who most need them.

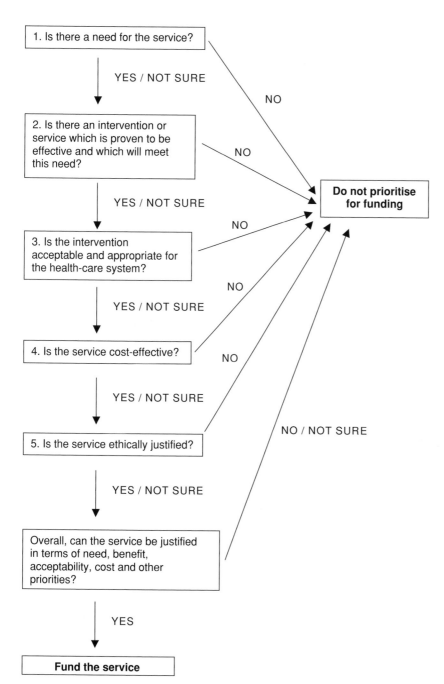

Fig. 9.1   A framework for setting priorities.

1. Is there a need for a smoking cessation service?

From the 2001 General Household [1] survey we know that across most of the UK the prevalence of smoking is around 25% and remains high even in children. Around 70% of smokers report that they would like to give up. There is plentiful evidence that smoking causes harm, including heart disease and several cancers. Thus, we have a population which has the capacity to benefit from smoking cessation services.

YES

2. Is there an effective intervention/service?

If an intervention doesn't work it shouldn't be provided. Evidence repositories such as the Cochrane Library can be searched and systematic reviews or evidence-based journals used (see Chapter 3). Critical appraisal skills ensure the best possible assessment of the effectiveness of potential services or interventions.

However, there can be practical difficulties in providing and using evidence for all services or interventions. Firstly, there are many areas of study where the quality and quantity of evidence is limited. Public health interventions often fall into this category as they may be multifaceted. Outcomes are due only in part to the intervention we are interested in (for example, how much of a reduction in lung cancer mortality in men is due to smoking cessation services and how much is due to treatment services and tobacco taxation?). Pragmatic solutions are often needed and evidence at the best available level is used to inform decisions (see Chapter 3 for the hierarchy of evidence and Chapter 4 for more details on how health promotion can be made effective). An example here is recent guidance from the National Institute for Health and Clinical Excellence which found poor-quality evidence for the effectiveness of pedometers in increasing physical activity levels. It has recommended that they are not used except as part of research studies [2].

Secondly, problems arise if the evidence base suggests that current services are ineffective. The evidence base changes over time and services which previously appeared effective may prove not to be when additional information becomes available. It can be difficult to reduce a service already in place and decisions such as these need careful implementation. For example, the evidence to support routine use of grommets in children with glue ear is limited. However, parents, and sometimes clinicians, need to be reassured that a useful service is not withheld. While the evidence suggests that use of grommets [3] should be restricted to children with persistent problems after a period of watchful waiting, it can be difficult to implement this.

> 2. Is there an intervention or service which is proven to be effective at helping people stop smoking and which will meet this need?

Certain models of supporting cessation work well. Smoking cessation services are likely to include pharmaceutical and behavioural interventions, brief interventions and those interventions which support smokers for longer periods of time but not acupuncture [4].

YES

3. Is the intervention acceptable and appropriate?

If services were provided which were not acceptable to patients or the public they would be less well used and potentially inefficient. Acceptability depends upon the context for an intervention, and the local situation needs to be considered. For example, studies may have examined cultural differences in attitudes to smoking cessation and a search for these could help determine which method would suit a particular population. When introducing new treatments, services or public health interventions the views of patients and the public on what services are needed should be taken into consideration. This helps to ensure that resources are committed where they are felt to be needed by patients and the public as well as where we see they could produce benefit. When introducing public health interventions which rely on people to change their behaviours (such as smoking cessation), the people who are targeted should be involved in the planning stages. Patients' views on what aspects of a service are important include adequate information, choice of practitioners, being taken seriously and treated confidentially, appropriate treatment and quick access to flexible services.

We discussed some ways that patients and the public can be involved in health needs assessment in Chapter 6. The same methodologies can be used to involve people in decision-making processes.

> 3. Is smoking cessation acceptable and appropriate for the health-care system?

Within the UK the provision of smoking cessation services in a variety of settings such as hospitals, general practices, community settings, over the telephone and pharmacies has proven acceptable to the public.

YES
↓

4. Is the intervention cost-effective?

In a system where health-care resources are limited, costs must be factored into decision-making. However, money is not the only cost and saving lives is not the only benefit. Costs and benefits should be measured accurately and can be compared between different interventions and outcomes. How do we determine whether one million pounds spent on coronary care to improve cardiac outcomes is more useful than one million pounds spent on cancer prevention? Here, the science of health economics comes into its own.

Health economics applies traditional economic theory to consider problems in health care. Economic evaluation helps decision making by considering the outputs of competing interventions in relation to the resources that they consume. To address these issues, relevant outputs must be defined, costs measured, and studies relating outputs to their costs undertaken. It is important, therefore, to have a basic understanding of techniques of economic evaluation.

Economic evaluation

Economic evaluation can be defined [5] as '. . . the comparative analysis of alternative courses of action in terms of both their costs and consequences'. In our smoking cessation example we would be comparing the costs (i.e. the consumed resources) and consequences (outputs or benefits) of having a smoking cessation service against the costs and consequences of not having one.

Costs are generally divided into direct and indirect costs. Direct costs can be easily identified as the expenditure associated with the activity (for example the cost of 10 minutes of a general practitioner's time and the cost of a nicotine replacement therapy (NRT) prescription). Indirect costs are more difficult to measure and might include items such as a share of the overheads (such as heating and lighting) for the building in which the doctor works. Opportunity costs are also often

Table 9.1. Types of economic evaluation

Type of evaluation	Costs measured in	Benefits measured in	Smoking cessation example
Cost minimisation	Money	Not measured	Cost of one clinic compared to cost of two
Cost effectiveness	Money	Natural units – units relevant to the intervention	Costs per additional quitter
Cost utility	Money	Comparable units – usually QALYs	Cost per additional QALY* gained for the quitters
Cost benefit	Money	Money	Here you would need to value the benefits in how much they were worth in financial terms – difficult to do

*See box 9.2.

Box 9.1 Opportunity cost

Opportunity cost is the amount lost by not using the resource (labour, capital) in its best alternative use. For example, the financial cost of admitting an elderly patient with influenza and respiratory problems to a surgical ward (due to lack of beds) is relatively low (cost of bed, nursing etc). However the opportunity cost of the admission may be much higher (for example, cancelled operations, increased waiting lists).

mentioned (see Box 9.1) and should be taken into account. This might include the loss of another clinic if we commit a health care worker to running a smoking cessation clinic.

Options are rarely simple and the concept of marginal or incremental costs is helpful. Increasingly, health care interventions make small, additional gains to health. Decisions are generally not whether to have a service or not but whether to improve the service in certain ways. Thus, while we could compare a smoking cessation service with none, we are more likely to compare the current service (say one nurse-led clinic per month) with an improved service (say two clinics per month). In this case we would compare the number of people who quit smoking from our original service with the number we predict for our improved service. We can then quote the benefits in terms of additional quitters per pound spent on the additional clinic. This is a marginal cost and tells us how much we could gain from our service improvement.

Table 9.1 illustrates the different types of economic evaluation.

Cost minimisation does not count what we gain but assumes the benefits of each option are the same. This type of analysis is often used in medicines management when alternative drugs having the same clinical indication and effect are compared according to price, and the cheapest prescribed. However, it is rarely the case that all consequences are equal. Within a cost-effectiveness analyses we measure the two sets of costs and compare the outcomes in units of relevance for the intervention. This is often lives saved or life years gained. With smoking cessation we might count the number of additional people who quit smoking. However, this does not allow us to say whether we should invest in smoking cessation in preference to exercise classes or weight management clinics as the outcomes are not comparable. This is where cost-utility analyses are useful as they measure all outcomes in terms of an index of benefit which is comparable across different types of service. The quality-adjusted life year (QALY) is the most commonly used index of benefit. This allocates a quality of life value (between 1 (perfect health) and 0 (death)) and combines quantity and quality of life to derive the QALY. Although the cost-utility method has the advantage that different interventions can be compared across a broad range of choices in resource allocation, a number of methodological problems remain (see Box 9.2).

Lastly, cost benefit analyses allow us as a society to choose between diverse uses of public money, for example on health care or education. However, allocating monetary values to all consequences is difficult (how much money is a life saved worth?) and requires complicated methodologies which are open to challenge.

Thus, types of economic evaluation vary in the way in which they measure benefits and the choice of which analysis to use for any particular service largely depends on which approach to benefit measurement is most practical.

A new drug enables patients to live for 5 years rather than dying within 2 years. However, they live with a minor disability and a quality of life equal to 80% of a full healthy life year. However, if they do not receive the drug their quality of life for the 2 years they live is only 60% of a full healthy life year. How many QALYs are generated by the intervention?
Five years of life at 0.8 QoL = 4, compared to two years of life at 0.6 QoL = 1.2. Therefore 4 − 1.2 = 2.8 QALYs generated.

Consider the following two health-improvement programmes. Which is the most cost-effective?
a. **Provision of home safety equipment for the elderly. This increases quality of life by 0.1 and the benefit lasts for 10 years. The extra cost is £1,500 per life year.**
b. **Intensive postnatal care for low-birth-weight babies. This improves quality of life by 0.8 and the benefits last for 35 years. The care costs £125,000.**

Box 9.2 How a QALY is constructed

A quality-adjusted life year (QALY) combines the quantity and quality of life.

It takes one year of perfect-health life expectancy to be worth 1 and regards one year of less than perfect life expectancy as < 1.

Patients, the public and professionals are asked to judge the quality value (utility) for one year of life lived with the relevant condition, and these values are then used multiplicatively with the number of years lived in this state to give the QALY.

For example, an intervention which results in a patient living for an additional 4 years rather than dying within 1 year, but where quality of life for treated and untreated fell from 1 to 0.6, will generate:

4 years extra life @ 0.6 quality of life values = 2.4

less 1 year @ reduced quality = 0.6

QALYs generated by the intervention = 1.8.

QALYs can therefore provide an indication of the benefits gained from a variety of medical procedures in terms of quality of life and additional years for the patient.

Disadvantages of QALY

- It is argued that seeking to compare the incomparable (different treatments, different states) with crude tools is methodologically flawed and that their use oversimplifies complex health care issues by reducing what should be a multifaceted assessment of option to simple quantitative values.
- QALYs are not based on an individual's assessment of value and the values determined by others may not reflect those of every patient.
- QALYs are controversial. They can be seen as 'ageist': reduced life expectancy results in lower QALY values so that interventions for elderly patients may compare poorly with those for young patients. Conversely, QALYs can be seen as 'insufficiently ageist' if one considers that the elderly have already had a 'fair innings' and the young are more deserving of treatment.
- QALYs may disadvantage those already disabled, as their quality of life is already lower; interventions for the disabled may yield fewer QALYs than those for healthier people.
- QALYs may lack sensitivity within a disease area: not every subdivision within or level of complex conditions will have been valued and one value may be applied to subdivisions with varying health states (for example the quality of life with a condition like depression might vary considerably depending upon the severity of the depression).

a. How many QALYs are gained? $10 \times 0.1 = 1$
    How much does it cost? $10 \times £1,500 = £15,000$
    What is the cost per QALY gained? $£15,000/1 = £15,000$ per QALY
b. How many QALYs are gained? $35 \times 0.8 = 28$
    How much does it cost? £125,000
    What is the cost per QALY gained? $£125,000/28 = £4,464$ per QALY

Health improvement programme b is the more cost effective as it gains the most QALYs for the cost. However, it does cost a lot more! Consider how you might persuade a health care organisation that programme b is worth investing in. While useful, this model does not reflect the complexities of measuring the impact of interventions on multiple outcomes.

The most useful health economic analyses for public health tend to be cost-utility studies. Ideally, analyses should be carried out alongside the original effectiveness studies but this adds to the cost of the study and is not always possible. It is well worth using a critical appraisal framework when considering an economic analysis and making a judgement about the reliability of the estimates of costs and benefits (see Chapter 3 for more details on critical appraisal).

---

4. Is the smoking cessation service cost-effective?

A health technology assessment carried out in 2002 estimated that smoking cessation interventions using NRT and/or bupropion are cost-effective as compared with many accepted health-care interventions. According to their estimates, the incremental cost per life years saved is about £1,000–2,300 for NRT, £640–1,500 for bupropion, and £900–2,000 for NRT plus bupropion [6]. Another study has estimated that the cost-effectiveness of advice during routine general physician visits ranges from $705 to $988 (£371–£519) per life year saved for men and from $1,204 to $2,058 (£633–£1,082) for women [7]. Modelling for NICE (National Institute for Health and Clinical Excellence) guidance has found that when only comparing the costs of brief interventions in primary care with no intervention, the estimated incremental cost per QALY gained varied from around £221 to around £9,515, depending on the assumptions used. When the health care savings were included (as smokers quit smoking and avoid preventable disease), these are offset by the cost of the intervention. Using this method, the incremental costs per QALY gained vary from £135 to £6,472, depending on the assumptions used [8]. This compares favourably to many interventions (for example hospital haemodialysis has been

estimated to carry a cost per QALY of over £100,000 at 1990 prices -see
www. jrz.ox.ac.uk/bandolier/painres/download/whatis/QALY.pdf).

YES

5. Is the service ethically justified when compared to other treatments?

There will always be competing needs to consider. Once we have assured ourselves
that the proposed services are needed, effective, acceptable and cost-effective,
we must still decide whether to fund them. We then judge their affordability
to us. This isn't as simple as asking 'Is there enough money to pay for this?'
Frequently, funding one initiative means something else cannot be funded – there
is an opportunity cost to pay. To make these kinds of judgements we typically
weight the options we have available. How we weight options is dependent upon
the ethical framework we use, implicitly or explicitly, to judge worth.

There are different ethical frameworks on which people base their decisions,
both in health care and in daily life.

- Decisions based on subjective perceptions of right and wrong – This approach
  is often seen in the popular press and media. Media headlines highlighting emotive issues around cancer treatments can make a dramatic impact
  on the public consciousness and influence the way in which decisions are
  made.
- Decisions made by people in power – There is a strong tradition, rapidly shifting
  now, of paternalism within health services. In a paternalistic system, decisions
  over treatment were pre-eminently the right of (mostly male) clinicians.
- Decisions made by professionals – Professionals abide by codes of conduct and
  it was the duty of the patient to abide by the doctor's decision. It is becoming
  increasingly unacceptable for clinicians to practice in this way, and another
  ethical framework is needed for both individuals and populations.
- Decisions based on the need for the greater good – Public health decisions may
  use a utilitarian framework, which aims to maximise the good consequences
  for a population. This does not mean that everyone gets the same service but
  that each receives health care based on his or her need. This is equity rather
  than equality and attempts to bring the greatest good to the greatest number.
  This implies that we are all willing to make sacrifices for the greatest good.
- Decisions based on 'What we have always done' – Health care decisions about
  what services to fund are often made on the basis of what was bought last year.

In these circumstances, services change very little and costs generally go up in line with inflation.

- Decisions around funding based on standards – We also tend to believe that everyone has the right to a minimum standard of service and many decisions are made based on guidance or targets set by others (such as NICE). In England interventions recommended in NICE technology appraisals must be funded by the health care system.
- Decisions made in emergencies – Another way of making decisions is by applying [10] the 'rule of rescue'. Why do we mount a rescue for the survivors of a disaster when their chances of survival are slim? Why do some people obtain a third transplant when the chances of success are higher with a first-time recipient? Why do we spend resources on critical care for patients where the effectiveness is limited? If we feel shocked by the circumstances of an individual and offer intervention based on this psychological imperative without thought for the opportunity costs, we are operating under the rule of rescue. For whole populations this kind of decision-making may take place in large-scale emergencies such as an influenza pandemic (see Chapter 10) when funds are diverted to controlling an immediate threat.

An ethical framework commonly used to guide clinical judgements is that of Beauchamp and Childress [11]. This can be adapted to form the basis of prioritising decisions made in health care settings. An example of such an ethical framework is given in Box 9.3a. The principles may conflict with each other. For example, the decision to offer an expensive treatment to one patient from a limited budget permits them autonomy and enables the health carer to do good for that individual. However, the treatment may have side effects that must be weighed against the benefits, and there may be insufficient funds left to treat others – thus unjustly restricting their right to treatment. Decisions around individual patient needs may conflict with the needs of populations and public health professionals are often involved in mediating over complex decisions.

---

5. Is the smoking cessation service ethically justified?

Use Beauchamp and Childress' principles to decide whether you think funding smoking cessation would be ethically justified.

You may have considered some of the following points:

Autonomy:

- smokers' right to choose when to stop or not to stop
- addictive nature of nicotine reduces smokers' autonomy
- advertising and peer pressure may reduce autonomy
- non-smokers' right not to be subjected to second-hand smoke.
- right to help quitting if wanted.

Non-maleficence:
- need to ensure non-smokers are not exposed to harmful tobacco smoke
- cessation may increase harm transiently (e.g. operative risk increases four weeks post-cessation)
- adverse effects of cessation therapies.

Beneficence:
- harms of smoking well documented so cessation is doing good
- smokers' friends and families are benefited by cessation.

Justice:
- Should we spend on this if we consider it self-inflicted?
- Should we fund one or several courses of treatment?

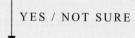

YES / NOT SURE

Box 9.3a Beauchamp and Childress principles (and rules) of biomedical ethics

Beauchamp and Childress posit four major principles of biomedical ethics and four minor rules:

Principles:
1. Respect for autonomy. This important principle is implicit in the requirement for consent for procedures. It can be difficult to apply this principle to those who are unable to make informed decisions, such as minors or those with learning difficulties.
2. Non-maleficence. Avoid harm. The need to avoid harm must frequently be weighed against the next principle when considering treatments with potential benefits and with some side effects.
3. Beneficence. Do good. Too much beneficence can be paternalistic! For example, our need to prevent the harm caused by obesity might lead us to coerce overweight people into lifestyle changes.
4. Justice. This principle reiterates the public health concept of equity in that a regard for fairness is important.

Rules:
1. Veracity. The truth. It is difficult to make decisions based on falsehood but the ability to be able to identify one common truth is debatable.
2. Privacy. The right of patients to withhold information is seen to be important but may hinder the diagnostic process.

3. Confidentiality. This is of increasing importance in modern health care and the need to handle patient-identifiable data sensibly is plain throughout many health care systems.
4. Fidelity. Trust. The relationship between clinician and patient requires trust; public health decisions which restrict treatments may jeopardise that trust.

Box 9.3b Example of an ethical framework based on Beauchamp and Childress

Ethical framework for making decisions relating to funding high-cost drugs (adapted from Suffolk West Primary Care Trust (PCT), England). The principles are based on those of Beauchamp and Childress.

Benefit vs. harm:

If there is insufficient evidence that a treatment confers a benefit its use should be questioned.

A treatment should not be offered unless a case can be made for its use in a particular circumstance.

Evidence of effectiveness should be sought for all treatments from a variety of sources including national guidance (such as NICE guidance) and repositories of clinical evidence (such as the Cochrane collaboration).

For low priority treatments, guidelines on their use are needed and exceptional decisions should be taken on a patient-by-patient basis.

Equity/justice

The PCT should aim to provide equity of access to treatments for all its patients based on need.

PCTs have a duty not to exceed their budgets. Decisions to limit access to treatments should, legitimately, include aspects of financial cost. Decisions to treat inevitably divert resources from other health care options.

Both cost-effectiveness and individual cost of treatments should be considered in deciding which treatments to limit and in making individual patient decisions.

In some cases the needs of a community for a range of treatments may outweigh the needs of an individual for a highly expensive treatment of unproven effectiveness.

Patient choice/autonomy

Patients should have a right to request treatments and have their case heard and considered.

The criteria and process for taking these decisions should be transparent and fair.

A differently constituted body to that making initial decisions should receive and hear appeals.

Conclusion

The last question in our framework is 'Overall, can the service be justified in terms of need, benefit, acceptability, cost and other priorities?' Using the smoking cessation example and working through the framework presented in this chapter, would probably lead you to fund smoking cessation services. In this case there is an effective service, which meets a need, is cost-effective and acceptable. Ethically, it would be very difficult to argue against the need for resources for this service and smoking cessation services are in place across the UK.

In practice such frameworks are applied to varying degrees. Priority setting committees frequently use frameworks to advise organisations on the use of funds. Alternatively, public health specialists may provide ad hoc answers to similar questions on an individual basis. The aim overall is to provide a more robust decision than would be achieved through a less systematic approach, to ensure that resources are used cost-effectively and to enable improvement in the health of individuals and populations.

REFERENCES

1. General Household Survey 2001–02. Colchester, UK Data Archive, 2002.
2. Public Health Intervention Guidance No. 2. Four commonly used methods to increase physical activity: brief interventions in primary care, exercise referral schemes, pedometers and community-based exercise programmes for walking and cycling. London, National Institute for Health and Clinical Excellence, 2006.
3. J. Lous, M. J. Burton, J. U. Felding *et al.*, Grommets (ventilation tubes) for hearing loss associated with otitis media with effusion in children. 2005. *Cochrane Database of Systematic Reviews*, 2006, Issue 4.
4. A. R. White, H. Rampes and E. Ernst, Acupuncture for smoking cessation (Cochrane review) The *Cochrane Library*, Issue 1, 2000.
5. M. F. Drummond, J. O'Brien, G. L. Stoddart and G. W. Torrance, *Methods for the Economic Evaluation of Health Care Programmes*. Oxford, Oxford University Press, 1997.
6. N. Woolacott, L. Janes, C. Forbes *et al.*, A rapid and systematic review of the clinical and cost effectiveness of bupropion SR and nicotine replacement therapy (NRT) for smoking cessation. York, NHS Centre for Reviews and Dissemination, 2002.

7. S. R. Cummings, S. M. Rubin and G. Oster. The cost-effectiveness of counseling smokers to quit. *Journal of the American Medical Association*, **261**; 1989, 75–9.

8. Public Health Intervention Guidance No. 1. Brief interventions and referral for smoking cessation in primary care and other settings. London, National Institute for Health and Clinical Excellence, 2006.

9. C. Phillips and G. Thompson, What is a QALY? 2001. Accessed via www.evidence-based-medicine.co.uk.

10. A. R. Johnsen, Bentham in a box: technology assessment and health care allocation. *Law Medicine and Health Care*, 1986, 172–4.

11. T. Beauchamp and J. Childress, *Principles of Biomedical Ethics*, 3rd edn, New York, Oxford University Press, 1989.

10

Health protection and communicable disease control

Key points

- The term 'health protection' covers immediate threats to health such as infectious diseases, environmental threats, e.g. chemical releases and radiological hazards, natural disasters and terrorism.
- Communicable disease control depends upon the nature of the infecting organism (pathogen), the transmission route and the response of the host. Individuals can help to protect themselves by being aware of the different modes of transmission of infectious diseases.
- Vaccines are an effective way to protect whole populations against many infectious diseases.
- Surveillance of infectious diseases is important to spot outbreaks, monitor levels of disease, plan control measures, monitor outcomes of control programmes and enable efficient targeting of resources.
- Communicable diseases are controlled through the prompt investigation of outbreaks and efficient implementation of control measures when outbreaks occur, or proactively.
- Environmental health involves the investigation and control of potential health hazards which arise from an environmental or man-made origin.
- Emergency planning is increasingly important as a mechanism to plan for and control the health effects of large-scale disasters and emergencies, including natural disasters and terrorist attacks.

Introduction

Health protection refers to immediate threats to health such as infectious diseases, environmental threats, e.g. chemical releases and radiological hazards,

Essential Public Health, eds. Stephen Gillam, Jan Yates and Padmanabhan Badrinath.
Published by Cambridge University Press. © Cambridge University Press 2007.

natural disasters and the threats from terrorist acts. However, this UK-based definition of health protection is not used worldwide; for example in the United States
health protection may include (as it used to in the UK also) legislative aspects of
promoting good health (see Chapter 4). These include, for example, workplace
smoking bans or speed restrictions and even lifestyle choices, and the health
issues of an aging population such as increasing levels of chronic disease. This
chapter will outline the public health aspects of communicable disease control
and touch on some of the other areas now included within health protection in
the UK. A glossary including important health protection terms is included on
the CD.

Principles of communicable disease control

Based on the demographic transition, it was widely believed until only a few years
ago that infectious diseases were an historic problem. The eradication of smallpox,
the development of new vaccines and other pharmaceutical advances appeared
to signal their continuing decline. However, the WHO Global Burden of Disease
project (GBD2002) portrays a different picture (see Chapter 17). The incidence of
infectious diseases is extremely high (over $5^1/_2$ million cases worldwide per year).
It is higher than the incidence of other diseases in all regions of the world, varying
from eight times higher than chronic conditions in Europe to 30 times higher in
Africa. Whilst interventions to moderate the burden of infectious diseases have
been shown to be cost effective (for example, a measles vaccination costs less
than $1 per vaccination and less than $25 per quality adjusted life year gained
[1]), the resurgence of diseases once thought to be coming under control, such
as tuberculosis (TB), illustrate an ongoing failure to tackle basic causes as well
as the natural ingenuity of causative micro-organisms. The lack of political and
pharmaco-industrial will to develop low-cost remedies for 'unprofitable' diseases
like leishmaniasis and TB also remains an obstacle. In the UK, the most dramatic
deterioration has been in the field of sexually transmitted infection. In addition to
human immunodeficiency virus (HIV), the incidence of chlamydia, syphilis and
gonorrhoea has risen remarkably over the last ten years.

New challenges continue to arise. Global pandemics such as HIV/AIDS (aquired
immunodeficiency syndrome) have graphically underlined the continued importance of health inequalities and poverty as determinants of ill health. Drug resis-
tances are emerging and linked in part to increasing use of antimicrobial agents;
examples here are malaria, tuberculosis, methicillin-resistant *Staphylococcus
aureus* (MRSA), salmonella and *Clostridium difficile*. Finally, more exotic threats
to human health such as variant Creutzfeld-Jakob's disease, avian influenza and
severe acute respiratory syndrome (SARS) have further fuelled media interest in
communicable disease.

Controlling communicable diseases

In many ways the public health challenges associated with infectious diseases are similar to those associated with other diseases: identify the burden of disease, consider how to prevent or treat it and take appropriate action. However, there are some elements of dealing with infectious agents which set this field apart. Causes of disease here have the ability to replicate, and interactions between the agent, the host and the environment are all important factors to consider. These agents are transmissible, can alter and evolve, as can the host's response to them. This host response is something we can use as a target for control when we utilise vaccines. Lastly, in contrast to much of public health, timescales in communicable disease control can be relatively short and there is often little time to initiate effective control measures. Thus, we often need to balance enforcement of control measures and education. The sporadic nature of outbreaks raises the importance of surveillance systems to spot problems early.

In the following section we will consider how communicable disease control systems work to prevent infection in individuals, prevent infection at the population level and prevent spread of infection when cases do occur. We also consider how these control systems are monitored. We will use influenza (flu) as an example to demonstrate the different types of control discussed.

Communicable disease control for individuals

Control of disease relies on the nature of the causal organism and determining opportunities to interrupt transmission from host to host. The organism causing the infection is termed an agent or pathogen and may be a protozoan (e.g. *Cryptosporidiosis*), a virus (e.g. polio, influenza), a bacterium (e.g. *Escherichia coli, Salmonella enteritidis*), a yeast (e.g. *Candida albicans*) or larger organisms (e.g. worms, ticks, mites).

The means by which agents are transmitted from host to host varies and determines what control methods are appropriate. Table 10.1 shows some modes of transmission with possible control measures.

So preventing transmission is easy in theory but not necessarily in practice. Box 10.1 shows how individual control might work for flu. Education is important to prevent outbreaks, to prevent further spread and to limit the chance of recurrence (e.g. educating health care staff in hand washing to prevent the spread of infection in hospitals).

Difficulties arise when preventing transmission. One of these is where reservoirs of infection exist in animals (for example, rabies, salmonella) or the environment (for example, cryptosporidium and legionella). Smallpox provided the WHO's

Table 10.1. Modes of transmission of communicable diseases and possible control measures.

Mode of transmission	Examples of agents transmitted in this way	Possible control measures
Physical contact with people	Sexually transmitted infections such as chlamydia Head lice	Isolation of cases Hygiene Barrier contraception Treat, cases e.g. with pediculocides
Physical contact with animals	Rabies	Avoidance Vaccination of animals Vaccination of humans
Physical contact with the environment	Tetanus	Hygiene Disinfection Vaccination
Respiratory	Flu Measles TB	Isolation of cases Treat cases Chemoprophylaxis Vaccination Hand washing
Faecal–oral	*Salmonella, E. coli* or *Campylobacter* Polio Typhoid Hepatitis A	Good hygiene Isolation of cases Separation of raw and cooked food, clean water and sewage Vaccination
Blood to blood	HIV Hepatitis B	Needle exchanges Safe sharps and clean-up practices Screening of blood products Sterilisation Safe operating practices Vaccination
Transplacental	HIV Hepatitis B Rubella Cytomegalovirus Listeria	Vaccination Chemoprophylaxis
Insect vector	Malaria Yellow fever Lyme disease West Nile virus	Eradication/control of vector Chemoprophylaxis Vaccination Barriers, e.g. mosquito nets
Contamination of food or water	Salmonella, Cryptosporidium, Legionella	Good hygiene practices for food safety (hand washing is of central importance) Destruction of contaminated goods Production controls assurance Legislation Good management of water-supply systems/effective cleaning and maintenance
Fomites (objects harbouring a disease agent)	Influenza Norovirus	Disinfection or destruction of fomites such as clothing or utensils

Box 10.1 Individual control of flu infection

The influenza virus has several features which make it an effective pathogen. It is a small virus easily transmitted in airborne droplets or from surface to surface (such as door handle to hand to nose). The symptoms it produces such as a runny nose and coughing promote this mode of spread and virus particles are transmitted before symptoms start. Thus individual methods of control include keeping away from crowded places and frequent hand washing.

greatest triumph partly because man is the only reservoir and an effective vaccine was available.

Control is problematic where it depends upon changing behaviours (e.g. controlling sexually transmitted infection relies on individual and cultural attitudes to behaviours such as condom use).

Organisms which have become resistant to some antimicrobial drugs are now being found in patients in both hospital and community settings. Organisms include MRSA, TB and certain strains of *E. coli*. While some organisms are naturally more resistant to antimicrobials (such as TB which has thick cell walls) resistance can also occur through changes in an organism's genes or be introduced by transmission of resistance genes from other organisms. Resistance is particularly problematic in the care of hospital inpatients who are especially susceptible to infections. It is still possible to treat most drug-resistant infections but the treatment options become limited and it is better to prevent the development of resistance.

England has higher rates of hospital-acquired MRSA infection than other European countries. Solutions to the reduction of health-care acquired infection (HAI) are multifactorial and include: surveillance, clear infection control standards, maintaining clean hospital environments, strict antibiotic prescribing practices and isolation of infected patients.

Controlling communicable diseases by protecting populations

Systems have to be in place to ensure that the control measures which prevent individuals transmitting or contracting infections are applied across large numbers of people. This type of control aims to reduce morbidity and mortality from these diseases in populations. Whilst it would be ideal from a human point of view to *eradicate* infectious diseases (as we have with smallpox), pragmatism dictates that our control objectives cannot always be so ambitious. In some cases we aim to *eliminate* infection by preventing transmission but accept that the organism still persists in our environment. We have achieved this to a large extent with the vaccination of chicken flocks to eliminate *S. enteritidis* in eggs from those flocks (eggs from salmonella-free flocks carry a 'Lion' mark), and pasteurisation to eliminate milk as a vehicle for transmitting TB and *E. coli* O157. Lastly, we may accept that a disease cannot be eliminated or eradicated but aim to *contain* it so that it does not present a significant public health problem. Winter outbreaks of influenza are an example of where a disease is contained to minimise its impact on the population.

Vaccination

The term vaccination derives from the historical origins of the process for inoculation with vaccinia virus against smallpox (first described by Edward Jenner in 1798). Whilst immunisation is, strictly speaking, the protection (making immune) of an individual by the administration of a vaccine, the terms 'immunisation' and 'vaccination' tend now to be used synonymously.

Vaccination is used to make large proportions of populations immune to bacterial or viral diseases. The agent administered (usually by injection) can be living but modified (e.g. yellow fever), a suspension of killed organisms (e.g. whooping cough (pertussis)) or an inactivated toxin (such as tetanus). The aim is to generate an immune response in those vaccinated which will protect them from serious disease should they later be challenged with that organism. Killed organisms provide a limited immunity and may have to be given as a starter dose with boosters to provide optimal protection. Vaccines can also be given in pulses (repeated doses over time) to maximise immunity. Live, attenuated vaccines such as the oral polio vaccine provide better cover. These tend to be for viral infections. Sometimes a temporary immunity can be generated by vaccination with antibodies, for example immunoglobulins against varicella are given to pregnant women who may have come into contact with chicken pox.

Immunisation may be mass or targeted. Mass vaccination aims to eradicate, eliminate or contain infection similarly to other control methods. For example the WHO has elimination targets for certified elimination of measles in every country in the European region by 2010. This will be achieved by mass vaccination, in the UK through the measles, mumps and rubella (MMR) vaccinations at 12–15 months and $3^{1}/_{2}$–4 years. However, targeted vaccine programmes can sometimes be more effective than mass vaccination. Box 10.2 shows that vaccination for flu is targeted to those most at risk and aims to contain infection. Smallpox is another example. When the incidence of smallpox was high then the dangers of vaccination (the vaccine causes death in approximately one in a million people) were vastly outweighed by the protection and reduction in mortality provided by the vaccine. As the likelihood of an outbreak is now small, mass vaccination is not warranted but in an outbreak situation vaccination would be targeted to cover all susceptible individuals in a prescribed area around an outbreak (termed ring vaccination).

Box 10.2 Protecting populations against flu

The flu virus is antigenically unstable with new strains and variants constantly emerging. This poses problems for vaccine development so that a new vaccine is needed for each new strain. A system of global surveillance is in place to monitor the movement of flu strains across the world and predict which vaccines will be needed for seasonal outbreaks, such as those in the UK in winter.

Once a vaccine is produced, susceptible individuals such as the elderly and health care workers are encouraged to take up the offer of vaccination.

Four flu pandemics have occurred since 1880. (Note: an epidemic is the occurrence of disease at higher than expected level and a pandemic is a worldwide epidemic.) History suggests that another pandemic is likely. A pandemic variant arises through mutation of an animal flu virus. However, a vaccine cannot be produced in advance as the particular variant is unknown until the pandemic occurs.

No vaccine is 100% effective as individuals mount different immune responses, which last varying amounts of time. However, it is not necessary for every person to be immune. *Herd immunity* is the degree to which a population is resistant to an infection as high general levels of immunity protect the non-immune. Herd immunity is an important concept in health protection and can be thought of as the immunity of a community. The reproductive rate is the mean number of new cases generated by each case of a disease. If there is adequate herd immunity (i.e. enough people have been vaccinated and had a good response), the reproductive rate is less than one and the incidence of cases falls. This is why the coverage rate for vaccinations is considered important. If fewer people are vaccinated the herd immunity drops and outbreaks of a disease occur. This is occurring in the UK with measles. Although the WHO recommend coverage above 95%[2], in the UK coverage falls below 90%. Low uptake and incomplete coverage of vaccination in earlier years (partly due to low vaccine stocks and partly due to public apprehension around the MMR vaccine fueled by negative media coverage) have resulted in an upswing in the number of measles outbreaks occurring in the UK.

The need for a vaccine is determined by consideration of the characteristics of the disease, and then vaccines are developed through clinical trials in much the same way as new drugs are. For example, a vaccine for meningococcal group C was introduced to the UK in 1999 because the disease, whilst quite rare (811 cases reported in England and Wales in 1998) is so devastating that a vaccine programme was considered cost-effective. The incidence has now fallen to less than 100 cases per year. The aims of vaccination programmes vary depending on the disease and whether the control intended is eradication, elimination or containment. In general, vaccine coverage in the more developed regions is higher.

Table 10.2. Vaccination schedule for the UK 2007

2 months old	Diphtheria, tetanus, pertussis (whooping cough), polio and *Haemophilus influenzae* type b
	Pneumococcal infection
3 months old	Diphtheria, tetanus, pertussis, polio and *Haemophilus influenzae* type b
	Meningococcal group C
4 months old	Diphtheria, tetanus, pertussis, polio and *Haemophilus influenzae* type b
Around 12 months old	Pneumococcal infection
	Haemophilus influenzae type b
	Meningococcal group C
Around 13 months old	Measles, mumps and rubella
3 years and 4 months to 5 years old	Diphtheria, tetanus, pertussis and polio
	Measles, mumps and rubella
13 to 18 years old	Diphtheria, tetanus, polio

This means that more booster vaccinations may be given in less-developed countries in attempts to improve coverage. Not all infectious diseases have effective vaccines and not all countries need programmes for all the vaccines available. For example, hepatitis B vaccination is currently given in many countries but not in the UK, as the incidence is low at less than 1,000 cases per year. The WHO hopes to eradicate polio and aims to provide as much vaccination as possible to those countries, such as India, which still have circulating polio virus (see Chapter 17). Thus, knowing the burden of diseases in various populations determines the vaccine policy developed. Ensuring adequate vaccine for targeted diseases is a major industry and public health can provide useful advice to those developing and manufacturing vaccines, through support for clinical vaccine trials as well as supporting the delivery of vaccines to target audiences (for example, by managing the maintenance of a cold chain where necessary). This can be particularly problematic in developing countries. Public health workers also have a role in educating the public and professionals about vaccination as well as managing immunisation programmes. At a national level the management of programmes also includes vaccine funding and surveillance to monitor vaccination uptake and programme targets.

Table 10.2 shows the current vaccination schedule for the UK and we suggest you use the internet to find current vaccination schedules for the USA and India. Think about what action would be needed if a new vaccine was to be added to the schedule. More information about immunisation can be found on the World Health Organisation website (see below).

Planning and monitoring control measures – surveillance

The practice of surveillance, monitoring diseases through measuring morbidity and mortality, arose in the fourteenth and fifteenth centuries with the Black Death. In this case authorities wanted to be aware of ships with infected people aboard in order to prevent them coming ashore and infecting others. Surveillance can be defined as the ongoing, systematic, collection, collation and analysis of data and the prompt dissemination of the resulting information to those who need to know so that action can be taken.

Surveillance is used to identify individual cases of disease so that action can be taken to prevent spread (for example, excluding food handlers from work if they contract food poisoning). This can also be used over time to monitor the incidence of disease so that rises in incidence can trigger an investigation. A microbiology laboratory, for example, might notice several cases of legionella infection and trigger an investigation into the possible source in order to prevent further cases. Trends in infection, which are continuously monitored through surveillance systems, can indicate changes in risk factors, or that certain elements of a population are at increased risk (for example, a rise in sexually transmitted infections in young women). This allows interventions to be targeted appropriately. Knowing the epidemiology of infectious diseases in close to real time through surveillance can help to evaluate current control measures such as vaccination programmes. A fall in incidence may allow control measures to be relaxed. For example, it is no longer necessary to vaccinate against smallpox. Lastly, and very importantly, surveillance allows new infections to be detected and hypotheses produced regarding their causes. Many countries have communicable disease surveillance programmes, which carry out these functions.

Surveillance is, however, resource intensive and it is important to make it as simple as possible to get the maximum amount of data reported (see Box 10.3). Reports generally come from individuals dealing with the diseases in question – clinicians and public health professionals – or from laboratory diagnoses. The type and importance of the disease determines the type of surveillance. In some cases reporting is mandatory; 'notifiable diseases' in the UK and the USA must be reported by doctors. It may, however, be preferable for surveillance to be voluntary and anonymous. Such is the case for HIV in the UK, which is monitored in annual surveys, and where it is not possible to identify an individual patient from the data collected. In some infections, as with the HIV surveillance, it is not practical to collect details of every case. Representative samples can be taken and the true rates of disease extrapolated from them.

Box 10.3 What makes a good surveillance system?

Clear objectives are needed for the system so that it can be evaluated and to ensure that it is relevant to the needs of the population to be covered.

Clear case definitions are required for the conditions under surveillance so that the same thing is counted accurately all the time. Data need to flow from clear sources to a clear collection point.

Easy reporting mechanisms maximise the number of cases reported and useful, timely feedback to reporters encourages participation and enables action. Not every case will be reported – for example, the incidence of gastro-intestinal infection can be up to 100-fold greater in the community than that reported. A clear understanding of *what proportion of cases are reported* is needed so that estimates of true incidence can be made. This may require population based surveys.

Data validation systems should be designed and used to maximise accuracy and enable efficient analysis and interpretation.

All of this requires adequate resourcing and aims to maximise the **completeness**, **accuracy**, **relevance** and **timeliness** of the system. More complex systems may be more sensitive, predictive and representative of the true disease status but they will be costly, take longer to operate, be less acceptable to those participating and lose flexibility. A balance is required.

Containing infection – outbreak investigation

When preventative measures fail (or when control was only ever going to contain the disease, not eradicate or eliminate infection), then control measures must be used retrospectively to contain the infection to as few people as possible. This is called outbreak investigation and aims to prevent spread of disease, ensure treatment for those infected and prevent similar instances in future. The management of an outbreak of a food-borne illness is a good example of how outbreaks are investigated, although the methods used can be applied to any infectious disease. How such an investigation might progress is summarised here and it highlights the stages and important points of such an investigation. Box 10.4 gives an example of how an outbreak investigation might work in practice.

- Initial investigation – is it an outbreak? An epidemic is the occurrence of disease at higher than expected levels. This could be an endemic disease (one which is always present in a population) at higher than usual levels or non-endemic disease at any level. An outbreak is a localised epidemic. Health protection professionals often look for two or more cases linked in time and place.

Box 10.4 An example of an outbreak investigation

On 6th August, cases of sickness and diarrhoea are reported to a local health-protection team. This is following a Sunday lunch party on 4th August at a local restaurant, The Golden Lion.

Firstly the team must decide if an outbreak has occurred to determine whether any action is necessary. For an outbreak there must be more than the expected number of cases linked in time and place. In this case the people who are reported ill have all eaten at the Golden Lion on the same day. An outbreak seems likely and an outbreak control team is formed. This includes membership from public health (health protection), environmental health (who are the most likely professional group to detect or report an outbreak), microbiology and communications. Immediate control measures may be needed, such as removal of contaminated foodstuffs; the potential source of infection (The Golden Lion) is visited and the staff's standards of hygiene examined. Case histories are taken. Any food which is left over from Sunday lunch is sent to the laboratory to be screened for food poisoning organisms.

It is decided that further investigation is warranted to find any more cases and to determine the exact source of infection so that future instances can be prevented. A clear case definition is needed so that cases can be found. This must include elements of time (accounting for the incubation period of the suspected disease, when might infection have occurred?), place (where it is believed the source is), person (who might be affected) and some definition of symptoms (so that cases can identify themselves). In this example the case definition might be, 'Any person who had diarrhoea and vomiting and who had eaten at The Golden Lion between 4th and 6th August'. Cases are then found (for example, by asking local doctors to report visits to their clinics) and a descriptive study carried out.

The descriptive study proposes a hypothesis for the cause of the outbreak and can usually be presented as an epidemic curve, which shows the number of cases over the time course of the outbreak. It is possible to use an epidemic curve to make hypotheses about the nature of the outbreak. The example in the chart shows a classic point-source epidemic. The graph shows number of cases occurring on each day. Here, there is one source of the disease, cases become infected from this source over a short period, and over the course of the disease's incubation period new cases become apparent. This epidemic tails off quickly. This occurs in a food-poisoning outbreak where only one foodstuff was contaminated, for example, undercooked meat at the Sunday lunch. It is also possible to spot a continuing source if cases continue to occur over a longer period. With food poisoning this indicates a source has not been eradicated, for example due to poor hygiene practices in a food preparation area. Several curves in succession indicate a single source but with secondary infection – for example, someone contracting food poisoning and then infecting their family, then a neighbour, followed by the neighbour's family, and so on. Each of these patterns provides useful clues to the management of the outbreak.

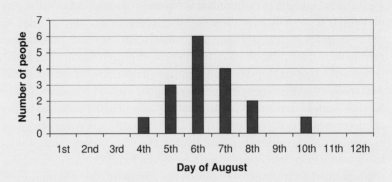

Epidemic curve for Golden Lion outbreak of vomiting and diarrhoea

In this example there is a single source of infection. In order to confirm that the cases have become infected from the restaurant, any organisms grown from the food samples must be linked to whatever organism is causing the illness. Stool samples are collected from cases and sent for microbiological investigation. The same organism is found in both food and stools and the evidence suggests that the roast beef cooked for Sunday lunch at the Golden Lion was the source. An analytical study can be used to test this hypothesis. A small-scale study examines the statistical likelihood of the illness being related to the consumption of roast beef. This is done by calculating relative risks or odds ratios as for any case–control or cohort observational study (see Chapter 2). An example of how this calculation can be made is included on the CD.

By this time is it usual to have instigated control measures and the analytical study confirms that these are appropriate or suggests other measures needed. In this example we would expect food remains to have been destroyed, the kitchen to have been thoroughly cleaned and food storage and preparation to have been inspected. Now that we are sure of the source, fuller and longer-term measures can be instigated. There may be issues of training for food-preparation staff, kitchen refit or redesign. Control measures vary depending upon the causal organism. *Escherichia coli 0157*, for example, is an important cause of food poisoning, and due to its high attack rate and serious nature is followed up carefully. All those who come into contact with a known case are investigated. In particular, food handlers, those caring for vulnerable people and those with poor personal hygiene are excluded from work or school until it is clear they are no longer carrying the organism.

Other important issues are considered throughout the investigation. Communication with the media is important, especially if the source of the outbreak is a public place. There may also be a need to prosecute (for example a butcher may have ignored regulations in the handling of the beef, permitting contamination), especially if this is a repeated offence. The investigation then forms legal evidence, and documentation and audit trails are of vital importance.

- Convene an outbreak control team. If a major outbreak has occurred a team is convened to carry out further investigations and to plan control. People involved are typically public health, environmental health, microbiology and communications experts (others may be needed, for example a representative from a water company if the outbreak is of a water-borne infection).
- Initial control – take early action, if necessary, to prevent further cases of disease.
- Descriptive study – generate a hypothesis about the cause of the outbreak.
- Control measures – throughout the investigation think about controlling spread.
- Analytical (environmental) study – confirm the source of the outbreak (in practice this may be the same as the descriptive study).
- Microbiological evidence – link the cases to the source through microbiological identification of the causal organism.
- Prevent further outbreaks – put in place long-term control measures to prevent the same thing happening again.

The hypothetical example here involves food poisoning but outbreaks of many communicable diseases are investigated in the same way.

Environmental public health

Environmental hazards to health include chemicals released into the air, contaminated water sources or industrial accidents. The medical model of control applied to communicable disease control serves less well in these circumstances. Here the environmental model (also called the pollution linkage model and source–pathway–receptor model) is used. Methods to control the hazard are determined by identifying the source, the pathway and the receptor (Table 10.3).

The receptor need not be human – it may be animal or vegetable. Pathways can be air, water or ground. An example might be the release of a toxic chemical into the environment due to a road accident and a tanker spillage. The crashed tanker is the source. Pathways for this hazardous chemical to become a problem may be

Table 10.3. Examples of sources, pathways and receptors for some environmental hazards.

Source	Pathway	Receptor
Chemical spillage from tanker crash	Air	Grazing cattle
	Ground	Man
	Rivers	Allotment vegetables
Oil dump into the ocean	Ocean water	Wildfowl
		Fish
Factory fire, ash and smoke	Air	Man
		Wildlife
		Crops

through the air if it is a fine powder or volatile liquid, through the ground if it leaks onto a porous surface such as fields, or through water if it enters a water course. From here it may reach a variety of receptors – plant life through soil or water, and then animal life, directly or via eating the plants. Animal life may also be affected directly from exposure to airborne matter. This model provides a methodology for considering where the path from source to receptor can be interrupted or contamination prevented.

So we can think about containing an environmental hazard in a similar way to containing the hazards from communicable diseases – consider how the hazard transmits its effects to us and find ways to interrupt this.

In addition to this there are more complex areas of environmental health that a public health practitioner might be called upon to contribute to, see the exercise below for examples of these.

Table 10.4 shows some environmental hazards which a public health practitioner may be called upon to control. In each case the receptor of interest is humans. For each hazard, what approaches to control might be relevant?

1. Specialist decontamination.
2. Provision of aid, clean or bottled water, drainage.
3. An analysis of the likelihood of an increase in disease may prove no link – this is similar to an epidemiological case–control study to assess whether the incidence of disease is significantly higher in the population hypothesised to be at risk.
4. Adequate emergency health facilities, search and rescue.
5. Relocation.
6. Mediation. Environmental/health impact assessment to ascertain the extent of likely health effects and mitigate these via new policy-making.
7. Workplace assessment, provision of supports such as foot rests.

Table 10.4. Environmental hazards

	Source	Pathway	Potential health effects
1.	Nuclear-waste spillage	Water, ground or air	Radiation poisoning
2.	Gastro-intestinal disease organisms in flood water	Water, food	Intestinal infection / food poisoning
3.	Radiation from radio masts	Air	Increase in leukaemia incidence
4.	Earthquake	Ground	Physical injury from falling buildings
5.	Volcanic ash	Air	Respiratory effects
6.	Loud neighbours or new airport runway	Air	Psychological distress
7.	Poor workstation posture	N/A	Repetitive strain injury
8.	Terrorist chemical attack	Air or water	Toxic effects dependent upon chemical used
9.	Poor building design	N/A	Low physical activity levels and adverse health effects
10.	Second-hand smoke in public places	Air	Increased lung cancer, coronary heart disease

8. See emergency planning section below for how emergencies are planned for and dealt with.
9. Impact assessment during planning stages to provide healthy building design.
10. Legislation.

It is important to note that some environmental hazards result from occupational sources and the effects of these and their modification are often dealt with by specialist occupational health practitioners. Some important areas of occupational health in the UK are:

- Vaccination of health care workers against infectious diseases they may acquire through their work, e.g. hepatitis C.
- Workstation assessment to prevent health effects due to poor posture for office workers.
- Care of substances hazardous to health where workers may be exposed to chemical hazards.
- The assessment and reduction of physical workplace hazards such as risk of slips, trips, falls, and hazards due to lifting.

In each case the tools needed are those already highlighted in previous chapters, the effective use of epidemiological methods and risk assessment.

Preparing for emergencies

Another specialist area within the field of health protection is disaster or emergency planning. There are a variety of interpretations of the words 'disaster' and 'emergency'. The UK Civil Contingencies Act of 2004 states that an emergency

Fig. 10.1   Disaster cycle.

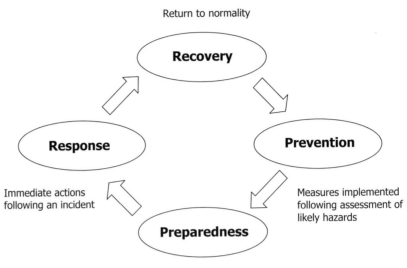

is an event or situation which threatens serious damage to human welfare; an event or situation which threatens serious damage to the environment; or war, or terrorism, which threatens serious damage to security. The United Nations International Strategy for Disaster Reduction states that a disaster must involve one or more of the following: ten or more people reported killed, 100 or more people affected, the declaration of a state of emergency or a call for international assistance. The common theme is a situation more serious than one organisation can cope with alone.

A somewhat different toolkit is needed here but it still draws heavily on basic public health skills. Figure 10.1 shows the disaster cycle, demonstrating the key stages in the lead-up and response to an emergency incident. Some of the examples listed earlier, such as terrorist acts or large-scale environmental disasters, fall into this area of work and require planning for in advance of their occurrence. Risk assessment is important, as is determination of the likely impacts of any disaster. Epidemiological skills are needed for this. Partnership working is key as plans and responses need to be co-ordinated across many agencies, public and voluntary. In many countries this process is highly organised. In the UK the Civil Contingencies Secretariat of the Cabinet Office co-ordinates the planning process and in the USA the Federal Emergency Management Agency is part of the Department of Homeland Security and leads the process. Other Governments have similar bodies such as the Indian Ministry of Home Affairs National Disaster Management Division.

In the process of planning for disasters the role of the health sector is to deal with mass casualties and deaths as well as, potentially, mass vaccination. With partners in the emergency services and those in the armed forces, health-care

Box 10.5   Disaster planning for a flu pandemic

We can use the disaster cycle to illustrate elements of how public health workers plan for an emergency such as a flu pandemic.

Prevention

Minimisation of opportunities for a highly pathogenic strain of animal influenza to acquire the ability to transmit to humans (e.g. slaughter or vaccination of bird flocks to prevent H5N1 transmission to humans)

Planning

Business continuity planning to deal with illness and absenteeism in the health care sector

Stockpiling of anti-viral drugs

Media awareness campaigns

Worldwide surveillance of circulating virus strains

Response

Rapid, co-ordinated development of case definitions and diagnostic tools

Rapid development of treatment guidelines, vaccines, etc

Identification of at-risk staff and implementation of increased safety measures

Isolation and treatment of cases

Development of supply chains for antiviral drugs and vaccines

Staff sharing to enable learning and cover of necessary functions

Development of alternative access for maintaining urgent care when some centres may be closed due to mass infection

Management en masse of infected casualties

Recovery

Additional services to manage increased waiting lists due to cancelled procedures

Cover arrangements for any staff who have worked overtime

Provision of counselling for staff

organisations form the front line in responding to a wide range of incidents, and have the primary responsibility for protecting health and maintaining health care services during the emergency, and restoring health afterwards. All agencies must also plan to maintain business continuity during times of disaster when the workforce may be significantly depleted due to illness, death or absenteeism. Box 10.5 illustrates how the health sector might plan for a flu pandemic, a disaster for planning purposes as it would kill large numbers of people.

Three main types of emergency are planned for: those which creep up on us like a rising tide, those that hit us with a 'big bang' and those which emerge completely out of the blue. Imagine how the disaster cycle could be used to deal with a range of disaster scenarios. You could think, for example, about floods, volcanoes, terrorist attacks, the emergence of a new disease, a breakdown in fuel supply, a hurricane.

Conclusion

In this chapter we have seen how the specialised public health field of health protection deals, in the UK at least, with communicable diseases, environmental hazards and emergency planning. Health protection is thus a setting which requires the use of many core public health skills to plan and respond to threats to health.

Further reading and sources of information

More sources of information are listed on the CD but a wide variety of information about health protection can be found in the following:
Centre for Disease Control: www.cdc.gov/node.do/id/0900f3ec8000e035
Health Protection Agency: www.hpa.org.uk/
World Health Organisation: www.who.int/topics/immunization/en/
J. Hawker, N. Begg, I. Blair, R. Reintjes and J. Weinberg, *Communicable Disease Control Handbook* Oxford, Blackwell, 2001.

REFERENCES

1. D. S. Shepard, J. A. Walsh, E. Kleinau, S. Stansfield and S. Bhalotra, Setting for the Children's Vaccine Initiative: a cost – effectiveness approach. *Vaccine*, **13**(8), 1995, 707–14.
2. Eliminating measles and rubella and preventing congenital rubella infection: European Region strategic plan 2005–2010. WHO European Region, 2005.

Part 2

The challenges of public health in practice

11

The health of children and young people

Rachel Crowther and Sarah Stewart-Brown

Key points

- Child public health is important in its own right, but also because children represent the future.
- Although child health has improved greatly over the last century, great disparities still exist between the health of children in different social groups and relative poverty remains a key determinant of child health both in the UK worldwide.
- Family relationships are an important determinant of risk factors for poor health across the life course and play a role in the transmission of social inequalities.
- The challenges facing child public health in the twenty-first century include the rise in emotional and behavioural disorders, childhood obesity, chronic disease and disability, and the continuing globalisation and commercialisation of children's lives.
- The promotion of child health requires action at the level of the individual, family, school and society and demands cross-disciplinary and intersectoral collaboration.

Children and their health

Why is child public health important?

Childhood is important in its own right, but children also represent the future: they are the adults (and the parents) of tomorrow. Because of their vulnerability children deserve particular care and protection from society, and their right to this protection, enabling them to enjoy life, health, identity, education and other

Essential Public Health, eds. Stephen Gillam, Jan Yates and Padmanabhan Badrinath.
Published by Cambridge University Press. © Cambridge University Press 2007.

fundamental goods, is enshrined in the United Nations Convention on the Rights of the Child. Although most countries are signatories to this convention many children worldwide – and some in the UK – are still denied basic rights through accident of birth, or through the ignorance or cruelty of adults. Another compelling reason to promote health in childhood is provided by the growing body of research showing the extent to which physical and emotional development in infancy and childhood influences adult health, and thus the health of the next generation [1].

At the end of the nineteenth and the beginning of the twentieth century, child public health was recognised as a vital aspect of public health practice. It slipped down the agenda in the latter half of the twentieth century when public health practitioners concentrated on improving adult health-related lifestyles, but it is now moving centre stage again. The goals of twenty-first century child public health include: ensuring a healthy start in life for all babies and reducing the gap in infant mortality rates between different sectors of society; increasing the chances of all children enjoying their childhood and developing and learning to their full potential; and seeing them on the way to becoming happy, healthy, productive adults.

Child public health shares many of the techniques, approaches and skills of other areas of public health practice but it is also a distinct subspecialty, reflecting the changing developmental stages of children and their dependence on adults for much of this period. Because adults are often keen to offer children conditions that they felt they deserved but were denied in their own childhood, and because children are rightly seen as vulnerable, child public health can also blaze new trails for the wider cause of public health. Social inequity is more obviously unfair to children, who play no part in creating the circumstances under which they live, and social inequity was a feature of child public health practice long before it was recognised as an important issue in adult public health. Sustainable development is important for the whole of society, but its relevance is nowhere more obvious than to child public health. Today, emotional and social well being are identified as appropriate goals for child public health in the UK in many policy documents (e.g. Choosing Health: making healthier choices easier [2] and the National Service Framework for children, young people and maternity services [3]), but it may take some time before such goals are similarly well recognised for adults.

Adapting Acheson's well known definition, Kohler [4] has defined child public health as 'the organised efforts of society to develop healthy public health policies to promote child and young people's health, to prevent disease in children and young people and to foster equity for children and young people, within a framework of sustainable development' [4]. It involves:

- *A concern for the health and well being of all children and young people in the population*, whether local, national or international, with a particular emphasis on less advantaged children whose experience of life and of health often differs markedly from their more fortunate peers.

- *Aiming to promote health in the broadest sense* captured in the World Health Organisation definition: 'a state of complete physical, mental and social well-being and not merely the absence of disease or infirmity.'
- *Understanding and responding to key child health problems*: studying patterns of health and illness in children; identifying factors which affect children's health and exploring ways in which these factors can be modified to improve health and well being; assessing health needs and providing guidance on ways of meeting them.
- *Identifying childhood antecedents of future disease or disability and developing preventive interventions.*
- *Seeing children in context*, as members of families, communities and wider social networks. Each different 'layer' of the environment has an influence on the child and his or her health, and thus provides a sphere of activity for child public health practice – e.g. seeking to improve family relationships, the local environment and social policy [5].
- *Implementing and managing a wide range of public health interventions*, including screening and immunisation programmes; advice on the commissioning of health care for children; and community-based health promotion initiatives such as Surestart, the Healthy Schools movement and support for parents and parenting.
- *Ensuring that child health remains in clear focus* in the fields of health, social and educational policy, and enabling children's voices to be heard in policy development and service planning.
- *Co-operation between a wide variety of individuals and organisations*, including specialist public health practitioners and many different professionals who work with individual children, in health, education, social services and a range of other fields. Many of this latter group are coming to recognise that the problems they see day-to-day reflect social, economic and political factors which need to be tackled collaboratively, at a population as well as individual level. Child public health seeks to bring together those from different disciplines and backgrounds who have a common interest in optimising the well being of young people – and within the health sector, it seeks to unite those working 'upstream' on the broader determinants of ill health in children and those who deal with the consequences 'downstream'. Most child public health initiatives involve collaboration between different organisations, sectors and departments at local and national level, including local authorities and voluntary sector organisations.

The child population

In 2001, there were 14.8 million children and young people aged 0–19 in Great Britain, of whom 11.7 million were dependent (under 16, or 16–18 and in full-time education). In common with most developed countries, Great Britain is currently witnessing a decline in its child population (see Chapter 1). The 0–19 population fell by almost 2 million between 1971 and 2001, and for the first time we now have more people aged over 60 than under 16. As a proportion, the under 16 population fell from 25% in 1971 to 20% in 2001, and is projected to fall to 17% by 2031 (see www.statistics.gov.uk).

According to the 2001 UK Census:

• one in three households in the UK contains dependent children and one in nine households contains children under 5
• 10% of children are from an ethnic minority group
• 19% of boys and 17% of girls have a minor disability (of which emotional and behavioural problems are the most common) or long-standing illness (of which asthma is the most common)
• 11 per 10,000 boys and 5 per 10,000 girls have a more severe disability (of which autism is the most common specific condition).

Worldwide, there were 2.1 billion children aged under 18 in 2001 and in many countries children make up 50% of the population. There are 1.2 billion children living in south and east Asia, 325 million in sub-Saharan Africa and 194 million in Latin America and the Caribbean. In other words, most of the world's child population lives in the poorest countries, where child and infant mortality rates are highest (Chapter 17). According to UNICEF, in the least developed countries in the world (which together have a child population of 340 million), 10% of children can expect to die before their first birthday and almost 16% before their fifth birthday – compared to 0.6% and 0.7% respectively for children in the UK.

Children all share basic needs, and with the progress of globalisation and information technology children across the world share values, experiences and cultural references to an extent which would not have seemed possible even a generation ago. However, different children live in very different circumstances, even within the affluent United Kingdom, and their experience of life and of health varies dramatically too.

Vulnerable children

'Vulnerable children' are the 20% or so of UK children whose circumstances substantially affect their experience of life and who may need help from public agencies to improve their life chances. (See for example the Quality Protects Programme, www.dfes.gov.uk/qualityprotects.) A high proportion of these children live in poverty and a disproportionate number come from minority ethnic backgrounds. They include children:

• with disabilities
• with behavioural and/or school-attendance problems

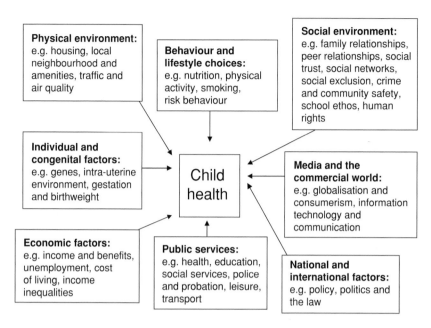

Fig. 11.1 Factors influencing child health.

- with caring responsibilities
- with mental health problems
- who misuse drugs
- who are teenage parents
- who are asylum seekers
- who are 'looked after' (in public care)
- who are at risk of abuse or neglect.

Determinants of health in children

Children's health is affected by a wide range of factors, from the intra-uterine environment and genetic inheritance to international business interests and cross-governmental agreements operating across the globe. Some of the main factors are illustrated in Figure 11.1 and explored in more detail below.

Individual and congenital factors

Genetic factors play a direct role in conditions such as cystic fibrosis, Down's syndrome and sickle cell disease. They have also been shown to be predictive of other conditions such as diabetes or juvenile chronic arthritis, but their contribution is minor compared to environmental factors. In some common childhood conditions (e.g. conduct disorder and depression) gene-environment interaction effects have been demonstrated [6]. Intra-uterine life also affects both child health (e.g. via birth weight or insults such as rubella virus or teratogenic drugs) and health in later life. David Barker has recently demonstrated that birth weight and weight at one year predict a range of common adult health problems and suggested that many chronic diseases originate in utero [7]. Even parental mental health problems during pregnancy have been shown to predict key health outcomes [8]. See Chapter 14 for more detail on this 'life course' explanation of adult health in the context of health inequalities.

Ethnicity

Children's ethnic background also plays a part in determining their health. Here socio-economic factors play a part (see below), but genetic and cultural determinants also have a role to play, together with the impact of racism, intolerance and stigma. Infant mortality rates in the UK are higher for babies of mothers born in Pakistan, the Caribbean, and most parts of Africa; but babies born into black and minority ethnic group families are more likely to be breastfed, and those whose mothers were born in Africa or Asia are less likely to die of sudden infant death syndrome. Risk factors and health status vary more between different ethnic groups than between specific groups and the white population. Children seeking asylum in the UK live in particularly difficult circumstances and have often experienced war, torture, separation from friends and relatives, and fear and danger in transit.

Families, relationships and parenting

The family constitutes a child's immediate environment and has a profound influence on health and well being. Maternal age and income, family structure, siblings and birth order all play a part, but relationships between parents and children are particularly important. The importance of parenting in the development of conduct disorder, delinquency, educational failure and criminal activity have been recognised for many years, together with its impact on emotional and social development. More recent long-term studies suggest a role in the development of poor mental health, lifestyles related to poor health, cardiovascular disease risk and premature mortality [9,10]. Studies in both man and animals show that early stressful experiences play a role in shaping the emotional and social brain, affecting future resilience and setting the scene for the quality of future relationships. Good relationships can buffer the detrimental health effects of stress and adverse life events. Parenting is to some extent socially patterned, but differences within social groups are greater than the differences between them. However, because of its role in supporting educational and social development, parenting plays a role in perpetuating social inequalities and cycles of disadvantage. Aspects of parenting which seem to play a role include parental behaviour (boundary setting, praise/derogation, encouragement and positive discipline) and relationship skills (sensitivity and attunement, especially in infancy, appropriate expectations, affection, hostility, conflict) as well as the more obvious components of offering children a range of experience and supporting their intellectual development. Clear, age-appropriate, consistent boundaries and sensitivity, encouragement, support and affection are important. Abuse and neglect are extreme examples of poor parenting and have the greatest long-term impact. Lesser degrees of suboptimal parenting are associated with less risk, but because such parenting is common, the population-attributable risk of parenting on health may be substantial.

Family break-up and conflict can seriously affect children's well being. In the UK 150,000 children experience parental divorce every year, of whom two-thirds are under 10. The outcome may be an improvement if conflict is resolved and children continue to receive loving care, but in many families break-up creates rather than solves conflict and it is this which is damaging [11]. Single-parent or reconstituted families (which now house 23% and 10% of children, respectively) have many disadvantages for some children, among which are poverty and lack of male role models.

Childcare and working patterns are changing too: the government's plans for 'wrap-around childcare' aim to support working parents and mean that more young children will spend more time in day care. There are benefits from contact with other children, but extended separation from the mother at an early age may also have less desirable consequences. Current evidence suggests that the quality of day care has a significant impact on children's emotional and social development [12, 13] and only a small proportion of the day care on offer in this country meets appropriate quality standards.

Later, when children go to school (and in some cases spend long hours in after-school care), peer relationships become increasingly important. The health effects of bullying frequently receive adverse publicity in the wake of teenage suicides, but long-term studies show an impact on adult mental health too [14]. Good relationships within the family provide a template for children to build good relationships with peers and protect them to some extent from the impact of bullying [15]. School ethos also has a role to play, and health-promoting school programmes with a focus on positive mental health can be important in supporting and enabling change [16].

Poverty and deprivation

Poverty has a profound influence on child health, in the UK and worldwide, and income inequality [17] accounts for much of the variation in morbidity and mortality in children across the country (Chapter 14). Both *absolute* and *relative* poverty are important. Absolute poverty is defined in terms of a family's ability to purchase essential goods (such as housing, heating, food, clothing and transport). There are various so-called 'consensus measures' of absolute poverty, which define a generally accepted minimum income for a family of a particular size. Relative poverty is defined in relation to the average income in a particular population: the European Union definition of relative poverty includes all families whose income is at or below 50% of the national average (sometimes called the 'poverty line'). Tackling absolute poverty by increasing the income of the very poor to minimally acceptable levels is potentially more straightforward than tackling relative poverty, which means achieving a more thorough redistribution of wealth. The effects of relative poverty, however, are generally accepted to be more powerful and more pervasive: their impact can be seen at every geographical level.

As average wealth has increased in the UK the distribution of wealth has become more unequal – and the numbers living in relative poverty have increased. The Joseph Rowntree Foundation has estimated that poverty costs 1,400 children's lives every year in the UK. The UK government has risen to this challenge, pledging to halve child poverty between 1998–99 and 2010, and eradicate it by 2020. While some progress has been made the risk of a child living in relative poverty today is still twice the level it was a generation ago [18]. As well as social policy interventions to support families, measures to redistribute wealth are likely to be needed if these goals are to be met.

Poverty and social deprivation are leading causes of ill health in children, and this is clearly illustrated by the social-class gradients which exist for almost all major causes of child mortality and morbidity in the UK (Chapter 14). For example:

- *Infant mortality (first year of life) and child mortality (1–15 years)*: the rate for social classes IV and V was almost double that for social classes I and II in 2000. (The gap in infant mortality rate between manual and non-manual groups is still rising despite a national target to reduce it.)
- *Low birth weight*: the rate for babies born to mothers living in the most deprived quintile of local authorities in England was roughly double that for those in the least deprived quintile of local authorities (data for 1996–2001) [19].
- *Prevalence of mental-health problems (ages 5–15)*: class V three times higher than class I in 1999 [19].
- *Sudden infant death syndrome (SIDS)*: three quarters of all SIDS cases now occur in socially deprived families [20].

Currently in the UK:

- 22% of children live in relative poverty.
- 18% live in households where there are no adults in work.
- 12% live in overcrowded households.
- Nearly 150,000 children provide unpaid care on a regular basis within the household, often for a parent with health (especially mental-health or substance-abuse) problems.

- Almost 60,000 babies and toddlers live two or more storeys above ground level (www.statistics.gov.uk).

The impact of socio-economic inequalities is apparent in differences in health between children in different countries – especially between the developing and developed world, as we have seen. But within the UK there is significant variation too – between north and south, and between deprived inner cities (where, in the worst wards, up to three quarters of children live in poverty), the more affluent suburbs, and rural areas (where there are also pockets of poverty, and isolation can be a real problem). Living in a deprived area adds to the disadvantage of poverty for individual families.

Communities, social capital and stigma

Most of the research on social capital relates to adult health (see Chapter 14), and shows that local community networks, social cohesion and social trust make a difference to health. These factors are likely to have an effect on children's health and well being too, if only through effects on their parents' health. Social capital describes the 'glue' which holds communities together and offers some protection against the adverse health effects of poverty and deprivation. However, strong social capital in one group may mean social exclusion and stigma for others and may thus adversely affect children from marginalised and minority groups. These include the very poor, travelling families, asylum seekers, ethnic and religious minorities, as well as children with disabilities or chronic illnesses, all of whom may be less able to access services and participate in community life.

Physical environment

Children's physical environment is important too. Damp housing increases the risk of asthma; overcrowding predisposes to infectious diseases, domestic violence and accidents [21]. Traffic danger and air quality are other important factors, and the condition of the local environment – buildings, streets, parks – has a profound influence on the lives children lead.

Behaviour and lifestyle choices

Changes in the quality and quantity of food consumed and the amount of exercise taken by children have generated the current epidemic of childhood obesity. Parents influence children's lifestyles both by making choices for them in early life and by shaping habits which children may follow later when choosing for themselves. Socio-economic and environmental factors also play a role: for example, local availability of food; the information on food labels; and local provision of safe outdoor play areas. These all significantly affect the choices made by parents and children. Many foods which are cheap and readily available are high in fat, calories, sugar and salt. Physical education provision can be poor in schools, especially where playing fields are absent, and parents are often reluctant to allow children to play outside because of fear of traffic or assault. Recently the amount of sleep children get and the hours they spend viewing television have been shown to be key predictors of childhood obesity [22].

Exposure to substances such as tobacco, alcohol and illegal drugs are also important factors. Smoking in pregnancy increases the risk of low birth weight, stillbirth and infant death, and smoking in the same household as a young child increases the risk of sudden infant death and respiratory problems. Many forms of risk behaviour are increasing among adolescents, including binge drinking, drug use, sexual behaviour, accidents and deliberate self-harm.

Media and the commercial world

The wider world has more and more impact on children as the broadcast and printed media, and particularly the internet, encourage the development of globalisation and consumerism. Examples include the marketing of unhealthy food and expensive consumer goods to children and the promotion of infant formula to mothers in the poorest countries.

Public services

Access to public services is important for children's health. As well as *health services* (including preventive, acute and community services), *education* has a significant impact on self-esteem and wellbeing in children and on later health; *social services* may provide vital support for families with difficulties, or protection for children at risk; *leisure services* such as sporting facilities and youth clubs can benefit physical, mental and emotional health; and *transport services* such as cycle lanes, traffic calming and safe routes to school also play a role in promoting health.

Main causes of mortality and morbidity in children

Over the last century, children in the UK have become healthier and their life expectancy has increased. Due to social and environmental – and to some extent medical – advances, many of the scourges of the nineteenth and early twentieth centuries have more or less vanished – but in their place are new problems and disorders which reflect changes in society over this period. Instead of life-threatening infectious diseases and high infant mortality rates, we now have life-threatening levels of obesity and high rates of survival for premature babies, many of whom will need care and support throughout their lives. Some of the leading concerns

Table 11.1. Key child public health challenges for the twenty-first century

Social and health inequalities. The UK has a poorer record on **child poverty** than most other European countries. Although Government action to tackle child poverty in the UK has met with some success, a child in the UK still has nearly twice the chance of living in a relatively low income family than was the case a generation ago.

Childhood obesity. Prevalence has increased sharply in recent years: between 1995 and 2000 the proportion of boys in England (age 2–19) who were overweight increased by 2% and the proportion of girls by 3%. In the same time period, the proportion of obese boys and girls increased by one per cent [19]. This trend threatens to curtail the life expectancy of current and future generations of children.

Emotional and behavioural / mental health problems. Prevalence is rising in children and young people [23]. Impacts may include educational failure, unemployment, unhealthy lifestyles and problems in interpersonal relationships in adulthood. These problems have implications (e.g. stress, violence) for parents and siblings, future partners and children, teachers and wider society (through their impact on social capital, delinquency and youth crime). **Suicide and self-harm** are also increasing: suicide accounts for a third of deaths in 15–24 year olds [19].

Substance misuse. This includes alcohol, tobacco, drugs and glue-sniffing. Binge drinking, and the continuing rise in smoking rates among teenage girls, are worrying trends (according to the Health Survey for England).

Teenage pregnancy. The UK has the highest rate in Europe, and little progress is being made in reducing it despite concerted action. The impact on health and well being is substantial, both for teenage mothers and their children. **Sexually transmitted infections** are a related problem [19].

Accidents and injuries. Despite considerable progress in recent years, injuries remain a significant cause of morbidity and mortality especially among adolescents, and the UK has the highest rates for injuries to child pedestrians in Europe. Non-accidental injury, and other types of **child abuse and neglect**, are also important – the NSPCC estimates that there are 100 fatal cases per year, and recent high-profile cases have made clear that identifying fatal abuse is fraught with difficulties.

Poor vaccine uptake. For example poor uptake of MMR, due to media scares about links to autism and mistrust of government advice, resulting in significant risk of outbreaks of measles and greater exposure of pregnant women to rubella.

Disabilities. These are increasing in prevalence, partly due to improved care and survival of premature and small-for-date babies, as are **chronic illnesses** such as asthma and diabetes.

for child public health today in the UK – and much of the rest of the developed world – are set out in Table 11.1.

Comparison of mortality rates and causes of death among children in different parts of the world puts child health problems in the UK into perspective and reveals the extent of the differences between the most and the least privileged children on the globe. Death rates for under fives are more than ten times lower in the UK than the worldwide average, and the main causes of death are very different too (see Table 11.2).

Causes of death for children in the UK vary a good deal by age and sex. Boys have a higher mortality rate than girls at all ages, but especially in adolescence, when they account for two thirds of deaths. Much of the steep rise in mortality rates in this age group is due to deaths from injury and poisoning. Leading causes of mortality among older age groups are shown in Table 11.3.

Table 11.2. Main causes of death among children under 5

UK	Worldwide
Population	**Population**
13.5 million children under 18 (0.6% of world child population)	2.1 billion children under 18
3.5 million under 5	613 million under 5
Deaths	**Deaths**
Around 5,000 deaths per year (under-5 mortality rate 7 per 1,000 live births)	10.6 million deaths per year (under-5 mortality rate 82 per 1,000 live births)
Causes of death	**Causes of death**
The commonest causes of death (excluding those occurring in the first 28 days) are:	Many of these deaths are potentially preventable by means of simple interventions – ensuring clean water supplies, and providing immunisation and basic health care (especially during pregnancy and childbirth). Overall, 54% of child deaths are due to infections, and many occur as a direct or indirect result of absolute poverty
• congenital anomalies (18%)	
• sudden infant death (14% – but 20% of deaths under a year)	
• prematurity, low birthweight etc. (perinatal conditions) (13%)	
• injury and poisoning (11%)	*70% of deaths are accounted for by six causes:*
• cerebral palsy and other diseases of the nervous system (9%)	• pneumonia (19%)
• respiratory disease (9%)	• diarrhoea (18%)
• infections (9%)	• neonatal infection (10%)
• cancer (5%)	• preterm delivery (10%)
	• malaria (8%)
	• birth asphyxia (8%)

Source: See refs. 2 and 24.

Health promotion and health policy for children

Child health promotion

Promoting and improving children's health across the population is a fundamental goal of child public health. In common with health promotion for adults, child health promotion involves action at national level (policy development, legislation etc) as well as local level (community development, family support, realignment of services). Some examples are given below for each of the five 'pillars' of the 1986 Ottawa Charter for Health Promotion:

Table 11.3. Main causes of death among older children in the UK

Rates per million	Cause of death	Boys	Girls
5–9 years:	Cancer	46	30
	Injury and poisoning	30	22
	Diseases of nervous system	20	20
	Congenital anomalies	12	8
	Respiratory disease	9	11
	All deaths	*141*	*111*
10–14 years:	Injury and poisoning	67	28
	Cancer	39	17
	Diseases of nervous system	21	23
	Congenital anomalies	11	11
	All deaths	*176*	*117*
15–19 years:	Injury and poisoning	329	114
	Cancer	53	34
	Diseases of nervous system	38	23
	Congenital anomalies	23	10
	Circulatory disease	16	13
	All deaths	*555*	*267*

Source: See ref. 2.

- *Building healthy public policy.* For example, health impact assessment for proposed new roads which takes into account child health concerns such as air pollution and asthma and the risk of road traffic accidents; banning physical punishment of children.
- *Creating supportive environments.* For example, encouraging walking and cycling to school, promoting food co-operatives and farmers' markets which make healthy food more easily available to local families, banning advertising of foods containing high fat and high sugar to children on television, clear food labelling.
- *Strengthening communities.* For example, enabling parents and children to contribute to decision-making about issues they feel are important to their health, such as community safety, leisure provision and the quality of the local environment (e.g. street lighting); supporting voluntary-sector provision and community development initiatives.
- *Re-orienting health services.* For example, reducing inequalities in access to child health services; ensuring services meet local needs and are child-centred; developing ambulatory care; increasing provision of support for parenting so

that all families can access it; increasing provision of mental health promotion initiatives in schools.

- *Developing personal knowledge and skills.* For example, offering programmes to support children's emotional and social development in schools, to offer some protection for those from homes where parenting is suboptimal; ensuring children are introduced to key health knowledge in sound programmes at an appropriate age.

Child health promotion can therefore operate in many different ways and at many different levels. It also involves a wide range of people working in partnership towards the common goal of improving children's health, including all those involved in health care as well as other fields of public and private life. Many child health promoting policies are essentially intersectoral – for example local Sure Start programmes and the future Children's Centres. Some activities led by different organisations or groups are set out in Table 11.4.

Child health promotion in practice is explored further in the sections below by focussing on:

- a setting (healthy schools)
- a determinant of health (parenting); and
- a key public health problem (childhood obesity).

Healthy schools

At the level of local communities and environments one of the most important influences on children is the school. The Healthy Schools movement aims to ensure that the school environment is a positive and supportive one which encourages children to develop healthy behaviour and helps to tackle health inequalities and promote social inclusion. The National Healthy Schools Programme (see www.wiredforhealth.gov.uk/cat.php?catid=842) defines a healthy school as one which 'promotes the health and well-being of its pupils and staff through a well-planned, taught curriculum in a physical and emotional environment that promotes learning and healthy lifestyle choices'.

The programme – which the UK government hopes will involve every school in the country by 2009 – encourages a whole-school approach in support of the five national outcomes for children set out in 'Every child matters [28]' and the Children Act (2004):

- being healthy
- staying safe
- enjoying and achieving
- making a positive contribution
- economic well being.

The programme follows a community development approach which encourages the involvement of pupils as well as staff, parents, governors and others. It

Table 11.4. Examples of health promotion activity in different sectors

Health professionals – including doctors, nurses, midwives, health visitors, dentists, pharmacists, orthoptists.

Roles include:
- Child health surveillance
- Immunisation and screening
- Advice and support to parents and carers

Other statutory agencies – including social services, education, transport, planning and leisure departments, Connexions (careers and training advice), the police and probation services.

Roles include:
- Supporting and protecting children and families
- Helping all children to reach their potential
- Ensuring that children live in safe and healthy environments
- Supporting and advising young people as they approach adulthood

Voluntary organisations – including UNICEF, NSPCC, Save the Children, National Children's Bureau, charities working with specific groups (e.g. children with disabilities, bereaved children, asylum seekers, travellers or young carers) and informal local groups (such as mother-and-toddler groups or youth drop-in centres); organisations offering parenting support.

Roles include:
- Supporting and protecting individual children
- Advocacy and lobbying for policy change and service improvement
- Identifying unmet needs (locally, nationally or internationally) and working with statutory agencies, communities and individuals to meet them
- Providing information and services (e.g. respite care, afterschool clubs, parenting programmes)

The commercial world – including employers, local retailers and multinational businesses, manufacturers, providers of leisure facilities.

Roles include:
- Offering family-friendly employment practices
- Helping to make healthy choices easier (e.g. enforcing age restrictions on the sale of tobacco and alcohol, reducing salt and fat content in processed food)
- Improving children's safety in public places
- Promoting physical activity

Local communities – including faith groups, residents' associations, parent–teacher associations (PTAs), parent support groups.

Roles include:
- Identifying local priorities (e.g. traffic-calming measures, parks and green spaces)
- Developing local networks and projects to support children and families
- Promoting community safety

National and international organisations – including governments, non-governmental organisations, UNICEF, WHO.

Roles include:
- Promoting healthy public policy
- Protecting and promoting children's rights across the globe

covers personal, social and health education, healthy eating, physical activity, emotional health and well being (including bullying). For schools as a whole, the observed and intended benefits include:

- improving the ethos of the school and staff health and well being
- improving emotional and social development, behaviour and attendance (Healthy Schools have been shown to have less fear of bullying)
- improving educational achievement (Healthy Schools have achieved better results at Key Stages 1 and 2 (ages 7 and 11 years))
- reducing and halting the increase in childhood obesity
- promoting positive sexual health and reducing teenage pregnancy
- reducing young people's drug, alcohol and tobacco use (Healthy Schools have less use of illegal drugs).

Many different projects might be developed by individual schools to help them achieve National Healthy Schools status. Some examples include:

- introducing a breakfast club and/or after-school care schemes
- building new play equipment in the playground
- introducing activities and clubs at lunchtime or after school – e.g. sports clubs, cookery classes – which might include parents as well as children
- creating a school council to ensure pupils' voices are heard when policy decisions are made
- introducing a peer counselling scheme.

Parenting

Because suboptimal parenting has important social as well as health consequences, research and development by those interested in preventing crime and delinquency has provided public health practitioners with a range of evidence-based programmes and initiatives. Health promotion is generally more effective when it combines action at several levels at once – targeting individuals, communities and policy decisions. Table 11.5 summarises approaches at different levels to promote child health by improving parenting.

Childhood obesity

The threat of the childhood obesity 'epidemic' to public health has been widely recognised in recent years. In the UK, prevalence rose by an average of 0.8% per year between 1995 and 2002, outstripping other European countries, and is now close to rates in the United States. If the increase continues, parents' life expectancy may exceed their children's, with obesity becoming the main cause of premature death in the UK. Some children are more at risk than others. Girls have higher rates than boys: up to 30% of girls aged 2–15 are overweight or obese in some areas of England. According to the Health Survey for England, Asian children are four times more likely to be obese than their white counterparts (data available at www.data-archive.ac.uk/findingData/hseTitles.asp).

Table 11.5. Health promotion action to promote child health through improving parenting

Individual level	A number of programmes exist which are proven to help promote attachment, especially for 'high risk' mothers and babies [25] (e.g. mothers who are very young or living in poverty and those with mental health or drug problems)
	Parents can be helped to improve their parenting, family relationships and children's health and well being [26, 27].
	Family support can prevent abuse in families where a risk has been identified [28].
Community level	Policy relating to Children's Centres envisages a major increase in parenting provision, but health service input to these centres is essential if services are to be non-stigmatising and provided very early in life, and this is not a foregone conclusion
	Some parenting interventions are offered with parallel programmes for children which seek to enhance their emotional and social development
	Some such programmes are offered through schools and may seek to change school ethos. They may be offered as part of Healthy Schools projects with wider benefits for health
Policy level	Physical punishment of children is an inappropriate aspect of parenting. The UK government recently debated, but rejected, legislation to ban physical punishment of children, even though the majority of the electorate supported such legislation, if parents could be protected from minor infringements. Current legislation thus defines how parents may hit their children and fails to give parents a clear message that physical punishment is inappropriate and ineffective
	All agencies working with children should have clear procedures for child protection in the event of suspected abuse
	Criminal Records Bureau checks are required for all staff working with children with the aim of preventing known abusers coming into contact with children

Changes in energy intake (diet) and output (physical activity) both play a part in creating this problem. Children in England eat on average double the required amounts of saturated fat, salt and sugar per day, and 40% of boys and 60% of girls get less than the recommended hour of physical activity a day.

Overweight and obesity affects children's physical, mental and social well being. The consequences may include:

- the development of risk factors for heart disease such as hyperinsulinaemia, high blood pressure and type 2 diabetes, previously only seen in adults, which is now seen (albeit rarely) in obese children
- low self-esteem, social isolation and bullying
- reduced participation in sport and physical activity, creating a vicious cycle
- poorer educational achievement
- up to 25% risk of becoming an obese adult, which carries serious long-term health risks. The risk is highest if both parents are overweight.

The UK government has set a national target to 'halt the year-on-year rise in obesity in children aged 2–10 years by 2010, in the context of a broader strategy to tackle obesity in the population as a whole' (Public Service Agreement 2004). How can public health measures contribute to achieving this target?

Table 11.6. Tackling childhood obesity: examples of action at individual, community and policy levels

Level	Input (food and nutrition)	Output (physical activity)
Individual	Classroom activities which focus on healthy eating and food preparation Programmes for parents	Exercise prescriptions, cycle proficiency training, wider provision of physical activities in school to appeal to 'non-sporty' children
Community	Community gardens, farmer's markets and local food co-operatives	Improved access to leisure facilities (e.g. free swimming for children)
Policy	Improved food labelling, reducing fat and sugar content of ready meals Ban advertising of high-sugar, high-fat foods to children	Transport policy measures to promote walking and cycling (e.g. cycle lanes, traffic calming)

Tackling childhood obesity

Childhood obesity is a complex problem which requires collaborative, multi-sectoral action to tackle both the input and output sides of the energy equation. The evidence on interventions to reverse or prevent obesity in individual children is not encouraging [29, 30]. Interventions which do show some impact include a component focussing on parenting and family relationships [31, 32]. The Health Development Agency's Evidence Briefing [33], 'Management of obesity and overweight', summarised evidence of effectiveness of strategies to tackle obesity, including those which aim to:

• prevent obesity and overweight in children (e.g. multifaceted family and school-based interventions)
• treat obesity and overweight in children (e.g. interventions which involve parents, including exercise and behaviour modification programmes).

Tables 11.6 and 11.7 illustrate how action might be planned at different levels, and by different agencies, to tackle childhood obesity.

The 2004 White Paper 'Choosing Health' set out details of the UK government's plans to prevent and treat obesity in children [2].

Health policy for children

A number of key documents shape health policy for children in the UK. Many of these – such as the Children Act and 'Every child matters' [34] – apply not just to the health sector but to all agencies working with children. Others – such as the recent Public Health White Paper 'Choosing Health'–include children but

Table 11.7. Tackling childhood obesity: examples of action by different agencies

Agency	Input (food and nutrition)	Output (physical activity)
Schools	Changing to healthy vending machines (selling fruit and other healthy snacks, not crisps and chocolate)	Developing safe routes to school and 'walking buses'
Local authorities	Allotment schemes to encourage local people to grow their own fruit and vegetables	Improving street safety and outdoor play spaces
Media	Campaign highlighting healthy eating – e.g. local restaurants with 'lite' menu; recipe ideas	Disseminating information about local sports teams' outreach programmes to young people
Commercial world	*Food manufacturers*: reducing sugar, salt and fat content of food *Supermarkets*: promoting 'Five a day' message and offering ranges of fruit and vegetables to appeal to children	*Leisure providers*: helping to widen access to sports facilities Sponsorship of local sports teams
National government	Food pricing policies to promote healthy rather than 'junk' foods; setting nutritional standards for school catering	Investing in school sport, cycle lanes, leisure facilities and sports clubs . . .

also cover the rest of the population. The National Service Framework (NSF) for children, young people and maternity services [3] sets out the government's vision for health and social care services for children and young people and includes eleven standards which should shape children's services in future. This is the first time that national evidence-based standards have been set for children's services. Standards 1 to 5 apply to services for all children and young people, Standards 6 to 10 apply to particular groups (such as those who are ill, those in hospital, those with disabilities, complex health needs or mental health problems) and Standard 11 covers maternity services.

Among the key aspects of the NSF are:

• introducing a Child Health Promotion Programme designed to promote the health and well-being of children from before birth to adulthood
• promoting physical health, mental health and emotional well being by encouraging children and their families to develop healthy lifestyles
• supporting parents to ensure that their children are healthy, safe and optimising their life chances
• improving access to services for all children according to their needs

- ensuring that services are child-centred, give children and families more choice and take account of their views
- tackling health inequalities and addressing the needs of children, families and communities who are at risk of poor outcomes
- promoting and safeguarding the welfare of children
- ensuring that young people have access to age-appropriate services which are responsive to their specific needs as they grow into adulthood.

'Toolkit' for the generalist practitioner

Promoting children's health and well being is the responsibility of everyone working with children, as well as those with a responsibility for health across the life course, but it is not always obvious how those with a caseload of individual children can make a difference to child health in general. The first step is to keep in mind the importance of child public health and the potential of individuals to influence children's environment and experience. The list below offers a starting point to identifying the opportunities available and the approaches which can be adopted so that practitioners can begin to broaden out from tackling the 'presenting problem' to considering and enhancing other aspects of health, and from a focus on the individual to the child population as a whole.

- Offer advice and support to parents and families – including health education and safety advice (e.g. cycle helmets, healthy eating).
- Recognise risk factors (e.g. obesity, smoking, suboptimal parenting) and respond with advice and/or referral or signposting to specialist services.
- Encourage the use of preventive and health promotion services such as immunisation, parenting programmes and support for vulnerable families.
- Be alert to and act on signs of abuse and neglect.
- Liaise and collaborate effectively with other agencies: know who does what (or who can do what) and appreciate the benefits of a partnership approach (e.g. drug action teams, family support groups).
- Lobbying and advocacy are important aspects of child public health which are open to everyone. Advocacy can be targeted at the individual level (e.g. supporting a request for a looked-after child to remain in the same school when changing foster placement), the community level (e.g. pressing the local council to do something about an accident black spot for child pedestrians) or the policy level (e.g. raising the profile of children's services within the NHS).

FURTHER READING

M. Blair, S. Stewart-Brown, A. Waterston and R. Crowther, *Child Public Health*, Oxford, Oxford University Press, 2003

REFERENCES

1. D. Kuh and Y. Ben-Schlomo, *A Life Course Approach to Chronic Disease Epidemiology*, Oxford, Oxford University Press, 2004.
2. Department of Health, Choosing Health; making healthier choices easier. London, H. M. Stationery Office, 2004.
3. National Service Framework for children, young people and maternity services. London, Department of Health, 2004.
4. L. Kohler, Child public health: a new basis for child health workers. *European Journal of Public Health*, **8**, 1998, 235–5.
5. U. Bronfenbrenner, *The Ecology of Human Development: Experiments by Nature and Design*, Cambridge, MA, Harvard University Press, 1979.
6. A. Caspi, K. Sugden, T. E. Moffitt *et al.*, Influence of life stress on depression; moderation by a polymorphism in the 5-HTT Gene. *Science*, **301**, 2003, 386–9.
7. D. Barker, *Mothers Babies and Health in Later Life*. Edinburgh, Churchill Livingstone, 1998.
8. B. R. Van Den Bergh, E. J. Mulder, M. Mennes and V. Glover, Antenatal maternal anxiety and stress and the neurobehavioural development of the fetus and child: links and possible mechanisms. *Neuroscience and Biobehavioural Reviews* **29**, 2005, 237–58.
9. R. Repetti, S. Taylor and T. Seeman, Risky families: early social environments and the mental and physical health of offspring. *Psychological Bulletin.* **128**, 2002, 330–6.
10. M. C. Rutter, Connections between child and adult psychopathology. *European Child and Adolescent Psychiatry*, **5**(Supplement 1), 1996, 4–7.
11. P. R. Amato, L. S. Loomis and A. Booth, Parental divorce, marital conflict and offspring wellbeing during early adulthood. *Social Forces*, **73**(3), 1995, 895–915.
12. A. C. Dettling, S. W. Parker, S. Lane, A. Sebanc and M. R. Gunnar, Quality of care and temperament determine changes in cortisol concentrations over the day for young children in childcare. *Psychoneuroendocrinology*, **25**(8), 2000, 819–36.
13. M. R. Burchinal, J. E. Roberts, R. Riggins, jr *et al.* Relating quality of center-based child care to early cognitive and language development longitudinally. *Child Development* **71**, 2000, 338–57.
14. L. Arseneault, E. Walsh, K. Trsesniewski *et al.*, Bullying victimisation uniquely contributes to adjustment problems in young children: a nationally representative cohort study. *Pediatrics* **118**, 2006, 130–8.
15. A. Sroufe, E. Egland and E. Carlson, One social world: integrated development of parent child and peer relationships. In *Relationships as Developmental Contexts. Minnesota Symposium on Child Psychology*, B. Laursen and W. A. Collins (eds.), London, Lawrence Erlbaum Associates, 1999.
16. K. Weare, *Promoting Mental Emotional and Social Health: a Whole School Approach*, London, Routledge, 2000.
17. D. Acheson and N. Spencer, *Poverty and Child Health*, Abingdon Radcliffe Medical Press, 2000.
18. D. Hirsch, *What Will it Take to End Child Poverty? Firing on All Cylinders*, York, York Publishing Services, Joseph Rowntree Foundation, 2006.

19. The Health of Children and Young People. www.statistics.gov.uk/children/ National Statistics report.

20. P. S. Blair, P. Sidebotham, J. Berry, M. Evans and P. J. Flemming, Major epidemiological changes in sudden infant death syndrome: a 20-year population based study. *Lancet* **367**, 2006, 314–19.

21. D. Wilkinson, Poor housing and ill health – a summary of research evidence. The Scottish Office, Central Research Unit, Housing Research Branch, 1999.

22. J. J. Reilly, J. Armstrong, A. R. Dorosty *et al.*, Early life risk factors for obesity in childhood: cohort study. *British Medical Journal*, **330**, 2005, 1357–9.

23. B. Maughan, A. C. Iervolino and S. Collishaw, Time trends in child and adolescent mental disorders. *Current Opinion in Psychiatry*, **18**, 2005, 381–5.

24. J. Bryce, C. Boschi-Pinto, K. Shibuya, R. E. Black, WHO Child Health Epidemiology Reference Group, WHO estimates of the causes of death in children. *Lancet*, **365**, 2005, 1147–52.

25. M. J. Bakermans-Kraneburg, M. H. van IJzendoorn and F. Jufer, Less is more; meta-analysis of sensitivity and attachment interventions in early childhood. *Psychological Bulletin* **129**, 2003, 195–215.

26. P. Moran, D. Ghate and A. van der Merwe, What works in parenting support? a review of the international evidence. London, Department for Education and Skills, Home Office, 2004.

27. Parenting and Public Health. Faculty of Public Health Briefing Statement. London, Faculty of Public Health, 2005 (healthpolicy@fph.org.uk).

28. J. Barlow, D. Simkiss and S. Stewart-Brown, Interventions to prevent or treat child physical abuse and neglect; findings from a systematic review. *Journal of Children's Services*, **In press**, **3** (1), 2007, 6–28.

29. C. D. Summerbell, V. Ashton, K. J. Campbell *et al.*, Interventions for treating obesity in children (Cochrane Review) *Cochrane Library*, Issue 4, 2003.

30. University of York NHS Centre for Reviews and Dissemination, The prevention and treatment of childhood obesity. *Effective Health Care*, **7**(6), 2002.

31. L. H. Epstein, R. R. Valoski Wing and J. McCurley, Ten year follow up of behavioural and family based treatment of obese children. *American Journal of Clinical Nutrition.* **264**, 1998, 2519–23.

32. M. Golan, A. Weizman, A. Apter and M. Fainaru, Parents as exclusive agents of change in the treatment of childhood obesity. *American Journal of Clinical Nutrition*, **76**, 1998, 1130–5.

33. Management of Obesity and Overweight. Evidence Briefing, Health Development Agency, October 2003.

34. Every child matters: change for children in health services. London, Department of Health, 2004.

12

Adult public health

Veena Rodrigues

Key points

- Adults aged 15 to 64 years account for a sizeable proportion of the population (over 60%) both worldwide and within the UK.
- Non-communicable diseases are the leading causes of death in developed countries whereas in developing countries, communicable diseases, maternal, perinatal and nutritional conditions and injuries are the leading causes of death.
- Within the UK, cancers, cardiovascular diseases, diabetes mellitus, mental illness and obesity are significant public health problems in this age group.
- Although national policies are already in place to tackle these conditions, concerted health improvement efforts with engagement of local populations are required to make a significant impact on the burden of ill health.

Introduction

Approximately 63% of the world's population in 2003 was estimated to be aged between 15 and 64 years, with a male : female ratio of 1.03. In developing countries as a whole, this age group comprises 64% of the total population whereas in Europe (central, eastern and EU countries) it was estimated to be just over 70% [1].

According to the 2001 Census, 65% of the population of England and Wales are aged between 15 and 64 years, with a male : female ratio of 0.98. Although the total population shows an increase of 2.6% on mid-1991 figures, the proportion of the population aged 15–64 years has remained constant. Within this age group, almost three quarters are young adults aged less than 30 years [2].

Essential Public Health, eds. Stephen Gillam, Jan Yates and Padmanabhan Badrinath.
Published by Cambridge University Press. © Cambridge University Press 2007.

Fig. 12.1   Determinants of
health.
Source: G. Dahlgren and N.
Whitehead, Policies and
strategies to promote social
equity in health. Stockholm,
Institute of Futures Studies,
1991; reproduced with
permission.

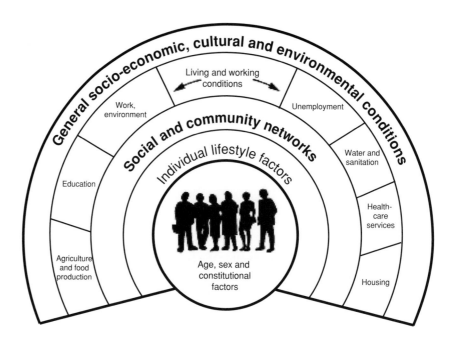

Determinants of health

There are several factors that determine the health of the adult population
(Figure 12.1). According to this model, determinants of health work at various
levels. These are:

- *Individual lifestyle factors* which can be grouped into fixed factors such as age,
  sex and genetics, and modifiable factors such as diet, physical activity, cigarette
  smoking and alcohol consumption. Personal behaviours and lifestyles adopted
  by individuals have the potential to promote or damage health and are therefore
  linked with a number of health outcomes.
- *Social and community networks* (interactions between friends, family, and other
  members of the community) play an important role in maintaining people's
  health and are particularly important in maintaining good mental health.
- *Living and working conditions* such as education, agriculture and food production, work environment, housing, water and sanitation, and unemployment
  also have a role as wider determinants of the health of the population. Compared to the rest of the population, people who experience material disadvantage, unemployment, homelessness, and lower educational attainment are
  more likely to have poorer health outcomes and a lower life expectancy.
- *General socio-economic, cultural and environmental conditions* such as standard of living, mean income levels, the place of women in society, employment

Table 12.1. Mortality among 15–64 year olds, 2004, England & Wales [4]

Underlying cause of death	Number of deaths (%)
Neoplasms	32,059 (38.9)
Diseases of the circulatory system	20,673 (25.1)
External causes of morbidity and mortality	8,807 (10.7)
Diseases of the digestive system	6,703 (8.1)
Diseases of the respiratory system	5,078 (6.2)
Other causes	8998 (11.0)
Total deaths	**82,318 (100.0)**

rates, levels of deprivation and inequalities prevalent in society as a whole have an impact on health.

The determinants represented within individual layers also have the potential to interact: a change in one layer could result in a change in another layer. Therefore, a non-health-sector initiative, such as a housing development, could have an impact on the health of the community by, for example, reducing parks and other opportunities for physical activity. Determinants such as lifestyle factors might impact directly on health whereas others, such as social support, food production and taxation policies, have an indirect impact on health.

Causes of mortality and morbidity

As described in Chapter 1, average life expectancy at birth has increased globally over the past five decades but there is still a gap in life expectancy between developed and developing countries [3] with life expectancy at birth actually decreasing in Africa and eastern Europe (former Soviet Union). This has been attributed to the HIV/AIDS in Africa and to the impact of social, economic and political instability on adult health in eastern Europe.

Similarly, adult mortality rates have been declining in most countries, but the relative importance of a range of causes differs across developed and developing countries, with non-communicable diseases predominating in developed countries and communicable diseases, maternal, perinatal and nutritional conditions, and injuries being leading causes of mortality in developing countries [3]. However, population ageing and changes in risk factor distributions in many developing countries have resulted in an acceleration of the epidemic of non-communicable diseases.

The leading causes of mortality among adults aged 15 to 64 years in the UK are shown in Table 12.1. Neoplasms account for 39% of the deaths, followed by diseases of the circulatory system, which constitute 25% of all deaths [4]. In terms

Table 12.2. Cancer deaths in the UK by country, 2004[a]

Country	Males		Females		Persons	
	Number	ASR[b]	Number	ASR[b]	Number	ASR[b]
England	65,945	216.7	60,116	153.5	126,061	179.2
Wales	4,497	231.3	4,035	160.2	8,532	189.2
Scotland	7,664	258.5	7,383	180.4	15,047	211.5
N. Ireland	1,938	222.9	1,819	156.1	3,757	183.5
UK	80,044	221.1	73,353	156.3	153,397	182.6

[a] Statistics are from the Cancer Research UK News and Resources website (2006), cancerstats, see info.cancerresearchuk.org.

[b] Age-standardised rate (European) per 100,000 population.

of the burden of ill health in this age group, apart from cancers and cardiovascular diseases, conditions such as obesity, diabetes and mental illness are significant public health problems.

Although the conditions discussed in this chapter are relevant to the young and older people, those included (cancers, cardiovascular disease, diabetes, obesity and mental health problems) have particular relevance for the large proportion of the population of working age. In each case, the burden of disease, risk factors and potential public health action is described.

Cancer

Burden of disease

Although the types of cancer diagnosed vary enormously across the world almost half of all cancer comprises cancers of the lung, breast, bowel, stomach and prostate. Each year 6.7 million people worldwide die from cancer and 10.9 million people are diagnosed with cancer.

In 2004, there were 153,397 deaths due to cancer in the UK. Table 12.2 shows the numbers and age-standardised rates for all cancer deaths in the UK by country. Overall, mortality from cancer is decreasing with a 4% reduction in the age-standardised mortality rates for all malignant neoplasms between 1995 and 2004. Cancer mortality is highest among people aged 65 and over but still significant in those under 65 (for example, breast cancer accounts for almost half of all cancers diagnosed in UK women aged 40 to 60 years). In younger age groups (15 to 24 year olds) the commonest cancers are lymphomas, testicular cancers, brain tumours, melanomas and leukaemia. Although trends may vary for individual cancers, mortality rates are decreasing for most cancers (Figure 12.2). Death rates

Table 12.3. Risk factors for cancers

Risk factor	Is a risk factor for
Smoking	Many cancers, particularly lung cancer
Ultraviolet radiation	Malignant melanoma and non-melanoma skin cancer
Physical inactivity	Colon cancer
Obesity	Breast cancer in post-menopausal women, endometrial cancer and colon cancer
Diet	Cancers of the colon, rectum, stomach and prostate
Alcohol	Cancers of the mouth, pharynx, larynx, oesophagus and liver
Infections	Human papillomaviruses linked to cervical cancer, and hepatitis viruses to liver cancer

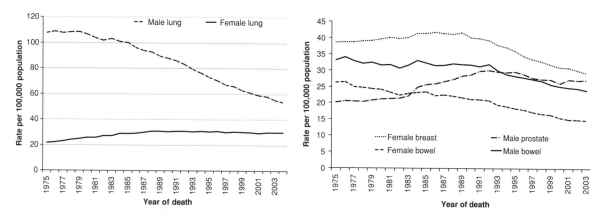

Fig. 12.2 European age-standardised mortality rates by sex for lung, breast, prostate and bowel cancer, UK 1975–2004. Figures from CancerStats, info. cancerresearchuk. org.

for lung, breast and bowel cancers have been decreasing. The decrease in lung cancer among males is largely due to declining prevalence of smoking. Among women, rates have been fairly stable since the mid 1980s but, over the last decade, rates among women in their 60s have fallen by about 18%. The decline in breast cancer has been attributed to several factors which include earlier diagnosis through screening and the availability of more effective treatment.

Risk factors

Many of the known risk factors for cancers are avoidable and cancer risk could be decreased further by making changes to individual lifestyles (see Table 12.3).

Prevention

Secondary prevention includes raising awareness of signs and symptoms, effective treatment and, importantly, screening. Screening was discussed in detail in Chapter 5 and has been estimated to save around 1,400 [5] lives per year in England due to breast cancer screening and 1,300 due to cervical cancer [6]. It is likely that screening can reduce bowel cancer mortality by 15% in those screened but the introduction of population screening for prostate screening is not supported by evidence of effectiveness. At the tertiary prevention level rehabilitation and palliative care are important aspects of health care.

Implications for policy

In England, the NHS Cancer Plan [7] describes a comprehensive strategy to tackle cancer through better prevention. It aims for reduction of smoking rates, early diagnosis, e.g. promoting screening, and provision of high-quality treatment and care throughout the country, e.g. establishing national standards for cancer services and specialist palliative care.

Cardiovascular diseases

Burden of disease

Cardiovascular diseases (CVD) are one of the leading causes of death within adults in the UK and accounted for 20,673 deaths in 2004. Of these, around half were due to CVD and another 25% due to stroke [8]. Mortality from CVD is falling in the UK, but despite this, the death rates are higher than rates in other developed countries. Only Finland, Sweden, and countries of eastern and central Europe have rates higher than the UK. Although death rates are falling, the burden of mortality and morbidity from CVD is still high. For example, it is estimated that there are around 2.68 million people living in the UK who have or have had either angina or heart attack and the Health Survey for England [9] and the General Household Survey [10] suggest that morbidity appears to be rising, particularly in older age groups.

There are inequalities in the cardiovascular mortality rates [8] with death rates from heart disease being highest in Scotland and the north of England, intermediate in Wales and Northern Ireland and lowest in the south of England. The highest mortality rates are concentrated primarily within urban areas. Premature death rates from heart disease also show socio-economic and ethnic differences with death rates being higher among manual workers as compared to non-manual workers among both sexes, and a higher death rate than average among south Asians living in the UK. Morbidity and treatment also show inequalities, varying by geography, socio-economic status and ethnicity. The prevalence of all heart disease is higher in the north of England and in Wales than it is in the south of England, and is also higher in lower socio-economic groups. Data from the Health Survey for England (2004) suggest that the prevalence of all heart disease is higher in Indian and Pakistani men as compared to the general population (there is less

Table 12.4. Risk factors for CVDs.

Non-modifiable risk factors for CVD	Modifiable risk factors for CVD
Older age	High serum cholesterol
Male gender	Hypertension
Ethnicity	Smoking (mortality is 60% higher in smokers and 80% higher in heavy smokers as compared to non-smokers [11]
Family history	Second-hand smoke
Genetic predisposition	Diet high in fat, salt and low in fruit and vegetables
	Obesity (particularly central obesity)
	Diabetes
	Physical inactivity (<2.5 hours moderate-intensity activity per week) [12]
	Hypertension
	High blood-cholesterol levels

ethnic variation in prevalence in women). Rates of coronary revascularisation and other procedures for CVD vary widely across the UK. In England, there was a greater than six-fold difference between the lowest and highest rates by local authority in 2002.

These inequalities have implications for the provision of both medical and preventative interventions [8] which include a high financial burden to health-care services, both for acute and chronic care. Overall, CVD are estimated to cost the UK economy just under £26 billion a year (around 57% is due to direct health-care costs, 24% to productivity losses and 19% to the informal care of people with CVD). As mortality decreases and morbidity increases, a shift in care from acute medicine to chronic disease management is required and new models of health care delivery may be needed to cope with this.

Risk factors

Although treatments for these diseases continue to be developed and improved, the proportion of people dying from heart attacks remains high and most heart disease is potentially preventable. Epidemiological studies have identified a number of risk factors for cardiovascular diseases (Table 12.4)

Prevention

The modifiable risk factors are of potential public health importance and hence national public health targets aim to reduce the prevalence of these risk factors in the population.

A key preventative intervention to reduce the impact of CVD is preventing smoking and stopping smoking. Ways to achieve this include smoking cessation interventions which support smokers to quit (see Chapter 9 for more details), tobacco taxation and legislation to ban smoking in public places. In 1994 the Committee on Medical Aspects of Food and Nutrition Policy [12] recommended targets for reducing *saturated fat, total fat* and increasing *fruit and vegetable consumption*. Progress towards the targets has been disappointing. *Salt* consumption also remains well above the levels (6 g per day) recommended. A reduction in the salt content of processed foods and drinks is required if the target is to be met. Apart from being an independent risk factor for heart disease, *obesity* is also a major risk factor for hypertension, raised serum cholesterol, and diabetes. See below for more details on preventing obesity. The Chief Medical Officer's report, [13] recommended that adults in England should participate in a minimum of 30 minutes of moderate-intensity activity (such as brisk walking, cycling or climbing the stairs) on five or more days of the week. Both drug treatment and lifestyle changes – particularly weight loss, an increase in physical activity and a reduction in salt and alcohol intake – can effectively lower blood pressure. Risk of heart disease is directly related to *blood cholesterol levels*; these can be reduced by drugs, physical activity and by reducing consumption of saturated fat. The National Service Framework for coronary heart disease [14] suggests a cholesterol target of <5.0 mmol per l for both primary and secondary prevention. *Diabetes* substantially increases the risk of heart disease in both sexes. It also magnifies the effect of other risk factors such as cholesterol levels, hypertension, smoking and obesity [8].

Implications for policy

In the UK, the National Service Framework (NSF) for coronary heart disease [14] sets standards for all levels of prevention, diagnosis, treatment and rehabilitation of heart disease, including fair access to high-quality services. This has led to significant improvements, e.g. faster treatment of heart-attack patients, higher numbers of revascularisation operations performed with shorter waiting times and the setting up of rapid-access chest pain clinics across the country to improve the speed with which people with suspected angina can be assessed. However, progress has been slower in other areas, e.g. prevention of heart disease, care of patients with heart failure and cardiac rehabilitation. Although CVD are a national priority warranting national targets and initiatives, additional local targets may be needed to address local need based on demographic and other factors.

Diabetes mellitus

Burden of disease

In 2004, it was estimated that about 1.8 million people in the UK had diabetes [15]; of these, the majority (about 1.5 million) had Type 2 diabetes. It was also estimated that up to a million more people could have undiagnosed Type 2 diabetes. The

Table 12.5. Risk factors for diabetes [15]

Ethnicity (African-Caribbean or South Asian)
Genetic predisposition
Overweight and obesity
Physical inactivity

number of people diagnosed with diabetes is rising and this is thought to be partly due to the ageing population and also the increasing prevalence of obesity in the UK.

Diabetes is a significant cause of morbidity and mortality. People with diabetes have a lower life expectancy and they are more likely to develop coronary heart disease and stroke. Diabetes is the leading cause of blindness among those of a working age in the UK and people with diabetes spend over a million days in hospital each year. If undiagnosed, untreated or not managed effectively, diabetes has a high risk of complications. Often complications begin before diagnosis (50% of individuals have evidence of complications on diagnosis of Type 2 diabetes) [15]. However, if managed effectively, complications of diabetes can be reduced considerably and life expectancy can be increased.

Risk factors

Type 1 diabetes almost always occurs in individuals under the age of 40 years, whereas Type 2 diabetes generally tends to occur in those over the age of 40. Changing lifestyle factors are resulting in Type 2 diabetes being detected in younger individuals. In the UK, the prevalence of diabetes is at least five times higher among individuals from Asian and African-Caribbean communities. Diabetes often appears before the age of 40 among these individuals. A genetic predisposition is known to exist in both types of diabetes, although the disease is determined by complex gene–environment interactions. Around 80–90% of individuals with Type 2 diabetes are overweight. The risk of developing diabetes is 10 times higher among obese individuals.

Prevention

The pattern of risk factors means that effective primary prevention should focus on increasing physical activity levels, improving diet and nutrition and reducing overweight and obesity. Secondary prevention includes increased awareness of symptoms, follow-up and regular testing of individuals known to be at increased risk of developing diabetes, and opportunistic screening of people with multiple risk factors for diabetes. The risk of complications due to diabetes is high which makes tertiary prevention important. Early detection and treatment of microvascular complications (retinopathy, nephropathy, neuropathy) can prevent impairment. Control of hypertension, reduction of cholesterol levels and smoking cessation in people with diabetes reduces their risk of developing both microvascular complications and cardiovascular disease, and regular recall and review of people with diabetes improves the subsequent outcomes.

Implications for policy

The National Service Framework for diabetes [16] sets out new standards and key interventions necessary to reduce the burden of diabetes and the associated health inequalities, as well as to raise the standards of diabetes care in the UK. Apart from prevention and early diagnosis and treatment of diabetes it recommends a structured, proactive care plan for each individual, drawn up in partnership with the individual and clinicians, in order to achieve the best outcomes.

Although, nationally, considerable improvements to service provision have been made and results are being delivered, treatment and care for people with diabetes still shows wide variation.

Obesity

Burden of disease

Obesity is caused by a sustained imbalance between the energy intake (higher) and energy expenditure (lower). The main measures for assessment of obesity are described below:

1. Body mass index (BMI) – This is measured as weight (kg) divided by height squared (m), and classified into four categories as shown in Table 12.6

   The risk of morbidity and mortality rises with increases in BMI over 25, the risk of co-morbidities being very severe in individuals with morbid obesity, i.e. BMI of 40 or more.
2. Waist circumference – Central obesity is also correlated with disease risk, with cut-off points indicating risk of co-morbidities as follows:

general adult population   >40 inches (men)   >35 inches (women)
south Asian population   >35 inches (men)   >32 inches (women)

3. Waist–hip ratio – This is calculated as the waist circumference (m) divided by the hip circumference (m). Values of 0.95 or more among men and 0.85 or more among women are correlated with a higher risk of disease.

Obesity is a significant public health problem in the UK and shows an increasing trend. Figures from the Health Survey for England [9] indicate that almost two thirds of adults are either overweight or obese with nearly a quarter of adults being obese. The levels of obesity have risen from 19.8% in 1993 to 23.7% in

Table 12.6. Classification of BMI

Classification	BMI (kg/m^2)
Underweight	<18.5
Healthy weight	18.5–24.9
Overweight	25.0–29.9
Obese	30.0 or more

Table 12.7. Effect of obesity on health

Greatly increased risk of:	Moderately increased risk of:	Slightly increased risk of:
Type 2 diabetes	Coronary heart disease	Breast cancer in post-menopausal women, colon cancer
Insulin resistance	Hypertension	Polycystic ovaries
Gall bladder diseases	Stroke	Risk of anaesthetic complications
Dyslipidaemia	Osteoarthritis (knees and hips)	Impaired fertility
Breathlessness	Hyperuricaemia and gout	Low back pain
Sleep apnoea	Psychological factors	Reproductive hormone abnormalities

2004. The relative increase is much higher among women as compared to men. However, many individuals are unaware that they may have a weight problem.

Obesity is associated with increased mortality and morbidity and a decreased quality of life. Health problems associated with obesity are shown in Table 12.7:

Risk factors

Table 12.8. Risk factors for obesity[17]

Older age
Female gender
Lower socio-economic status
Black Caribbean and Black African ethnicity (obesity is low in Chinese populations)
Physical inactivity

The rise in global obesity has been linked to environmental and behavioural changes (e.g. sedentary lifestyle, easy access to high-calorie, low-cost foods) brought about by economic development, modernisation and urbanisation.

The metabolic syndrome, a condition characterised by obesity and insulin resistance, confers an increased risk of diabetes, heart disease and stroke. Almost a quarter of the adult population in the UK are estimated to have this condition.

Prevention

The *population* approach to primary prevention seeks to lower the risk of becoming overweight or obese in the whole community. It consists largely of two elements: promoting a balanced diet and increasing physical activity levels in the community. The UK Government recommendations on diet are based on the recommendations of the Committee on Medical Aspects of Food Policy. These include advice to eat at least five portions of fruit and vegetables per day, decrease consumption of saturated fats to less than 11% of total energy consumption, decrease salt to less than 6 grams per day, and increase dietary fibre to 18 grams per day.

United Kingdom Government recommendations on physical activity for adults are a total of at least 30 minutes of physical activity (moderate intensity) per day at least five times a week. This could be achieved through everyday activities such as walking, gardening and swimming or through sport or structured exercise.

The *high risk* approach to primary prevention concentrates on individuals who have an increased chance of becoming overweight or obese, such as individuals from lower socio-economic classes, individuals from south Asian communities (increased risk of diseases caused by obesity), Black Caribbean and Black African individuals (higher prevalence of obesity), people with physical disabilities affecting mobility and people with learning difficulties.

For secondary prevention in those already overweight or obese, for *weight management* to be effective and sustainable, a combination of advice on diet and physical activity, and motivation and support to make and maintain these changes, are essential. For some individuals, drug treatment and surgery may be additional options to be considered.

Implications for policy

Obesity is becoming increasingly important in UK health policy. Guidance on the management of overweight and obesity in primary care in the UK was published in early 2006 by the Department of Health [18]. Clinical guidelines on the prevention and managements of obesity (including drugs and energy) has been published by the National Institute for Health and Clinical Excellence (NICE) [19].

Local action should focus on developing or reviewing strategies to tackle obesity using a 'whole-systems' approach to promote a balanced diet and to raise levels of physical activity, through multi-agency working involving the NHS, local authorities, voluntary and private sector, patient groups and the community.

Mental health

Burden of disease

Definitions of mental health include concepts such as psychological well being, autonomy, competence, inter-generational dependence, and actualisation of one's intellectual and emotional potential. Although it is difficult to define mental health comprehensively, it is generally agreed that mental health is broader than a lack of mental disorders.

The World Health Organization defines mental health as 'a state of well-being in which the individual realises his or her own abilities, can cope with the normal stresses of life, can work productively and fruitfully, and is able to make a contribution to his or her community'.

The terms mental illness or mental disorder refer to health conditions characterised by alterations in thinking, mood or behaviour associated with distress and/or impaired functioning.

Mental illness is a leading cause of morbidity worldwide and in the UK. Mental disorders constitute four of the ten leading causes of disability worldwide. By 2020, it is projected that mental and neurological disorders will account for 15% of the total disability-adjusted life years lost due to all diseases and injuries. The WHO estimates that a quarter of all people suffer from mental and behavioural disorders at some time during their lives, with a prevalence of about 10% among the adult population at any time [20]. Among adults living in Great Britain, the prevalence of common mental illness such as anxiety and depression was 7% of women and 6% of men in 2003 [21]. There do not appear to be differences in those conditions diagnosed most often (depression, anxiety and substance misuse) in primary care in developed and developing countries (21).

Risk factors

Table 12.9. Risk factors for mental health problems (20)

Age
Female gender for depression
Exposure to violence, conflict and disasters
Stressful life events
Ethnic minority status
Low socio-economic status
Genetic predisposition

Age is an important determinant of mental disorders and the prevalence of some mental disorders (for example, depression) rises with age, with a high prevalence among the elderly. Most studies report no difference in overall prevalence of mild to moderate mental disorder by gender. This is also true for severe mental disorders, except depression, which has a higher prevalence among women, and substance misuse, which has a higher prevalence among men. The gender difference in some mental disorders could also be due to a higher exposure to domestic and sexual violence among women. The lifetime prevalence of domestic violence ranges from 16 to 50%. It is estimated that 20% of women suffer rape or attempted rape in their lifetime [20]. Research suggests the existence of a genetic predisposition to mental disorders such as schizophrenia, depression and dementia [20]. Common mental disorders are twice as high among the lowest socio-economic categories as compared to the highest category. This is true for both developing and developed countries. Disorders such as schizophrenia are reported to be higher among British-born ethnic-minority populations. Explanatory factors suggested include increased vulnerability due to social isolation and fewer social networks, and that people from these communities may be more likely to be singled out. Mental and behavioural disorders such as schizophrenia, depression, suicide show an association with life events (job insecurity, bereavement, relationship breakdown, change of residence, business failure, etc.) particularly if they occur in quick succession. War, civil strife and natural disasters affect several million people worldwide and have a huge effect on the mental health of the people affected. Common mental health disorders reported include mental distress, post-traumatic stress disorder, depression and anxiety [20].

Prevention

The prevention of mental disorders is discussed in more detail below.

Implications for policy

In many parts of the world, mental health and mental illness have a low priority as compared to physical health, with only a minority receiving any treatment. Among adults living in Great Britain, around 23% of the population reported receiving some treatment for a mental health problem [21]. However, women were more likely to have received treatment or used services as compared to men (29% vs. 17%). The onset and recovery of common mental disorders were associated with unemployment, financial problems and difficulties with activities of daily living. There is a disproportionate relationship between the burden of mental illness and spending on mental health. According to the WHO, although mental and behavioural disorders constitute 12% of the global burden of disease, the mental health budgets of many countries is less than 1% of their total expenditures [20].

Health promotion

This chapter has outlined some diseases and conditions which are public health problems among adults aged 15 to 64 years. It is recognised that primary prevention of these conditions through health promotion is a key component of any strategy to tackle these issues. It is, therefore, worth a brief consideration of the ways in which this preventative or health improvement action can be delivered. Chapter 4 considers health improvement as a key public health tool. Some of the themes of that chapter are illustrated here.

There are several approaches to adult health promotion. These are outlined below drawing on major health issues of adults as examples. It is possible to prevent many diseases at once by working within certain settings, e.g. the workplace. Another approach is to modify a determinant of health, such as housing, in order to improve adult health. Lastly, public health often works through vertical programmes (see Chapter 17) tackling single health conditions; this is illustrated using mental illness as an example.

1. A settings approach – Healthy workplaces

Productivity is influenced by the health of individuals, which is in turn affected by conditions in the workplace. Adverse health-related outcomes can therefore be reduced by improvement of the working environment within organisations.

In the UK, sickness absence is a growing concern to employers and costs around £12 billion each year. Common causes of reported sickness absence from work are musculoskeletal disorders such as back pain, and stress related conditions. A recent survey showed that 5% of the working-age population had taken time off work during the previous month because of back pain. Overall, 40% of adults reported suffering from back pain in the previous year, with a higher proportion among skilled, partly skilled and unskilled workers as compared to professional, intermediate and skilled non-manual workers (44% and 37% respectively). [22].

To tackle ill health in the workplace, the Department of Health in collaboration with the Department for Work and Pensions and the Health and Safety Executive has launched a health, work and well being strategy [23]. It covers the prevention of work-related illness and accidents, and ensures that access to occupational health is available when needed. It also emphasises the need to create healthy working environments in order to ensure delivery of the workplace health commitments outlined in the strategy.

Benefits of a healthy workplace include increased productivity, reduced sickness-absenteeism, and a decrease in injuries and accidents, with a positive impact on staff morale and retention.

Elements of health promotion that are relevant to this setting are:
- *Creation of a safe and healthy workplace* through increased awareness of employer responsibilities, carrying out risk assessments, and provision of occupational health services for employees.
- *Good recruitment and retention policies* including options such as flexible working arrangements and policies for managing sickness absence.

- *Promotion of mental wellbeing and reduction of stress* through identification of problem areas and taking action to address these, and raising awareness of mental health issues among employees.
- *Prevention and management of musculoskeletal disorders* through risk assessment, provision of training, good reporting systems, early identification and follow-up of symptoms.
- *Smoke-free policies* in the workplace to prevent exposure to tobacco smoke and referral to smoking cessation services for those who need it.
- *Prevention and management of substance misuse including alcohol* through the development of policies for the organisation and increasing employee awareness of issues involved.
- *Encouraging physical activity and healthy eating by* increasing awareness, encouraging cycling and walking to work, providing vending machines with healthy options, etc.

2. Approaching a determinant of health – Housing

Tackling the health of homeless people

Some examples are given here of how a range of agencies might improve the health of homeless adults. At a community level, neighbourhood watch schemes are useful vehicles to develop social capital (see Chapter 14) and local people can become involved in development of local policies. Local authorities have a role to play in many areas including the enforcement of housing standards, assessment of health and safety hazards, housing policies for vulnerable adults, provision of temporary housing and permanent re-housing to those who need it, advice to home owners regarding health and safety issues, pest control, inspection of council properties and repairs. Private tenancies can provide safe housing and have supportive tenancy agreements. Publicity campaigns to raise awareness of housing issues and the impact on health can reinforce work going on across a community. The NHS can contribute to local partnerships for prevention of accidents and ill health and modification of housing environment for vulnerable people. Voluntary agencies can run schemes to engage with homeless adults and resource support groups for disabled people and/or carers. At a national level: legislation on housing standards can help provide healthy environments; housing-benefit schemes and schemes to offer funding/assistance to voluntary organisations can support local work; and taxation policies can improve house-buying opportunities.

3. Approaching a public health problem – Mental illness

According to the WHO [20], in countries with sufficient resources, actions required to prevent mental illness include the following: raising public awareness, provision of effective drug therapy and psychosocial interventions, development of good mental health information systems and initiation/extension of research on service delivery and prevention of mental disorders.

Health promotion in the prevention of mental illness is essentially concerned with making changes that will promote people's mental well being. It covers a variety of strategies which can be delivered at three levels: individual, community and national. Promotion of interventions that increase coping and life skills work at an individual level. For example, supporting new parents and relationship education helps improve maternal and child mental health [20]. Workplace initiatives, for example raising awareness of mental health issues among employees, can provide opportunities for those suffering from mental health problems to seek help [25]. Increasing social inclusion and cohesion, developing support networks, promoting mental health in workplaces and neighbourhoods are examples of measures that can be undertaken to promote mental health at the community level. Workplace initiatives could include increasing employers' awareness of mental health issues, creating a balance between job demands and occupational skills, social-skills training, provision of counselling services and early rehabilitation strategies. As unemployment is a significant issue, mental health promotion strategies could seek to improve employment opportunities, through programmes to create jobs or the provision of vocational training. Reducing barriers to mental health through national policies to reduce discrimination, promote access to employment, and support for vulnerable citizens, are examples of action that can be taken at a national level

The Mental Health National Science Framework [24] aims to improve the quality of adult mental health services through mental health promotion, improved access to mental health services in primary care, effective care for people with severe mental illness, and better support for carers of people with mental illness in England. The initial focus has been on improving specialist care, and provision of intensive support for people with the most complex needs. The focus is now being extended to the mental health needs of the whole community. For this to be effective, emphasis on multi-agency working (health and social care; the voluntary and private sectors; housing, employment, and training; and the community) is essential – not only to tackle mental illness but also to promote mental well being and independence.

REFERENCES

1. Human Development Report 2005. United Nations Development Programme, 2005.
2. Office for National Statistics, *Population Trends*, **112**, 2003, 2–4.
3. The World Health Report 2003: Shaping the future. Geneva, World Health Organization, 2003.
4. Office for National Statistics, *Mortality Statistics: Cause.* Series DH2 no. 31, 2005.

5. Advisory Committee on breast cancer screening, Screening for breast cancer in England: past and future. NHSBSP Publication No. 61, Sheffield, NHS Cancer Screening Programmes, 2006.

6. National Statistics, Cervical screening programme, England 2004–05 Statistical Bulletin 2005/09/HSCIC, NHS Health and Social Care Information Centre, Health Services Community Statistics, 2005; see www.ic.nhs.uk/pubs/cervicscrneng2005/sb0509.pdf/file.

7. The NHS cancer plan: a plan for investment, a plan for reform. London, Department of Health, 2000.

8. Coronary heart disease statistics: British Heart Foundation Statistics Database, 2003. London, British Heart Foundation.

9. Health Survey for England 2004. London, Department of Health, 2005.

10. Office for National Statistics, General Household Survey. London, HMSO, 2004.

11. R. Doll, R. Peto, J. Borcham and I. Sutherland, Mortality in relation to smoking: 50 years' observation on male British doctors. British Medical Journal, **328**, 2004, 1519–27.

12. Department of Health, Nutritional aspects of cardiovascular disease. Report of the Cardiovascular Review Group of the Committee on Medical Aspects of Food Policy. London, HMSO, 1994.

13. Chief Medical Officer, At least five a week: evidence on the impact of physical activity and its relationship to health. London, Department of Health, 2004.

14. National Service Framework for Coronary Heart Disease. London, Department of Health, 2000.

15. Diabetes in the UK 2004. London, Diabetes UK, 2004.

16. National Service Framework for Diabetes. London, Department of Health, 2001.

17. K. Swanton and M. Frost, Lightening the load: tackling overweight and obesity. London, Faculty of Public Health and National Heart Forum, 2006.

18. Care pathway for the management of overweight and obesity. London, Department of Health, 2006.

19. Obesity: the prevention, identification, assessment and management of overweight and obesity in adults and children. Clinical guideline 43. London, National Institute for Health and Clinical Excellence, 2006.

20. The World Health Report 2001: mental health: new understanding, new hope. Geneva, World Health Organization, 2002.

21. National Statistics, Better or worse: a follow-up study of the mental health of adults in Great Britain. London, H. M. Stationery Office, 2003.

22. The prevalence of back pain in Great Britain, 1998. London, Department of Health, 1999.

23. Health, work and well-being: caring for our future: a strategy for the health and well-being of working age people. London, Department of Health, 2005.

24. National Service Framework for mental health. London, Department of Health, 1999.

13

Public health and ageing

Lincoln Sargeant and Carol Brayne

Key points

- The population of older people has been increasing in numbers and as a proportion of populations worldwide.
- The prevalence of physical and cognitive frailty increases with age and as a result older people develop disabilities that prevent them from living independently as they age.
- Primary, secondary and tertiary prevention strategies can be effective for specific conditions that are common among older people.
- Where the scope for prevention is limited, as for example in dementia, provision needs to be made to provide support through health and social care.
- Informal carers, who are often relatives, provide the majority of social care for older people with more formal arrangements possibly becoming necessary as disability levels or health status deteriorate.
- Policy responses to ageing populations need to promote independent living, financial and physical security, as well as health and social care provision, in order to encourage older people to be active participants in society.

Introduction

At the start of the twentieth century a child born in the United Kingdom could expect to live for less than 50 years. Now life expectancy at birth averages about 80 years. This substantial change could well be seen as proof of the triumph of public health (broadly defined); but the success has also brought challenges.

Essential Public Health, eds. Stephen Gillam, Jan Yates and Padmanabhan Badrinath.
Published by Cambridge University Press. © Cambridge University Press 2007.

> ### Box 13.1 Old-age categories
> Young old – 65 to 74 years
> Middle old – 75 to 84 years
> Oldest old – 85 years and over

In this chapter we will examine the factors that lead to ageing populations and explore the health, social and economic consequences of the change in the population structure. We will then outline the preventive strategies that can lead to healthy ageing and the public health actions that could help to manage the challenges posed by the relative and absolute increase in the numbers of older people.

The demography of old age

'Old age' is often defined as beginning at age 65 years but there is no biological rationale for this cut-off. It may be possible to define old age in terms of economic activity. In the UK, 65 years has been the age of retirement for men since 1908 but before then it was 70 years. Between 1950 and 1995 the average age of retirement in men had fallen in developed countries but in the last decade there has been a small increase. Recent analyses, such as those of the UK Pensions Commission, suggest that an increase in the state pension age may occur in the near future. Defining old age in terms of economic activity is therefore flexible. Nevertheless, old age is often categorised as shown in Box 13.1.

The proportion of the population living into old age has been increasing worldwide. There are several factors that contribute to the changing structure in populations. Falling fertility rates and increased infant survival since the late nineteenth and early twentieth century have contributed to a larger proportion of the population surviving to middle age. The population structure resembles a pyramid in a young population but becomes more cylindrical as the population ages, see Figure 13.1.

Adult survival has also increased since the mid-twentieth century following improvements in prevention and treatment of major premature causes of death such as heart disease. More people survive to age 65. Improved life expectancy has also occurred in the older age groups. It is estimated that more than 70 per cent of the rise in the maximum age at death in Sweden, which rose from about 101 years during the 1860s to about 108 years during the 1990s was attributable to reductions in death rates above age 70 [1]. Together these trends have led to relative and absolute increases in the population at older ages, most marked in the oldest old.

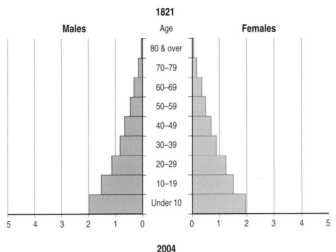

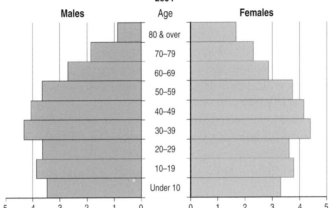

Fig. 13.1 Population pyramids; population (in millions) in Great Britain, by gender and age, 1821 and 2004. Source: Office for National Statistics; General Register Office for Scotland.

Another phenomenon occurring in the mid-twentieth century indicates that further marked increases in the older population can be expected in developed countries in the next few decades. A rapid increase in fertility rates beginning with the end of the Second World War lasting into the 1960s gave rise to the 'baby boom' generation. This generation is now middle aged and will further exaggerate the ageing population profile in those developed countries.

The economic activity of the working population supports children and economically inactive adults such as retired older people. Dependency ratios are used to summarise the balance of economically active to inactive members of a society. The total dependency ratio is the ratio of children and people aged 65 and over to economically active adults. One constituent of this, the old age dependency ratio, has been increasing steadily since the 1960s in the UK and, despite a fall in the youth dependency ratio in the same period, is expected to cause a rise in the total dependency ratio from about 2010 onwards.

A high dependency ratio has the potential to limit the available funds for pensions and health care of the elderly, and can have a profound impact on societies.

However, the experience of old age varies greatly. People over 65 years can and do continue to contribute economically and are not necessarily dependent on the 'working-age population'. In light of this, the UK government has introduced legislation to remove age discrimination in employment practices so that age does not limit opportunities for older people. Furthermore, many older individuals support economically active younger family members through child care and provide social care as unpaid carers for frail or disabled family members. The challenge for public health is to understand the relation between ageing and health in order to prevent the disability and subsequent dependency that is often associated with growing old.

Ageing and health

Ageing is related to ill health in one of three main ways:

- Some conditions are associated with ageing in that they can be expected to occur with all individuals as they age. High-frequency hearing, for example, declines predictably with age.
- Ill health can occur in the elderly because resilience decreases with age. Hence a fall in an elderly person is more likely to lead to fractures because of bone loss than in a young person.
- Some diseases are very closely associated with ageing such as Alzheimer's disease.

Cognitive and physical frailty increase with age and so does the number of chronic conditions that affect an individual. Together, these factors increase the likelihood of disability in the elderly patient (see Box 13.2). The prevalence of disability in the elderly increases steeply with age. This means that increasing proportions of people as they age need more support to perform activities of daily living such as bathing and dressing (Box 13.3). Figure 13.2 shows the prevalence by age of disability (difficulty with one or more activities of daily living) from the English Longitudinal Study of Ageing [2].

The strong association of ill health and disability with age has led to concerns that as the population ages so will the burden of ill health. It should be noted, however, that the burden and costs of ill health are concentrated at the end of life, irrespective of the age of death.

There are limited data on the overall effect of a longer life span on time spent in ill health. The worst-case scenario (see Figure 13.3) is that with increased life expectancy a greater proportion of time is spent in ill health. Between 1981 and 2001 in the United Kingdom, both life expectancy and

Box 13.2 Three dimensions of disability

In 1980 the World Health Organization published the International Classification of Impairments, Disabilities and Handicaps that provides a conceptual framework for disability which is described in three dimensions – impairment, disability and handicap:

Impairment. In the context of health experience an impairment is any loss or abnormality of psychological, physiological or anatomical structure or function.

Disability. In the context of health experience a disability is any restriction or lack (resulting from an impairment) of ability to perform an activity in the manner or within the range considered normal for a human being.

Handicap. In the context of health experience a handicap is a disadvantage for a given individual, resulting from an impairment or a disability, that limits or prevents the fulfilment of a role that is normal (depending on age, sex, and social and cultural factors) for that individual.

Box 13.3 Activities and instrumental activities of daily living

Activities of daily living

Dressing, including putting on shoes and socks

Walking across a room

Bathing or showering

Eating, such as cutting up food

Getting in or out of bed

Using the toilet, including getting up or down

Instrumental activities of daily living

Using a map to figure out how to get around in a strange place

Preparing a hot meal

Shopping for groceries

Making telephone calls

Taking medications

Doing work around the house or garden

Managing money such as paying bills and keeping track of expenses

healthy life expectancy have increased but life expectancy has increased faster. The result is that the expected time lived in poor health from age 65 onwards for men increased from 3.1 years in 1981 to 4.3 years in 2001. For women in 1981 the corresponding figure was 5.0 years, rising to 5.8 years in 2001 (Office of National Statistics (www.Statistics.gov.uk), 2004).

Fig. 13.2   Prevalence of
difficulty with one or more
activities of daily living, in the
English Longitudinal Study of
Ageing, by age.

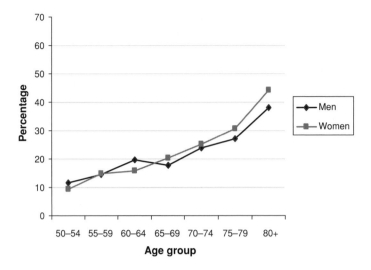

Fig. 13.3   Scenarios for
healthy-life expectancy.

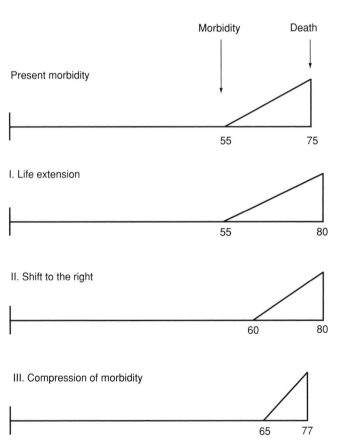

Strategies for healthy ageing have aimed at keeping people in good health as long as possible. Since the 1990s the World Health Organization has adopted the term 'active ageing' to signal that the ageing process can be so. Active ageing is defined as 'the process of optimizing opportunities for health, participation and security in order to enhance quality of life as people age.' This clearly includes broader themes than just health.

A key factor for promoting active ageing relates to the role of the social environment. Both individual and neighbourhood deprivation are associated with poor health but the specific mechanisms are not understood. An investigation of English middle-aged civil servants [3] found no evidence of adverse health consequences of being poor in an affluent neighbourhood. However, being poor in a poor neighbourhood was associated with low self-rated health. It is postulated that the collective material and social resources of the neighbourhood provide protection against the adverse consequences of personal material deprivation. These observations are supported by results of a survey of people aged 65 years and over [4]. Perceptions of good-quality facilities in the area were associated with good self-reported health while perceptions of problems such as noise and crime were associated with poorer health.

Prevention

Promoting active ageing has many facets but any public health approach to active ageing needs to consider the major preventable health threats in old age. The major chronic conditions are listed in Box 13.4.

Box 13.4 Health conditions affecting the elderly

- Cardiovascular disease (such as coronary heart disease)
- Hypertension
- Stroke
- Diabetes
- Cancer
- Chronic obstructive airways disease (COPD)
- Musculoskeletal conditions (such as arthritis and osteoporosis)
- Mental health conditions (mostly dementia and depression)
- Blindness and visual impairment

Note: The causes of disability in older age are similar for men and women although women are more likely to report musculoskeletal problems

   Source: the World Health Organization.

Primary prevention

Prevention of chronic disease starts with promotion of healthy lifestyles in earlier life but is also beneficial in old age. The Cardiovascular Health Study [5] investigated risk factors for five-year mortality risk in older people living in four communities in the United States. Physical inactivity, a history of smoking and high blood pressure were among the modifiable factors identified to increase risk of death. Promoting physical activity in older people is an effective primary prevention strategy for conditions such as heart disease, diabetes and dementia. Other primary prevention strategies such as blood pressure control are also highly effective in the elderly in preventing heart disease and stroke.

   Primary prevention is also relevant for acute illnesses in the elderly. During the winter months the number of deaths among older people reaches higher levels than observed in the summer months. This excess winter mortality is mainly due to acute respiratory illnesses, of which influenza is the most important. Primary prevention of excess winter mortality among the elderly is achieved through vaccination against influenza.

Secondary prevention

For other conditions, the opportunity for primary prevention in old age may be limited. In this context, secondary prevention may be appropriate where the condition can be detected and treated at an early stage. Screening is a public health measure where a suitable test is used to detect a disease before it causes symptoms or signs. The disease is then treated with the expectation of prolonging life expectancy. For example, colorectal cancers develop slowly and prevention in older people often depends on early diagnosis through screening. There is limited evidence for primary prevention of breast cancer, and screening by mammography is the most effective method for reducing breast-cancer mortality in older women (see Chapter 5).

Tertiary prevention

Where primary or secondary prevention are not possible the aim is to reduce the complications of disease. Many chronic illnesses have their onset in middle age but have their greatest impact in old age. Rehabilitation is therefore the mainstay of prevention for many older people.

   As mentioned above, disability from physical and cognitive impairment limit the potential of older people to enjoy optimal health. The older population is susceptible to injury from falls and this is a major cause of disability and mortality in those aged over 75 years. Falls prevention strategies make use of rehabilitation to reduce the disability that can occur with fractures that result from falls in this age group. Dementia, the leading cause of cognitive impairment in the older population, is also a key threat to active ageing. Falls prevention and the management of dementia are examined in greater detail to highlight the different approaches that are necessary to deal with two of the major causes of frailty in the elderly.

Prevention example 1. Falls

The challenges of prevention in the elderly can be illustrated by falls prevention. Falls are common in the elderly, estimated to occur in about 30% of the over-65 population. Although less than one fall in 10 results in a fracture, a fifth of fall incidents require medical attention.

A Cochrane review [6] has reported that multidisciplinary interventions targeting multiple risk factors are effective in reducing the incidence of falls in older people with and without a history of falling. This review found no randomised controlled trials but summarised evidence from five controlled population-based intervention studies. Muscle strengthening combined with balance retraining, individually prescribed at home by a trained health professional, is effective in preventing falls; so is home hazard assessment and modification by a health professional, especially in those with a history of falling. The National Institute for Health and Clinical Excellence (NICE) concluded in 2004 that there was a lack of cost-effectiveness evidence for falls prevention in the UK. However, they found through a modelling study that multifactorial assessment and intervention programmes, as well as exercise programmes for older people living in the community, were likely to be cost-effective in preventing falls.

Older people at risk of hip fractures often present initially with a fall. One strategy that has been tried involves the fitting of hip protectors. These consist of plastic shields or foam pads fitted in pockets within specially designed underwear and aim to reduce the impact of a fall on the hip, and thus the risk of a hip fracture. However, there is no compelling evidence of any benefit from hip protectors for the majority of older people living in their own homes.

After a hip fracture, many older people are not able to return to independent living, with about 20% requiring nursing home care. Mortality is high with estimates of up to 40% within the first year after the fracture. Tertiary prevention seeks to reduce this heavy burden and several approaches to rehabilitation have been investigated. A Cochrane review [7] found that patients receiving co-ordinated in-patient rehabilitation tended to do better in terms of survival or need for institutional care but the results were inconclusive. Similarly, there was not enough evidence from randomised trials to show the effects of different strategies for helping people walk after hip-fracture surgery or of exercise programmes to improve and maintain mobility after discharge from hospital.

Prevention example 2. Dementia

Dementia is another condition that is common in the elderly and for which there is limited evidence for prevention. The commonest form is Alzheimer's disease for which there are few modifiable risk factors. On the basis of observational studies and short-term trials it is possible that addressing vascular risk factors, for example, by treating high blood pressure, increasing physical activity and memory training may offer benefit in preventing Alzheimer's disease as well as vascular dementia.

There is an on-going debate about the role of secondary prevention in dementia. Mild cognitive impairment (MCI) refers to a subtle but measurable impairment in memory that can be detected using standardised cognitive tests. There is no consensus on which tests should be used and what criteria to use to define the condition. Although some people with MCI progress to dementia and have pathological evidence of Alzheimer's disease at post mortem, studies have shown that up to 40% revert to normal over two to three years. Furthermore, similar pathological changes may be present in people who showed no signs of dementia during life.

Some cholinesterase inhibitors show promise in people with mild to moderate Alzheimer's disease but long-term clinical benefit is unproven. It is not clear whether active case finding alters the life-course of demented individuals. Cognitive rehabilitation involves recovery of deficits through restoration and compensation through guided therapy to learn (or relearn) ways to cope with cognitive impairment. However, whilst there is some evidence for short-term benefit of multi strategy approaches to in-patient and residential-home rehabilitation [8], there is insufficient evidence for cognitive rehabilitation [9].

With increasing age the burden of chronic conditions and physical and mental frailty increase and the scope for prevention declines. The oldest old typically need more and more support, initially in their own homes but eventually a substantial proportion require institutional support. This varies between countries and is influenced by policies for social-care provision and the cultural context.

Health and social care

The increasing prevalence of cognitive and physical frailty with age means that older people are more likely than younger age groups to use health and social care services. According to the 2002 English Longitudinal Study of Ageing (ELSA), the need for help because of limitations in activities of daily living or mobility increased with age with 42% of those 80 years and over having difficulty with one or more activities of daily living [2]. Assistance with activities of daily living included help with dressing, bathing or showering, eating, getting in or out of bed, preparing a hot meal, shopping for groceries or taking medication. In the Medical Research Council Cognitive Function and Ageing Study [10], the prevalence of severe cognitive impairment rose from 1% in men and 0.9% in women aged 65–69 years, to 18.4% and 40.5%, respectively, in those aged over 90 years.

The support needed can be provided formally by health and social services, voluntary organisations and community projects, or informally by spouses, extended family, neighbours and friends. In the 2002 ELSA, family members accounted for most of the help provided to people aged 60 and over, with spouses or partners most likely to provide help to those aged 60 to 74. For those aged 75 and over caring was mostly provided by the younger generations such as children, children-in-law or grandchildren. In addition to family, privately paid employees, social- or health service workers and friends or neighbours provided some help.

The burden of providing care for the elderly is considerable. The 2001 census in the UK reported 5.7 million unpaid carers, half of whom were caring for someone over 75 years old. Ninety per cent of carers were caring for relatives. A quarter of carers were caring 20 or more hours per week. In addition to the time required to care for an elderly relative there are health consequences for the carer. Carers were more likely than the general population to report health problems and 39% reported that their physical or mental health was affected by caring.

Despite the input of unpaid carers there is a substantial economic cost to supporting older people in their homes as they become increasingly frail. In 2004–5 older people (those aged 65 and over) accounted for 44% of spending by local authorities in England on personal social services, which include home help and home care. This was the single largest portion [11].

Based on 1995–6 admission rates [12], the risk of future admission to a residential home at age 65 years was 20% for men and 36% for women. Physical and mental health problems predominated as reasons for admission to a care home but carer-related problems were also important, accounting for 38% in a survey of social workers. The majority were admitted from hospital. This is important because illness requiring hospitalisation often makes it difficult for the older person to return to independent living.

People admitted to a care home as a supported long-stay resident were typically aged in their 80s, female and unmarried. Those living alone, or, where living with others, living in *their* home or living in a house rented from the local authority or housing association, were at increased risk of care home admission. Other risk factors included receipt of income support and housing benefit, residence in poorer neighbourhoods, being multiply disabled and the presence of a limiting long-standing illness.

End of life care

The majority of deaths in most developed countries occur in old age. It is important to recognise and deliver high-quality care to older people with terminal conditions in a way that relieves suffering and maintains the autonomy and dignity of the individual and their families. Cancer, heart failure and dementia are among the most common conditions requiring palliative care among older people.

There is evidence of lack of access to specialist palliative care for older people in many countries. For example, there is inequality in the provision of hospice care in the UK. As of January 2004 about 80% of specialist palliative services were provided by voluntary agencies (National Council for Palliative Care; see www.ncpc.org.uk/palliative carehtml). The location of such services is often determined by historical factors rather than by needs assessment. Studies from Australia, the USA and the UK suggest that people with terminal conditions other than cancer are less likely to be admitted to hospices where specialist palliative services are offered. This diverts the provision of specialist care towards younger cancer patients. Heart failure, despite having a five-year prognosis that is comparable to or worse than several cancers, is more likely to be overlooked as a reason for specialist palliative care.

Policy responses

The WHO identifies several challenges posed by ageing populations. In developing countries there is a double burden of disease, where diseases associated with old age are emerging alongside traditional health problems of infectious diseases and malnutrition. The second challenge relates to the increasing prevalence of disability associated with old age and this in turn puts additional pressure on health care systems to provide adequate care. Women typically outlive their spouses and this places them at great risk especially where social support systems are not well developed.

The other challenges arise because of the economic and social sequelae of old age and the associated dependency. The WHO highlights the need for new paradigms that view older people as 'active participants in an age-integrated society and as active contributors as well as beneficiaries of development.' The policy framework for active ageing therefore rests on three pillars: participation, health and security.

In addition to prevention and provision of adequate health and social care support, including the needs and training of carers, the WHO advocates steps to increase participation of older people in the wider society. This can be achieved through emphasis on lifelong learning and on opportunities for economic and social participation through formal or informal work and voluntary activities. Security issues are also highlighted to defend the rights of the elderly and to protect against elder abuse. These concerns may become particularly pressing at the end of life if the older person's autonomy is not respected in decisions about their health and financial affairs.

The UK has set out standards for health and social care of older people in its National Service Frameworks (NSFs). There is an NSF for older people that sets out standards for health care but also addresses age discrimination, mental health issues in the elderly and the promotion of health and active life in old age [13]. Other NSFs also address health issues of older people such as the NSF for long-term conditions as well as more specific conditions like heart disease and diabetes that affect older people.

In order for older people to age actively, broader issues of housing, transport and income support must be considered. The UK government [14] has set out its policy for promoting active ageing in a white paper 'Opportunity and security throughout life'. The values of active independence, quality and choice are emphasised.

There is the need to provide the appropriate evidence base to underpin policy. This is particularly challenging in the case of older people. The presence of co-morbidity often means that older people are excluded from clinical trials of interventions that could prevent ill health in this population. The Medical Research Council Cognitive Function and Ageing Study (MRC CFAS) found that individuals who refused participation in the follow-up phase were more likely to have poor cognitive ability and had less years of full-time education compared with those followed up [15]. This suggests that long-term studies of ageing and health may underrepresent the disadvantaged and disabled.

Conclusion

Longevity is a reasonable goal for public health but brings about a new set of challenges. Health in old age, as at any age, is not 'merely the absence of disease'. However, age is strongly associated with disease and disability. The role of prevention may be progressively limited at increasing ages and this means that public health must seek to support and care where prevention is not possible.

The phenomenon of ageing also illustrates the wider determinants of health that must be addressed if older people are to remain active and independent participants in their communities. This demands flexibility in approaching the definition and expectations of 'old age'.

FURTHER READING AND SOURCES OF INFORMATION

P. Babb, H. Butcher, J. Church and L. Zealey (eds), *Social Trends No. 36*. London, Palgrave Macmillan for the Office for National Statistics, www.ic.nhs.uk, 2006.

NHS Health and Social Care Information Centre, 2006.

The Pension Commission (Turner Reports). The Pensions Commission, chaired by Adair Turner, was set up in 2002 to review the UK private pension system and long-term savings and produced three reports that can be accessed from: www.pensionscommission.org.uk/index.asp.

Royal College of Nursing. Clinical practice guideline for the assessment and prevention of sfalls in older people. Guidelines commissioned by the National Institute for Health and Clinical Excellence.

Active ageing: a policy framework. WHO/NMH/NPH/02.8, World Health Organization, 2002.

Better palliative care for Older people. Copenhagen, World Health Organization (Europe) 2004 (www.euro.who.int/document/E82933.pdf).

REFERENCES

1. J. R. Wilmoth, L. J. Deegan, H. Lundstrom and S. Horiuchi, Increase of maximum lifespan in Sweden, 1861–1999. *Science*. **289**, 2000, 2366–8.

2. M. Marmot, J. Banks, R. Blundell, C. Lessof and J. Nazroo (eds), *Health, Wealth and Lifestyles of the Older Population in England: The 2002 English Longitudinal Study of Ageing*. London, Institute of Fiscal Studies, 2002.

3. M. Stafford and M. Marmot, Neighbourhood deprivation and health: does it affect us all equally? *International Journal of Epidemiology*, **32**, 2003, 357–66.

4. A. Bowling, J. Barber, R. Morris and S. Ebrahim, Do perceptions of neighbourhood environment influence health? Baseline findings from a British survey of aging. *Journal of Epidemiology and Community Health*, **60**, 2006, 476–83.

5. L. P. Fried, R. A. Kronmal, A. B. Newman *et al.*, Risk factors for 5-year mortality in older adults: the Cardiovascular Health Study. *Journal of the American Medical Association*, **279**, 1998, 585–92.

6. R. McClure, C. Turner, N. Peel *et al.*, Population-based interventions for the prevention of fall-related injuries in older people. *Cochrane Database of Systematic Reviews* Issue 1, 2005, CD004441.

7. I. D. Cameron, H. H. Handoll, T. P. Finnegan, R. Madhok and P. Langhorne, Co-ordinated multidisciplinary approaches for inpatient rehabilitation of older patients with proximal femoral fractures. *Cochrane Database of Systematic Reviews*, Issue 3, 2001, CD000106.

8. A. Holm, M. Michel, G. A. Stern *et al.*, The outcomes of an inpatient treatment program for geriatric patients with dementia and dysfunctional behaviours. *The Gerontologist* **39**, 1998, 668–76.

9. L. Clare, R. T. Woods, E. D. Moniz Cook, M. Orrell, and A. Spector, Cognitive rehabilitation and cognitive training for early-stage Alzheimer's disease and vascular dementia. *Cochrane Database of Systematic Reviews*, issue 4, 2003, CD003260.

10. C. Brayne, F. E. Matthews, M. A. McGee and C. Jagger, Health and ill-health in the older population in England and Wales. The Medical Research Council Cognitive Function and Ageing Study (MRC CFAS). *Age and Ageing* **30**, 2001, 53–62.

11. Personal Social Services expenditure and unit costs: England 2004–2005. NHS Health and Social Care Information Center, Social Care Statistics Bulletin: 2006/01/HSCIC.

12. A. Bebbington, R. Darton and A. Netten, *Care Homes for Older People Volume 2. Admissions, Needs and Outcomes. The 1995/96 National Longitudinal Survey of Publicly-Funded Admissions.* University of Kent, Canterbury, Personal Social Services Research Unit, 2001.

13. National Service Framework for Older People's Services 2001. London, Department of Health, 2001.

14. Opportunity Age – Opportunity and security throughout life (First report). London, Department of Work and Pensions.

15. F. E. Matthews, M. Chatfield, C. Freeman, C. McCracken and C. Brayne; MRC CFAS. Attrition and bias in the MRC cognitive function and ageing study: an epidemiological investigation. *BioMed Central Public Health*, **4**, 2004, 12.

Tackling health inequalities

Chrissie Pickin

Key points

- Many diseases show a strong and consistent social gradient.
- Socio-economic inequalities in health are widespread in developed countries and are increasing in some countries.
- They are caused by the unequal distribution of health determinants affecting individuals across their life-course with prenatal and early life influences having a large impact on people's health experience later in life.
- Differences in lifestyle and health behaviours and access to care account for some of the observed differences between groups.
- Economic factors are key determinants of health inequalities but differences in the distribution of psycho-social stressors are increasingly acknowledged as contributory.
- Tackling health inequalities requires action at multiple levels involving many agencies with government playing a pivotal role.

Introduction – what are health inequalities?

Different people experience different health. That my health is better or worse than yours does not necessarily indicate the presence of health inequalities. At an individual level it is hard to predict one's health experience. The term 'health inequality' refers to differences observed between groups due to one group experiencing an advantage over the other group, rather than to any innate differences between them. In some countries the term 'health inequity' is used. The Commission on the Social Determinants of Health of the WHO defines health equity as 'the absence of unfair and avoidable or remedial differences in health among populations or groups defined socially, economically, demographically or geographically'.

Essential Public Health, eds. Stephen Gillam, Jan Yates and Padmanabhan Badrinath.
Published by Cambridge University Press. © Cambridge University Press 2007.

Most people would expect the health of a group of 20 year olds to be better on average than a group of 80 year olds; so differences in health due to age are not considered inequalities and in any of our comparisons we adjust for age differences. There are differences between the health experience of men and of women. In developed countries men tend to die younger although this has been reducing recently, in part due to better treatment of heart disease. However, women tend to experience more ill health throughout their lives. This is partly related to genetic and innate cultural differences between men and women but much of the observed difference is related to discrimination, which varies between countries and between societies. The nature and causes of women's health experience is touched upon in Chapter 11. The determinants of ethnic variations in health are not considered here; except to say that much past work has overemphasised the importance of culture and underplayed the importance of discrimination and socio-economic influences [1]. Other work identifies how to tackle ethnic inequalities [2].

This chapter will focus on inequalities between groups of people in developed countries with different socio-economic circumstances. One hundred years ago the dominant causes of death were infections, not heart disease, and child mortality was high. As countries develop economically and material living standards rise we see changes in the patterns of death and disease (see Chapter 1). In countries which have not experienced this 'epidemiological transition', health inequalities can mostly be explained through differences in levels of material deprivation and education. The picture is more complex in richer, developed countries.

Repeated enquiries in the United Kingdom and in continental Europe [3–6] have found that socio-economic inequalities in health are widespread and have been widening over the last few decades. They challenge policy makers and health professionals everywhere. The Whitehall studies of civil servants referred to in Chapter 2 [7] show that there is a social gradient in health, not a bimodal distribution. Socio-economic inequalities in health thus affect all of us – not just the poor. Wherever we are in the social hierarchy, our health will be better than those below and worse than those above us. The real challenge is not only to identify those in poor health and focus our attention on them but to address the underlying causes of the inequality, i.e. the slope of the graph (Figure 14.1).

Trends

In most developed countries the overall health of the population has been steadily improving for decades. However, the health of some socio-economic groups has been improving at a faster rate than others which means that health inequalities have been increasing. In the UK and many other European countries health inequalities widened substantially in the last decades of the twentieth century and similar changes were seen in many other developed countries (Figure 14.2).

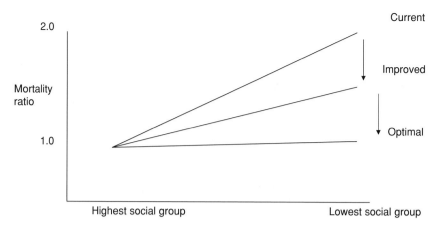

Fig. 14.1   Reducing/
Eliminating the social gradient in
mortality.

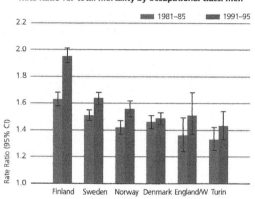

Rate Ratio for total mortality by occupational class: men

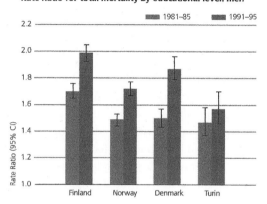

Rate Ratio for total mortality by educational level: men

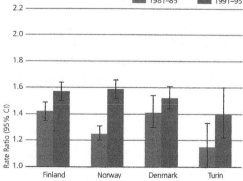

Fig. 14.2   Inequalities in mortality by educational level and occupational class, 1981–1985 and 1991–1995. Finland, Sweden, Norway, Denmark, England/Wales, Turin. Note: 95% CI = 95% confidence interval. This is an indication of the influence of random variation, and gives the range of values which, with 95% probability, contains the true value. Source: J. P. Mackenbach, V. Bos, D. Anderson *et al.*, Widening soio-economic inequalities in mortality in Six Western European Countries. *International Journal of Epidemiology,* **32**, 2003, 830–37.

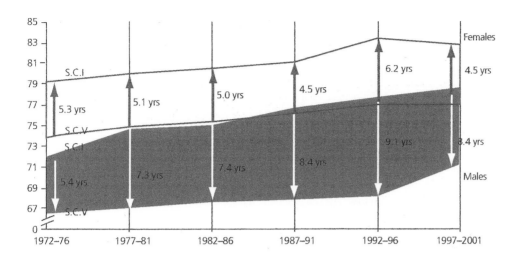

Fig. 14.3 Inequalities in life
expectancy at birth by
occupational class in England
and Wales 1972–2001. Source:
Office of National Statistics
Longitudinal Study.

There are now wide variations in health in many countries including the USA, UK, continental Europe and Australia. The fact that health inequalities have widened suggests that they are not fixed and should be amenable to intervention. There is evidence that they are beginning to reduce in some countries (Figure 14.3).

Which diseases contribute to health inequalities?

The incidence of many diseases shows a social gradient. A few diseases such as breast cancer, prostate cancer and leukaemia show an inverse relationship. Cardiovascular disease accounts for a significant element of the difference in mortality between social groups but, in addition, people from lower socio-economic groups experience excess deaths and morbidity from type II diabetes, many cancers, chronic respiratory disease, mental illness, suicide, infectious diseases, accidents and violence, homicides and digestive diseases including liver disease. The excess deaths are experienced at all ages but particularly in childhood and in adults of working age. What is it about being poor in a rich country that puts you and your family at such a consistent disadvantage healthwise? Table 14.1 identifies determinants of health the unequal distribution of which has been shown to be important in causing and/or sustaining health inequalities in developed countries.

Which determinants are most important in explaining health inequalities and how do they interact?

Research has identified a number of models for the interplay between health determinants and health inequalities [8–11]. These models include several common elements in explaining health inequalities:

Table 14.1. Determinants of health important in sustaining health inequalities in developed countries

Economic determinants
- Level of income relative to others
- Money worries
- Unemployment

Social determinants
- Level and quality of individual social support
- Extent and quality of social networks
- Level of social cohesion of the community in which the individual lives
- Social capital or social resources through trust, civic engagement, reciprocal relations and community participation
- Educational attainment
- Early life experience
- Place in the social hierarchy/social status

Psychological determinants
- Perception of autonomy and control over one's life
- Ability to cope with demands/stressors at home and work
- Balance between effort and reward – particularly at work
- Perception of one's social status relative to others

Environmental determinants
- Level of pollution
- Quality of housing
- Extent of environmental hazards such as busy roads, railway lines
- Access to safe, green spaces for play and recreation
- Quality of the built environment – a 'proper' place to live

Lifestyle and personal behaviour
- Smoking
- Diet
- Pattern of drinking alcohol
- Level of physical exercise
- Risk-taking behaviour including drug use, speeding

Access to medical treatment and care
- Particularly to high-quality, extended primary care and to effective treatments

- the stratification of society – the distribution of power, wealth and risk and the consequent social position of the individual within this
- the social environment within which the individual is born, grows up, lives and works
- material conditions such as working and housing conditions
- psycho-social stressors
- health behaviours/lifestyle
- access to health care and other services.

Box 14.1 The Whitehall Studies

The first Whitehall study was started by Professor Michael Marmot in 1976. It studied the health experience of 18,000 men working in the British civil service. The men were classified according to their employment grade – at the lowest end porters and messengers all the way through to the most senior civil servants – the permanent secretaries (the Sir Humphreys made famous by the television programme '*Yes Minister*'). The second study known as Whitehall II was started in 1985 and this time included women. Follow-up studies have continued for over 20 years and a large number of papers and reports based on data from the studies have been produced. The data from these studies have been crucial in developing our understanding of the social gradient in health and the determinants of socio-economic health inequalities.

Recent work [12, 13] has particularly highlighted the importance of psychosocial stressors, i.e. the psychological impact of the social environment in which we live and work. This is not to dismiss lifestyle and personal behaviour as important determinants but the Whitehall studies (see Box 14.1) suggest that lifestyle differences account for only 30% of the health differences between social groups [7].

Richard Wilkinson identifies the level of income inequality within any society as a key determinant of health inequalities [13–15]. Michael Marmot suggests that one's position in the social hierarchy within which one lives predicts one's health relative to others [12]. This research suggests that it is the experience of being poor in a rich society that affects your health through its impact on your actual and perceived social status. Marmot and Wilkinson both hypothesise how this might lead to poor health. They have collated research from a range of disciplines including sociology, anthropology, evolutionary psychology and social epidemiology. This leads them to suggest that in a society in which social status differentials are marked and obvious those with lower social status experience:

- more adverse, unpredictable and stressful events and less control (perceived and actual) over them
- more maternal and early life stress
- access to fewer social resources and poorer quality social relations
- a stronger sense of social shame and consequent attempts to gain higher social status and respect among near peers, sometimes associated with violence (including domestic and racial violence) over them.

How these may affect the health of individuals has been made much clearer as our knowledge of responses to stressors has developed – through research in primates [16, 17] and also in humans [18, 19]. All of the above stressors raise blood levels of the 'stress hormones' in humans – fibrinogen, catecholamines and glucocorticoids. In addition, there is some evidence that they can reduce serotonin levels. This chemical response is entirely appropriate in the presence of an actual physical threat to life and helps the body's 'fight or flight' response. If the perceived threats are short-lived and the body's hormone levels can return to normal quickly then no harm is done. It appears that living in a state of sustained tension/stress leads to high levels of circulating stress hormones; it is this that affects health, particularly if this stress occurs in early life [20, 21]. The effects of these chronic stressors can be direct through this hormonal response but can also be mediated through health behaviours such as smoking, alcohol use and drug taking.

There is a strong body of evidence on the protective effect on health of access to social resources – social support, strong social networks and living in a community with high social capital [22–24, 41]. However, there is evidence of less social cohesion and lower social capital (lower social trust, reciprocity, participation in civic life) in societies who are particularly at risk [25].

The workplace can be a source of great stress, increasing rates of heart disease and depression in mid and later life [26]. Three factors that particularly impact on health in relation to work are

- the balance between the demands of the job and the control one perceives oneself to have to address these demands
- the level of job insecurity
- the balance between the effort expended and the rewards of the job.

Living in poorer quality housing, in localities with depleted local facilities and with high rates of violence and crime lead to poorer physical and mental health throughout the life-course through the impact this has on sustained levels of stress hormones and the associated increased risk of heart disease, high blood pressure, central obesity, diabetes, depression, violence and cancers.

Differences in access to treatment cannot explain the differences in the *incidence* of diseases between social groups but can explain some of the differences in survival rates – particularly for cancers. Extrapolating from research on the contribution of health spend to health improvement in industrialised countries, access to health care probably determines no more than 10 to 20% of the difference in health outcomes overall – although the OECD (Organisation for Economic Co-operation and Development) study showed that health care seems more important for women's health [27]. This study also showed that public spending on health care predicted outcomes better than spending in the private system. Other studies would suggest that access to medical care has contributed significantly to improved health outcomes – particularly over the last 30 years [28, 29].

The importance of the life-course and the 'probabilistic cascade'

The unequal distribution of health determinants influences health throughout the life-course. In early life this leads to more childhood accidents, more life-threatening infections, more behavioural problems and more disability. However, health determinants in early life do not just affect health in childhood. Prenatal and early life influences cast a long shadow over people's health experience [30]. Low birth weight is a predictor of illness in middle and old age [20]. A child born thin or who has poor growth in the first year is at much higher risk of high blood pressure, heart disease, stroke and diabetes in later life. This appears to be due to high levels of stress within the mother during pregnancy leading to the foetus being exposed to high levels of cortisol, which programmes the child's metabolic pathways and thus their biochemical response to stressors in later life [31].

The unequal nature of determinants influences the older child's experience at school, and their level of educational achievement will have a huge impact on their future career and income. The unequal distribution of determinants in young adults' lives leads to more drug misuse, poorer mental health, more suicides, more deaths and injuries from accidents and violence, and more teenage pregnancies which, in turn, can lead to social isolation and reduced income.

Adults of working age are differentially affected by unemployment, workplace stress or poor working conditions. Older people are differentially affected by social isolation, poorer living environments and less access to effective health care (see Chapter 13).

Childhood and prenatal experiences, early social environment, working conditions, adult social position and the physical environment within which we live all affect our health experience. The effects of the unequal distribution of these health determinants are cumulative – a 'probabilistic cascade' [32]. Proponents of a 'life-course' approach argue for interventions at critical points (prenatally, early years, transition from primary to secondary school, entry into the labour market, becoming parents, retirement) to prevent this accumulation of risk.

The causal pathways linking poor health and health inequalities are shown in diagrammatic form in Figure 14.4.

Interventions to reduce health inequalities

Three possible policy frameworks have been proposed to tackle socio-economic health inequalities [33]. These are:
1. improving the health of poor people
2. narrowing the health gap or 'raising the health of the poorest, fastest'

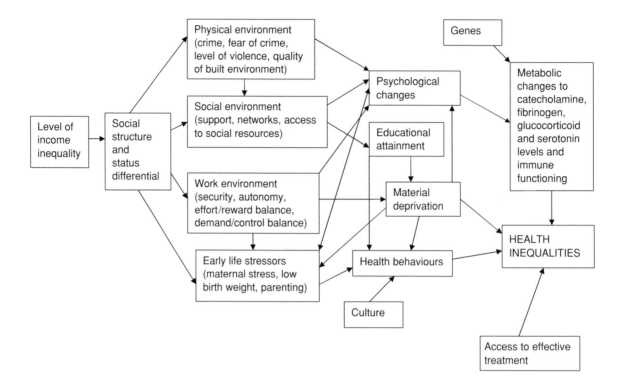

Fig. 14.4　Proposed causal pathway for health inequalities in developed countries.

3. reducing the social gradient in health – reducing the slope (see Figure 14.1).

All three are potentially effective ways to alleviate the unequal burden of illness experienced by socially disadvantaged groups; however, they differ significantly in their underlying value base and their implications for programme development and implementation.

Initiatives to reduce health inequalities act at four different levels [34]:
- strengthening individuals
- strengthening communities
- improving access to essential facilities and services
- encouraging macro-economic and cultural change.

Which level we focus on depends on which of the three policy approaches above we are adopting. The first two approaches target individuals and communities. These enable us to align action with more general, usually area-based efforts to tackle disadvantage but geographical approaches can miss a significant proportion of those in need [35]. Tackling the social gradient in health requires a more population-wide and comprehensive approach that will involve major structural and cultural change. The three approaches are not mutually exclusive, however, and can build on each other.

Strengthening individuals

The constraints on people living in disadvantaged circumstances limit the effects of individual approaches. For example, untargeted health education messages can actually increase health inequalities because of differential uptake by more advantaged groups. Many lifestyle interventions fail to recognise the context within which disadvantaged people live. Unhealthy lifestyles are often symptoms of inequality as much as causes and in some cases can be seen as rational responses to the chronic stressors being endured [36]. Targeted approaches to support disadvantaged people to stop smoking, improve their diet and increase levels of physical exercise need to be carefully delivered so as not to further contribute to the perceptions of the disadvantaged individuals' low social status.

Interventions which aim to strengthen individuals need to be geared towards

- improving the individual's social status in relation to peers and others
- improving the perception of the individual's social status
- strengthening their abilities to cope with demands
- improving their social networks.

The 'independent inquiry into inequalities in health' report [37] suggested that work with individuals should focus on children and parents including expectant mothers, adults at work and older people. The best ways to do this at an individual level are through education, empowerment and improving access to material and social resources. Appropriate interventions therefore focus on

- improving the quality of school-based education (including health education) in disadvantaged areas
- promoting adult education and life-long learning and supporting access to it through benefits, child care, etc.
- providing access to cheap, high-quality preschool education
- providing support for parents, particularly new, lone and young parents
- providing youth support schemes that educate and empower young people and delay pregnancy (including access to emergency contraception)
- encouraging social clubs, groups and associations and ensuring easy access to them (including public transport)
- improving social welfare benefits and pensions to narrow the gap between those who depend on them and average incomes
- improving individual access to financial resources, e.g. credit unions and community-based financial institutions
- improving access to high-quality work (with an appropriate demand/control and effort/reward balance)
- increasing individual autonomy in the workplace particularly in those places where many disadvantaged individuals work, e.g. factories, call centres, hospitality, retail, agriculture
- supporting disabled people's entry back into jobs.

Strengthening communities

Individual social support and community social cohesion are important in protecting health [22]. Therefore policies which promote these and reduce social exclusion of disadvantaged groups and communities are an important part of any strategy to address health inequalities.

Social capital is a term used to denote the level of resources made available through co-operation, trust and networks. Robert Putman [38], who popularised the concept of social capital, calls it 'the connections among individuals – social networks and the norms of reciprocity and trustworthiness that arise from them' [39]. Other work distinguishes between *bonding, bridging* and *linking* social capital.

Bonding social capital relates to the strength of social ties within a given area or community; bridging refers to social links and networks between communities; and linking social capital refers to social connections between the community and its power structures. In most developed countries the power structures which impact most on people's lives are government and public services. Research suggests that, in general, bonding social capital – shown by a strong sense of identity and strong social bonds within the community – is not associated with community health. It is often higher in disadvantaged communities with poor health [25]. It is now thought that bridging and linking social capital – i.e. weaker, wider social ties and a more equal relationship with organisations that impact on the community – seem to predict community health better.

In the UK the multisite Social Action Research Project (SARP) of the Health Development Agency (now part of the National Institute for Health and Clinical Effectiveness) aimed to explore how the growing research on the importance of social capital for community health might impact on the way we work with disadvantaged communities. In Salford we found that increasing social capital meant involving citizens in developing policies that affect them and in designing and delivering the services they use. Doing this in ways that increased bridging and linking social capital, which improved the social status of individuals and perceptions of that community by outsiders, required a change of mindset from both community members and public service organisations (see Box 14.2). This kind of action research makes it clear that *how* we work with disadvantaged communities is as important as *what* we do if we are to tackle health inequalities.

Ensuring access to essential facilities and services

Efforts to strengthen individuals and communities are likely to have a limited effect on health inequalities. They often alleviate the symptoms rather than the causes of inequality. Broader policy initiatives aimed at improving living and

Box 14.2 Lessons learned from the Salford Social Action Research Project

When working with disadvantaged communities it is important to:

- Focus on identifying the existing and potential assets of that community rather than simply their needs and deficits. Focus on the positives!
- Move away from the idea that we need to *build* capacity to the idea that we need to identify and *release* capacity within the community. This forces us to look at the resourcefulness within the community and to the barriers to those resources being utilised effectively. It forces us to look at the barriers we impose and how we may remove them.
- Develop more equal and *reciprocal* relationships between community members and service providers and local government, e.g. co-mentoring schemes, local exchange trading schemes (LETS), employing community members as researchers, participatory democracy models, etc.
- Shift the focus from working with individuals and groups within the community to stimulating collective community action. This means identifying the community's 'burning issues' and supporting the community to take collective action to address these issues themselves.
- Challenge assumptions on all sides through dialogue and enquiry. This means spending time to get to know each other's worlds.
- Move away from offering training to developing shared learning opportunities.
- Recognise that the organisational development of government and public service organisations to help them change their ways of working is as important as any community development.

The author acknowledges the Salford SARP steering group in the development of this learning; in particular Jennie Popay, Gerry Stone, Anne-Marie Pickup, Emma Rowbottom, Owen Gilliker, Kelly McElroy, Diane Plamping, Julian Pratt, Steve Cropper, Alan Higgins, Steve Young and Diana Martin.

working conditions will be vital for major sustained reductions in health inequalities. Very often the facilities and services in areas of, or for groups in, greater need are worse than those in lesser need: 'the inverse care law [40]'. Services and facilities that are required by all to promote health include a decent living and working environment and access to goods and services deemed to be essential today. What constitutes 'essential' varies from culture to culture and over time. Economists have always recognised that this is relative. Adam Smith said over 200 years ago that what was necessary was what the 'customs of the country renders it indecent for creditable people' to be without. In his time this was a linen shirt. Today's economists define poverty in terms of the capabilities required to lead a proper, fulfilling life [41].

What constitutes a 'proper' living environment today?

We expect where we live to include:

- clean, graffiti-free public space
- provision of clean, safe, play areas for children and traffic calming measures in residential streets
- clean air and water
- high quality, well designed, affordable housing
- safe environments designed to reduce crime and the fear of crime
- environments that encourage leisure, walking and cycling
- efficient and affordable public transport
- affordable leisure opportunities
- access to appropriate local shops. (Out of town shopping centres usually discriminate against those without cars, those who can't drive, disabled and older people.)

All of these impact on health both directly and indirectly through their impact on our sense of self-control and self-worth. Their unequal distribution will contribute to health inequalities.

List factors that, if universally available at work, would contribute to a reduction in health inequalities:

- strong health and safety policies and practices
- appropriate job intensity, variety and job control
- management practices that encourage more autonomy at work
- jobs with a good balance between effort and reward
- anti-discrimination policies at work
- economic development that reduces unemployment and job insecurity
- access to high quality training and learning.

Universal access to which essential services would also reduce health inequalities?

- high quality, affordable child care
- affordable, high quality pre school education
- high-quality schools
- facilities for life-long learning and adult education
- parental support services
- contraceptive services including access to emergency contraception
- high-quality, affordable primary care services especially in disadvantaged areas and for disadvantaged groups, e.g. homeless, refugees, prisoners, drug users.
- high-quality, community-based mental health care.
- high-quality care services for vulnerable and looked-after children
- effective and efficient secondary and tertiary care health services
- appropriate services for older people.

What should the health service do to address health inequalities?

- be funded publicly with resources distributed according to need rather than by activity levels
- ensure access to high-quality primary care for all
- understand and reduce the potential barriers to access for disadvantaged groups – costs of care, travel and time off work, lack of child care, culture, language etc
- ensure equal uptake of treatment for those conditions amenable to intervention.

Ensuring equitable access to these essential goods, facilities and services is important in tackling health inequalities. However, even this will not be enough without major macro-economic and cultural change.

Encouraging macro-economic and cultural change

National, provincial, regional and international policies influence the distribution of many of the determinants of health, and have a major impact on the extent and nature of health inequalities within a country, state and region (see Chapter 16). In order to tackle the root causes of health inequalities within a society and the social gradient we need to tackle income inequality and resulting differentials in social status. A strategy of narrowing those income inequalities through taxation, welfare benefits, pension entitlements, and the setting and monitoring of decent wages is likely over time to impact significantly on health inequalities. Manipulating direct taxation is an effective strategy to redistribute wealth within a society and to reduce income differentials. Indirect taxation (e.g. value added tax, goods and services tax) increases income differentials.

Other fiscal action likely to have an impact on health inequalities includes:

- equitable distribution (i.e. according to need not demand) of resources for public services
- laws that affect the quality of work, e.g. in the European Union – the Working time Directive, which restricts excessive work hours
- setting and monitoring building and design standards for urban planning and housing, particularly social housing
- producing laws and incentives to reduce environmental pollution and rigorously enforcing them
- antidiscrimination laws.

Conclusion

The nature of the society in which we live and work is crucial for reducing, sustaining or widening health inequalities. Encouraging a co-operative and collective approach to society versus fostering an individualistic, competitive approach to life is central to tackling health inequalities. How successful governments are at creating a co-operative society will be reflected in that society's attitudes to women, ethnic minorities, people with disabilities and older people. Intolerance in general and racist violence in particular are markers of a society in which social-status differentials predominate and low-status communities seek to achieve some sort of dominance over their near equals. Anti-discrimination laws and policies and ways to promote tolerance are all important in addressing inequalities. Participatory forms of democracy help foster this collectivism.

REFERENCES

1. J. Y. Nazroo, Genetic, cultural or socioeconomic vulnerability? Explaining ethnic inequalities in health. *Sociology of Health and Illness*, **20**, 1998, 714–34.
2. C. Pickin, S. Karlsen, C. McLean, and G. Randhawa, Ethnicity and health inequalities. *INpho* issue 2, Cambridge, Eastern Region Public Health Observatory.
3. Inequalities in health: report of a research working group (Black report). London, Department of Health and Social Security, 1980.
4. M. Whitehead, *The Health Divide*. London, Pelican Books, 1988.
5. M. Whitehead, P. Townsend and N. Davidson, *Inequalities in Health: the Black Report/ the Health Divide*, London, Penguin, 1992.
6. J. P. Mackenbach, Health Inequalities: Europe in Profile. London, Department of Health, 2006.
7. M. G. Marmot, and M. J. Shipley, 'Do socioeconomic differences in mortality persist after retirement? 25 year follow-up of civil servants from the first Whitehall study'. *British Medical Journal*, **313**, 1996, 1177–80.
8. M. Whitehead and G. Dahlgren, What can be done about inequalities in health? *Lancet*, **338**, 1991, 1059–63.
9. J. P. Mackenbach, Socioeconomic inequalities in health in the Netherlands: impact of a five year research programme. *British Medical Journal*, **309**, 1994, 1487–91.
10. M. G. Marmot and R. G. Wilkson RG (eds.), *Social Determinants of Health*, Oxford, Oxford University Press, 1999.
11. F. Diderichsen, T. Evans and M. Whitehead, The Social Basis of Disparities in Health. In *Challenging Inequities in Health – from Ethics to Action*, T. Evans, M. Whitehead, F. Diderichsen and A. Bhuiya (eds.), New York, Oxford University Press, 2001.
12. M. Marmot, *Status Syndrome*, London, Bloomsbury Publishing, 2004.
13. R. G. Wilkinson, *The Impact of Inequality – How to Make Sick Societies Healthier*, New York, The New Press, 2005.
14. R. G. Wilkinson, *Unhealthy Societies: the Afflictions of Inequality*, London, Routledge, 1996.
15. B. P. Kennedy, I. Kawachi and D. Prothrow-Smith, Income distribution and mortality: cross sectional ecological study of the Robin Hood index in the United States. *British Medical Journal*, **312**, 1996, 1004–7.
16. R. M. Sapolsky, Endocrinology al fresco; psychoendocrine studies of wild baboons. *Recent Progress in Hormone Research*, **48**, 1993, 437–68.

17. C. A Shively and T. B. Clarkson, Social status and coronary artery atherosclerosis in female monkeys. *Arteriosclerosis and Thrombosis*, **14**, 1994, 721–26.

18. M. Kristenson, Z. Orth-Gomer, B. Kucinskiene, *et al.*, Attenuated cortisol response to a standardised stress test in Lithuania versus Swedish men: the LiVicordia Study. *International Journal of Behavioural Medicine* **591**, 1998, 17–30.

19. E. J. Brunner, M. G. Marmot, K. Nanchahal, *et al.*, Social inequality in coronary risk: central obesity and the metabolic syndrome. Evidence from the Whitehall II study. *Diabetologia*, **40**, 1997, 1341–9

20. D. I. W. Phillips and D. J. P. Barker, Association between low birth weight and high resting pulse in adult life: is the sympathetic nervous system involved in programming the insulin resistance syndrome? *Diabetic Medicine*, **14**, 1997, 673–77.

21. D. I. W. Phillips, B. R. Walker, D. E. H. Reynolds *et al.*, Low birth weight predicts elevated plasma cortisol concentrations in adults from 3 populations. *Hypertension* **35**(6), 2000, 1301–6.

22. L. F. Berkman and T. Glass, Social integration, social networks, social support and health. In *Social Epidemiology*, L.F Berkman and I. Kawachi (eds.), Oxford, Oxford University Press, 2000.

23. M. G. Marmot and S. L. Syme, Acculturation and coronary heart disease in Japanese Americans. *American Journal of Epidemiology*. **104**(3), 1976, 225–47. Sep.

24. S. Cohen W. J. Doyle, D. P. Skoner, B. S. Rabin and J. M. Gwaltney, Social ties and the susceptibility to the common cold. *Journal of the American Medical Association*, **277**, 1997, 940–4.

25. C. Campbell, R. Wood and M. Kelly, *Social Capital and Health*. Oxford, Blackwell, 1999.

26. H. Kuper, M. Marmot and H. Hemingway, Psychosocial factors in the aetiology and prognosis of coronary disease. A systematic review. *Seminars in Vascular Medicine* **2**(3), 2002, 267–314.

27. Z. Or, Determinants of health outcomes in industrialised countries: a pooled, cross country, time series analysis. Paris, Organisation for Economic Co-operation and Development, 2000.

28. J. P. Mackenbach, A. Looman, A. E. Kunst *et al.,* Post 1950 mortality trends and medical care: gains in life expectancy due to decline in mortality from conditions amenable to medical intervention in the Netherlands. *Social Science and Medicine*, **27**(9), 1998, 889–94.

29. J. P. Bunker, H. S. Frazier and F. Mosteller, Improving health care: measuring effects of medical care. *Milbank Quarterly*, **72**, 1994, 225–58.

30. D. J. P. Barker, *Mothers, Babies and Health in Later Life*, Edinburgh. Churchill Livingston.

31. R. Gitau, A. Cameron, N. M. Fisk and V. Glover, Foetal exposure to maternal cortisol. *Lancet*, **352**, 1998, 707–8.

32. M. Bartley, D. Blane and G. Davey-Smith (eds.), *Sociology of Health Inequalities*, Oxford, Blackwell, 1998.

33. H. Graham and M. P. Kelly, Health inequalities: concepts, frameworks and policy. Briefing paper, NHS Health Development Agency, 2004.

34. M. Benzeval, K. Judge and M. Whitehead (eds.), *Tackling Inequalities in Health – an Agenda for Action*. London, Kings Fund, 1995.

35. G. Smith, Area Based Initiatives CASE paper 25. London, Centre for Analysis of Social exclusion, London School of Economics, 1991.
36. H. Graham, *Hardship and Health in Women's Lives.* London, Harvester Wheatsheaf, 1993.
37. D. Acheson (chair), Independent enquiry into inequalities in health report. London, H. M. Stationery Office, 1998.
38. R. Putnam, Bowling Alone. The Collapse and Revival of American Community, New York, Simon and Schuster, 2000.
39. M. Woolcock and D. Narayan, Social capital: implications for development theory, research and policy. *World Bank Research Observer*, **15**, 2000, 225–49.
40. J. Tudor Hart, The inverse care law. *Lancet*, **297**, 1971, 404–12.
41. A. Sen *Inequality Reexamined*, Oxford, Oxford University Press, 1992.
42. I. Kawachi, B. P. Kennedy, K. Lochner and D. Prothrow-Smith, Social capital, income inequality and mortality. *American Journal of Public Health*, **87**, 1997, 1491–8.

15

Health policy
Richard Lewis

Key points

- Public policy goes beyond the formal decisions of government and is also determined by what governments choose not to do.
- The social, political and cultural context within which policy is developed is an important determinant of policy content.
- Health care policy is strongly influenced by the existence of 'structural interests' (such as the medical profession) that enjoy significant power to influence policy goals.
- Policy-making and policy implementation are intertwined and policy development continues during its implementation.
- Health policy in England is seeking to improve efficiency, cost containment and service quality through the use of market incentives.
- The Labour governments since 1997 have been more successful in improving health services than they have in improving longer-term trends in population health.

The policy process

Introduction

This chapter considers the nature of health policy with special reference to public health. An understanding of how policy is made is an important means by which the health practitioner can comprehend the service within which they work – and perhaps change it. The policy process is the means by which particular policies emerge and are pursued by governments and government agencies. Policy-making is also influenced by the wider political and social environment (or 'context') within which it is developed and implemented.

Essential Public Health, eds. Stephen Gillam, Jan Yates and Padmanabhan Badrinath.
Published by Cambridge University Press. © Cambridge University Press 2007.

The nature of 'policy' and how it should best be studied is highly contested. Some political scientists seek to understand the policy process by studying institutions and their formal rules and procedures; some by examining the actions of those involved in policy through empirical study; others by seeking to identify how power is distributed to provide dominance over the policy process itself.

The task of the student is not to select one optimal approach (and there are many more than have been touched on here), but rather to understand when one approach or another is particularly helpful in illuminating a particular question within a particular context. Indeed, policy may be best understood as the consequence of the interrelation of 'actors' (those people or organisations that populate the process), the wider context, the process by which policy is made and the content of the policy itself – i.e. what it is designed to achieve [1].

What do we mean by 'policy' and the 'policy process'

There is much confusion over the use of the term 'policy'. A common-sense approach might be to equate public policy with the formal decisions or explicit proposals of governments or public agencies. Yet to focus on explicit decisions misses a more subtle picture – one in which 'a forceful implicit policy' may emerge from a series of apparently unrelated decisions [2], or in which governments or public agencies do not control the outcomes of intended policies with any great certainty. In fact, government policy may be as much about what they choose not to do as with what they choose to do [3].

Descriptions of the policy process as a system have tended to be dominated in recent years by two opposing schools of thought – the 'rationalists' and the 'incrementalists'. 'Rational' models of the policy process attempt to describe it in terms of a series of linked, but distinct phases and types of activity that together produce 'a policy'. Such an approach is 'technocratic' rather than political – fundamentally based on the application of a logical and apparently sequential set of functions and technical skills that will ensure that an appropriate and feasible response is generated to a 'policy problem'.

The World Health Organization famously produced a description of the process for health services development with eight sequential stages [4]. Walt [2] simplified this rational approach to four key stages: problem identification and issue recognition; policy formulation; policy implementation; and policy evaluation.

While such a rational model is attractive in that it identifies the types of activities that are very likely to be present in the policy process, Charles Lindblom has criticised the notion that values and objectives (i.e. the policy 'ends') can be identified separately to any consideration of the policy 'means' [5]. In actual decision-making, he suggested, policy makers should not set prior aims but should seek only to move from the status quo by small steps and by reaching agreement among competing interest groups – human beings simply do not possess the ability to process all necessary information to make 'rational' decisions.

Lindblom's analysis was itself challenged. Would not incremental change risk taking policy endlessly round in meaningless circles [6] or be inadequate as a means of coping with dynamic societal change [7]? Nevertheless, the importance of incrementalism is that it emphasised the value of empirical studies of what actually happened in practice. It also served to open the door to a more complex consideration of the interplay between policy actors and the policy process.

The context for policy making

Policies exist in a context which reflects both constraints and opportunities within the broader environment within which any policy is located [8]. Leichter [9] identified four distinct sets of contextual factors that would impact on national health policy:
1. situational factors (transient conditions such as war that allow governments to introduce policies otherwise considered out of bounds)
2. structural factors (relatively unchanging elements in society such as the political regime)
3. cultural factors (reflecting the values within society)
4. environmental factors (those that impinge on states from their contact with other countries).

At a more practical level, context will include factors such as the existing relationships between organisations and local interest groups and the local population's health status.

One important contextual factor of particular interest to those studying health policy is that of 'professionalism'. Professionals wield power by virtue of their specialist knowledge, ability to control the supply of their membership and to regulate their own affairs. As a result professionals enjoy high degrees of autonomy and discretion.

Robert Alford's classic study of the New York health system [10] identified key interests within the policy process. 'Professional monopolisers' (the medical profession) were the dominant power within the system, challenged only by 'corporate rationalisers' (managerial interests) who sought to exert control over the medical professionals. The interests of community groups and patients exercised little power within the health care system and were described by Alford as 'repressed'. Importantly, Alford suggested that professional power allowed the medical interest group to control the ideological and cultural environment that supported their dominant position. Alford was able to invert a long-held view of professional power [10]:

several writers have argued that it is the high esteem in which physicians are held by society which provides them with the leverage they have to influence the content of legislation . . . If I am correct in asserting the importance of dominant structural interests, then the causal order may be precisely the reverse. Rather than a societal consensus giving the doctors power, it is the doctors' power which generates the societal consensus.

The position of the medical profession within the British policy process has been described as a 'state-licensed elite'. The predominance of medical interests since the formation of the NHS has been held to represent a form of 'ideological corporatism,' where governments and the profession share a similar world view [11].

However, a number of conflicts have emerged recently between government and the medical profession. For example, the introduction of market-based reforms to the NHS since the 1980s have been a source of on-going public tensions between government and the British Medical Association and Royal College of Nursing. Successive governments have also changed the contractual terms which bound both independently contracted and employed professionals to the NHS. The fact that many of these reforms were pursued in the teeth of opposition from professional interests suggests that the prevailing corporatist accommodation between government and professions is weaker now than it once was [12].

Implementation as part of the policy process

In the rational models of the policy process described above, implementation featured as a distinct phase that would occur once the formal 'policy' had been created. This was based on an assumption that implementation was somehow simply a 'technical' or 'managerial' process unconnected to the more vital issue of policy content.

This essentially 'top-down' conceptualisation of the policy process (where administrators faithfully implement policy coming down from a political policy-making cadre) has been challenged by a welter of empirical policy studies. These studies suggest that policy implementation is fundamentally intertwined with 'policy-making'. In this view, policy is made 'bottom-up' by those responsible for implementation.

The bottom-up approach is based on two propositions: that the selection of policy solutions may occur during implementation (i.e. policies may not always be clearly defined prior to their operationalisation); and that the behaviour of implementers may mediate the policy content or its outcome.

Lipsky [13] identified a key role for 'street-level bureaucrats' who were able to alter policy outcomes through the way in which they chose to respond to pressures from above. An examination of Dutch policy on heart transplants showed that national policy was deliberately subverted by health service providers [14]. A study of implementation of primary care policy in London demonstrated that front line managers were able to reinterpret policy instructions from government to fit more closely with their own values. Their power derived, in part at least, from their expertise that was required during implementation [15].

Health care institutions therefore may pursue their own organisational strategies and policy-making agenda and are unlikely to see themselves as passive implementers of government policy. Indeed, NHS organisations have their own collective interest group (the NHS Confederation) that actively promotes policy and seeks to influence government opinion.

Governments may be more active in pursuing their own aims in the face of this mediation where:

- the policies in question are core to their political programme
- there is a high degree of public concern over the issue
- governments have their own sources of technical expertise
- interest groups are poorly mobilised [15].

Conclusion

From this theoretical discussion of the policy process we can infer a number of things that may be useful to the student seeking to understand the dynamics of health policy in the UK or abroad.

There is likely to be only limited use in focusing attention on formal policy documents or government decisions. In the 'real world' policy is far more complex than that set out in official papers, and the policy process is far more dynamic. Important policies may not even be acknowledged with their own dedicated prospectus, emerging instead from a series of apparently unrelated activities. Governments have a tendency to introduce bold policies that aim to transform one realm of activity or another. In practice, their ability to achieve change on the ground is rather more constrained in many cases.

The government of the day is, of course, a hugely important actor in making policy but it is by no means the only actor. Some interests, particularly the medical profession, enjoy significant structural power – that is, their views are always listened to and they enjoy a privileged position within the policy process. However, as recent history has shown, they do not always win the day. The power of those charged with implementation should not be underestimated. Implementation is no technical afterthought, but a vital part of the policy-making process where bargaining over policy content continues.

Contemporary health policy

This section considers briefly some of the main features of health policy in England since the election of the Labour government in 1997. The fact that it is necessary to identify exactly which part of the British health service is under consideration points to a very important feature of policy-making in the post-devolution era. England, Wales and Scotland have adopted very different paths to health service policy, notwithstanding that the Labour Party dominates government in all three countries. Britain is in the midst of a natural experiment on how best to run a national health service.

According to one of its architects the Labour government's reform agenda can be divided into three overlapping strategies [16]. The first dimension of reform was to improve the provision of care through a mix of initiatives such as increasing the supply of professionals, supporting learning and innovation, and improving the physical infrastructure. This was supported by a giant leap forward in NHS funding announced in 2000. Current commitments to NHS spending increases suggest that UK spending on health (both public and private) will have risen from around 7% of gross domestic product (GDP) in 2000 to reach about 10% by 2009, a proportion of GDP approaching that of the European average [17].

The second dimension of reform was referred to as 'hierarchical challenge' – setting national standards and targets, introducing inspection of providers, intervening in local provision where required, and publishing information on performance. The third dimension of reform focused on a 'localist challenge' through the development of the 'commissioning' function in local health agencies, giving patients rights to choose their provider and introducing a diverse market of providers supported by new financial incentives.

Of course, such a neat exposition of the government's programme is partly a post hoc rationalisation of what was in reality a rather more reactive and negotiated process. What is clear is that the Labour government's approach to health policy has relied on both top-down and highly directive central planning while simultaneously creating a mechanism designed to drive change from the bottom-up. Moreover, a new political consensus around the management of the NHS has emerged – at the 2005 general election the similarities between the major political parties in terms of their plans for the NHS was striking.

The drive for efficiency and cost containment

The Labour Party came to power in 1997 advocating an end to competitive markets and private-sector involvement in clinical services, promoting instead a more cooperative planning approach [18]. An early, and highly symbolic, act was to abolish GP fundholding (where general practitioners received budgets with which to purchase some of their patients' care).

Yet the main architecture of the quasi market was retained, notably the split between purchasing and providing and, by 2006, the Labour governments had gone further in introducing market-inspired reforms than their Conservative predecessors would have dared. The main features of this market-based system include:

- new financial incentives (fees for each hospital treatment given) designed to promote competition between providers
- rights for patients to choose from among at least four providers for most consultant-led services, and an unlimited choice of providers that meet NHS standards and prices by 2008
- diversification of supply in hospital and primary care with national and local procurement of independent-sector provision
- greater autonomy of NHS providers through the replacement of central accountability of NHS hospitals to the Department of Health with accountability of 'foundation trusts' to local people and to an independent regulator.

So what can explain this apparent volte face? The move towards markets was inspired by a number of concerns. Firstly, the substantial investment in NHS services since 2000 had seen productivity fall, at least as measured by the NHS 'efficiency index' (put simply, rises in clinical activity have not matched the rises in funding). There emerged an increasing concern that an abundance of funds had led to inefficient practices and only modest gains for patients. However, there was also a parallel concern that the public-monopoly nature of the NHS had led to a lack of responsiveness to the needs of individual patients. Without challenge, and the potential for patients to 'exit' the system, providers might lack motivation to listen to their customers. The 'patient choice' policy, underpinned by new financial incentives designed to reward hospitals that attract more patients and punish those that lose custom, is intended to improve responsiveness to the needs of patients.

It is not clear at the time of writing whether these policies will achieve these objectives. Whether the reform prescription is the right one is highly contested. Proponents of health care markets point to evidence of improvements in efficiency at the time of the introduction of the quasi market in the 1990s [19]. However, there is a clear danger that 'supplier-induced demand' will result from the introduction of fee-for-service incentives leading to an oversupply of expensive hospital care [20]. Furthermore, hospitals may prioritise those services from which they make a financial surplus, rather than those that might most benefit their population's health.

Even the government has admitted that unless the commissioning function within primary care trusts and general practices is significantly and rapidly improved, hospitals are likely to increase activity and hospital spending. For this reason, the government has now switched its focus to strengthening the commissioning function.

Tackling professional power – the drive to improve quality

As was noted above, the relationship between government and the professions has not been uniformly smooth. While the Conservative government of 1990 imposed new contractual conditions on general practitioners and dentists, these new contracts were deemed to have failed by the mid 1990s with still little influence being wielded by government over the activities of professionals or the quality of care they provided.

The groundwork for a radical overhaul of general practice was laid by the Conservatives in the mid 1990s and the Labour government inherited and enacted the Primary Care Act of 1997. This Act served to end the national monopoly of independently contracted general practitioners, allowing new entrants to the previously closed market place. It also undercut the power of the national negotiating machinery by introducing for the first time local contracts negotiated directly between providers and local health service authorities [17].

This implicit challenge to the medical profession has continued so that, by 2004, 37% of general practitioners held contracts negotiated with local primary care trusts rather than the national contract [22]. An increasing number of general practitioners are now employed on a salaried basis rather than holding the traditional status of independent contractor. New regulations mean that private corporations are able to bid for contracts and the Department of Health is tendering to diversify the market place [23]. Attempts to reform the working practices of hospital doctors have proved harder to achieve in practice, although a new contract was implemented in 2003 after protracted negotiation.

The desire to tackle professional autonomy also had its roots in a growing public disquiet about quality of care that affected a number of developed countries. In 1991 an important research study in the USA discovered an alarming rate of 'adverse incidents' in which patients were harmed, and sometimes killed, by the treatments intended to help them [24]. A similar finding emerged from Australia [25]. Evidence also came to light in the 1990s that children were dying due to poor quality of heart surgery at the Bristol Royal Infirmary [26]. Worse still the culture of secrecy and self-protection among doctors and managers meant no action was taken to prevent this harm once it came to light. The arrest for murder in 1998 of Dr Harold Shipman added to this change in the climate of public opinion.

One result of this exposure of medical 'dirty linen' was the demand for greater public accountability. The case for reform of the machinery of professional self-regulation was made, in particular to increase lay representation. The Chief Medical Officer was instrumental in a campaign to end the myth of professional infallibility, exhorting the NHS to acknowledge mistakes and to learn from them [27].

The government's response was to introduce a raft of new structures and requirements of professional staff in the NHS to secure quality [28]. New national service frameworks set out expected quality standards for a number of major clinical conditions (see Chapter 16). A National Institute for Clinical Excellence was introduced to draw up care guidelines based on the best available evidence. Professional staff were instructed to take part in 'clinical governance', a new form of professional accountability to ensure the maintenance and improvement of clinical standards, and doctors are now to face periodic 'revalidation' of their competence to practise [29].

The Commission for Healthcare Improvement (now the Healthcare Commission) was established to inspect NHS providers and more recently general practices. The Department of Health subsequently developed a range of care standards that all NHS providers are expected to comply with.

As a consequence of this package of reform, the behaviour of clinicians in the NHS is now directed, monitored and accredited more than ever before. While these reforms may begin to address concerns relating to variations in clinical practice, potential new hazards, such as 'defensive medicine' (where patients face over-treatment) and high costs of regulation, may emerge.

Better health as well as better health services?

While much of the public's attention has been drawn towards the debate over how best to improve health services, the government has also developed a substantial public health agenda. One of the first major policy statements made by the Labour government was 'Saving Lives: Our Healthier Nation [30]'. This made an avowed effort to focus on the outputs of the health system – reduced health inequalities, better survival rates for diseases such as cancer and heart disease.

The financial as well as health benefits of securing a healthier population were brought into sharp relief by the report by financier Sir Derek Wanless commissioned by the Chancellor, Gordon Brown [31]. In his projection of health expenditure, Wanless calculated that a population that was uninvolved in promoting its own health would be significantly more expensive than one that was 'fully engaged'.

Other policies developed the theme of public health. The new general practice contract in 2004 provided a wide range of financial incentives to encourage GPs to prevent, identify and manage a number of chronic diseases. In 2005, a further public health white paper, 'Choosing Health', was launched (see Box 15.1 for details). This paper demonstrated a shift in emphasis by the government: less about delivering public health interventions at the population level and more about supporting health-promoting choices by individuals (such as in relation to smoking, alcohol and obesity).

Box 15.1 Government priorities for public health

Priorities for action in 'Choosing Health – making healthy choices easier'
- Reducing the numbers of people who smoke
- Reducing obesity and improving diet and nutrition
- Increasing exercise
- Encouraging and supporting sensible drinking
- Improving sexual health
- Improving mental health

This theme was continued in 2006 with the publication of 'Our health, our care, our say' [23]. This white paper contained a number of new (and rather more recycled) policies designed to improve health. In particular, it proposed that patients should receive more help in managing their diseases in the shape of education and information. All people should be offered the opportunity to complete a health questionnaire on-line, with those most at risk receiving the services of a 'health trainer'. Greater integration between health and social services is to be promoted and the Director of Public Health is to have a new role in assessing the overall health and well being of the local population. Cross-cutting activity, involving a range of public services, is seen as a key to improving health.

Against its own targets, the government can claim to have been broadly successful. Targets for reduced deaths from cancer and heart disease look set to be met. Yet when looked at more critically, many of the achievements are simply in line with longer-term trends in disease prevention and survival.

Perhaps more worryingly, progress on dealing with health inequalities has been elusive. The government has continually stressed its commitment to reduce inequalities between the richest and poorest populations. A key target was set in 2001 – by 2010 to reduce by at least 10% the gap between the fifth of local authority areas with the lowest life expectancy at birth and the population as a whole. The government has established a range of different strategies to tackle health inequalities, including an independent inquiry chaired by Sir Donald Acheson, a review and a programme for action. However, evidence so far suggests that health inequalities are continuing to widen [32].

The government cannot yet claim to have delivered the transformation that its policies and its own financial projections require. Improvements in health status by their very nature are likely to take time to be established and recorded. Whether the range and effectiveness of government interventions will be sufficient to deliver the anticipated impact on health spending that was projected by Sir Derek Wanless remains to be seen.

From public sector to public service

The reform of the health service has become a highly visible and contentious policy arena (notwithstanding a high degree of consensus over broad policy instruments shared by the major political parties). At the heart of the reform process has been a reformulation of the very meaning of the 'public sector'. In England, NHS services are decreasingly supplied by providers owned and controlled by the Department of Health; indeed, such providers will be in a minority if current policies continue to be implemented. Instead, the NHS is gradually being redefined as an entitlement (to comprehensive services free at the point of delivery) rather than as a coherent mechanism of service delivery.

Tony Blair came to power claiming that 'what counts is what works'. In health services, 'what works' can now be sourced from either the public or private sector. However, such pragmatism is not unconstrained. Limits to the involvement of the private sector have been imposed by successive secretaries of State (between 10 and 15% of NHS elective surgery). In addition, foundation trusts were created with elaborate governance structures designed to create at least the appearance of local public control [33].

This points to an unresolved tension at the heart of the Labour government's new public management. If what matters is the ability to access care free at the point of use, rather than the maintenance of NHS services within state control, why has it been necessary to create foundation trusts to offer 'local ownership' of hospitals through membership and rights to elect governors?

The government is seeking the right balance between a consumerist model of delivery based on 'choice' and one based on 'voice'. In the former, the efficient and responsive providers are ensured by the acts of individual patients making choices in the health market place. In the latter, the actions of health care providers are shaped in accordance with the collective interests of patients and the public elicited through an essentially political process.

The challenge for the government now is to develop a coherent system where both these models of provider motivation can operate simultaneously; choice where this is possible, 'voice' where choice is weak.

However, the search for the right form of public accountability continues. The advent of foundation trusts means that the recent secretaries of State are no longer formally accountable for the actions of all NHS hospitals (and will refuse to answer questions in Parliament about 'operational matters' relating to foundation trusts). However, there is little evidence so far that foundation trust 'local ownership' has resulted in significant powers for their members [34].

To bolster local accountability, local authorities have been given an increasing role in holding local health services to account. Alongside this, new forms of 'direct democracy' are to be experimented with, including local 'petitions' by patients in response to apparent service failures [23].

Conclusion

The NHS in England has undergone significant change under the Labour government. This government, like its Conservative predecessor, has shown a clear preferment for market incentives over central planning (indeed the three main political parties share a significant degree of consensus over the main features of their health policy). Unlike the Conservative government that went before, however, the present government has been less hamstrung in introducing such reform. If current plans are implemented fully, the NHS will have changed markedly in a relatively short period of time.

It is too early to tell what impact these new policy solutions will have on the very familiar problems that they are designed to resolve – rising demand and indifferent productivity. These issues have haunted previous governments for many decades and look set to remain for some time to come. Supporters of the NHS were stung by the relatively low ranking (18th) awarded to the British NHS by the WHO when constructing international 'league tables' for health systems [35].

Yet, even if the current government is successful in terms of more effective services delivered with greater efficiency and resulting in better health outcomes, will the fruits be evenly distributed across different populations? In particular, will the government halt the apparently inexorable widening of health inequalities? The early evidence is not encouraging.

REFERENCES

1. G. Walt and L. Gilson, Reforming the health sector in developing countries. *Health Policy and Planning*, **9** (4), 1994, 353–70.
2. G. Walt, *Health Policy: an introduction to process and power*, London, Zed Books.
3. T. Dye, *Top Down Policymaking*, London, Chatham House Publishers, 2001.
4. Guiding principles for the managerial process for national health development. Geneva, WHO, 1980.
5. C. E. Lindblom, The science of muddling through. *Public Administration Review*, **19**, 1959, 79–88.
6. A. Etzioni, Mixed scanning: a 'third' approach to decision-making. *Public Administration Review*, **27**, 1967, 385–92.
7. Y. Dror, Muddling through – science or inertia? *Public Administration Review*, **24**, 1964, 153–7.
8. C. Collins, A. Green and D. Hunter, Health sector reform and the interpretation of policy context. *Health Policy*, **47**, 1999, 69–83.
9. H. M. Leichter, *A Comparative Approach to Policy Analysis: Health Care Policy in Four Nations*, Cambridge, Cambridge University Press, 1979.
10. R. R. Alford, *Health Care Politics*, Chicago, University of Chicago Press, 1975, p. 17.

11. P. Dunleavy, Professions and policy change: notes towards a model of ideological corporatism. *Public Administration Bulletin*, **36**, 1981, 3–16.

12. R. Klein, *The New Politics of the NHS*, 3rd edn, London, Longman, 1995.

13. M. Lipsky, Towards a theory of street-level bureaucracy. In W. D. Hawley, M. Lipsky, S. B. Greenberg *et al.* (eds.), *Theoretical Perspectives on Urban Politics*, Englewood Cliffs, New Jersey, Prentice-Hall, pp. 196–213.

14. A. De Roo and H. Maarse, Understanding the central-local relationship in health care; a new approach. *International Journal of Health Planning and Management*, **5**, 1990, 15–25.

15. R.Q. Lewis, Improving London's primary care – centre–local relations in the implementation of national policy objectives. Ph.D Thesis, London School of Hygiene and Tropical Medicine, University of London, 2001.

16. S. Stevens, Reform strategies for the English NHS. *Health Affairs*, **23** (3), 2004, 37–44.

17. J. Appleby and T. Harrison, *Spending on Health Care – How Much is Enough?* London, King's Fund, 2006.

18. New Labour because Britain deserves better – Britain will be better with new Labour. London, Labour Party, 1997.

19. J. Le Grand, N. Mays and J. Mulligan (eds.), *Learning from the NHS Internal Market – a Review of the Evidence*. London, King's Fund, 1998.

20. R. Lewis and J. Dixon, *NHS Market Futures – Exploring the Impact of Health Service Market Reforms*, London, King's Fund, 2005.

21. R. Lewis, S. Gillam and C. Jenkins (eds.), *Personal Medical Services Pilots – Modernising primary care?* London, King's Fund, 2001.

22. Statistics for general medical practitioners in England: 1994–2004. London, Department of Health, 2005.

23. Our health, our care, our say: a new direction for community services. Cm6737. London, HM Government and Department of Health, 2006.

24. T. A. Brennan, L. L. Leape, N. M. Laird *et al.*, Incidence of adverse events and negligence in hospitalized patients. Results of the Harvard Medical Practice Study I. *New England Journal of Medicine*, **324** (6), 1991, 370–7.

25. R. M. Wilson, W. B. Runciman, R. W. Gibberd *et al.*, The Quality in Australian Health Care Study. *Medical Journal of Australia*, **163** (9), 1995, 458–76.

26. The Report of the Public Inquiry into children's heart surgery at the Bristol Royal Infirmary 1984–1995: Learning from Bristol. Cm 5207. London, H. M. Stationery Office, 2001.

27. Department of Health, An Organisation with a memory: report of an expert group on learning from adverse events in the NHS chaired by the Chief Medical Officer. London, The Stationery Office, 2000.

28. Department of Health, *A first class service. Quality in the new NHS*. London, Stationery Office, 1998.

29. L. Donaldson, Good doctors, safer patients – proposals to strengthen the system to assure and improve the performance of doctors and protect the safety of patients. London, Department of Health, 2006.

30. Department of Health, Saving lives, our healthier nation. London, Stationery Office, 1999.

31. D. Wanless, Securing our future health: taking a long-term view. Final report. London, HM Treasury, 2002.

32. M. Shaw, G. Davey Smith and D. Dorling, Health inequalities and New Labour: how the promises compare with real progress. *British Medical Journal*, **330**, 2005, 1016–21.

33. A short guide to NHS foundation trusts. Department of Health, London, 2003.

34. R. Lewis and L. Hinton, *Putting Health in Local Hands – Early Experiences of Homerton University Hospital NHS Foundation Trust*. London, King's Fund, 2005.

35. The World Health Report 2000: Health systems: improving performance. Geneva, World Health Organisation, 2000.

16

Quality measurement and improvement in health care
Nicholas Steel

Key points

1. Good quality health care makes a large contribution to public health, both by increasing life expectancy and improving quality of life.
2. Quality can be defined; it is multidimensional. The different dimensions of quality can be measured, but some (e.g. clinical effectiveness) are easier to measure than others (e.g. professionals' empathy and respect for patients).
3. Problems with quality of care are widespread, with many people either not receiving effective health care, or receiving care that is ineffective or harmful.
4. Quality of health care for populations can best be improved by change at health-system level.

Introduction

If you had asked a public health professional working in an industrialised country in the late twentieth century whether health care was important for public health, they would most likely have told you that health care contributed very little to population health. In the 1970s McKeown's work showed that improved nutrition had been responsible for most population health improvement from about 1700 up to the middle of the twentieth century (see Introduction). Health care first had an effect on national mortality trends following the introduction of sulphonamides in 1935[1]. The second half of the twentieth century was very different, with many effective health care interventions being developed and coming into routine use for the first time. This has led to a reappraisal of the potential benefits of health care at both an individual and population level.

Modern, effective health care makes a large and increasing contribution to preventing disease and prolonging life, by reducing the population burden of

Essential Public Health, eds. Stephen Gillam, Jan Yates and Padmanabhan Badrinath.
Published by Cambridge University Press. © Cambridge University Press 2007.

disease. Bunker has estimated that about half of the $7\frac{1}{2}$ years of the increase in life expectancy seen in the USA and UK in the second half of the twentieth century can be attributed to health care, with additional benefits in terms of improved quality of life[2]. Increased life expectancy attributable to treatment of a specific condition was estimated from three calculations: the decline in death rates for specific conditions; the increased life expectancy seen with treatment in clinical trials; and an estimate of the proportion of the relevant population receiving effective treatment in routine practice. Changes to the health of populations resulting from the delivery of effective health care can be estimated using measures such as population health impact[3]. However, only the right kind of healthcare can improve health. Health care interventions that are powerful enough to improve population health are also powerful enough to cause harm if incorrectly used.

What is quality and can it be measured?

The science of quality measurement in health care is still young, but it is already generally accepted that quality of health care can be defined, and that elements of quality can be measured. Some dimensions of quality, such as clinical effectiveness, are more straightforward to define and measure quantitatively than 'softer' dimensions such as patient-centred health care. As quality measurement becomes commonplace in health care, there remain concerns that attempts to measure something as complex as quality will inevitably undermine professionalism and the doctor–patient relationship. Thus, paradoxically, measurement may reduce overall quality of care. A more widely held view is that measurement is an essential component of quality improvement. If we do not measure quality, we cannot know whether health services are achieving the level of population health benefit of which they are potentially capable.

Quality has been defined as: 'the degree to which health services for individuals and populations increase the likelihood of desired health outcomes and are consistent with current professional knowledge'[4]. 'Desired health outcomes' is a key phrase as it deliberately does not specify who is doing the desiring. It implicitly accepts that different people will want different outcomes. Desired health outcomes may be different for managers, patients, and clinicians [5]. Managers may be rightly concerned with efficiency, and seek to maximise the population health gain through best use of an inevitably limited budget. Clinicians are usually more focused on effectiveness, and want the treatment that works best for each of their patients. Patients clearly want treatment that works, and also place a high priority on how the treatment is delivered. Coulter [6] has described the following health care aspirations of patients:

> **Box 16.1 A question to think about. . . .**
>
> A 72 year old woman with osteoarthritis of her left hip is booked for a total hip replacement operation. She also suffers from diabetes and mild high blood pressure.
> - List as many aspects of good quality of care in this situation as you can.
> - Who should be involved in assessing quality of care?
> - Describe the likely concerns of the different individuals and groups involved in this situation

- fast access to reliable health advice
- effective treatment delivered by trusted professionals
- participation in decisions and respect for preferences
- clear, comprehensible information and support for self-care
- attention to physical and environmental needs
- emotional support, empathy and respect
- involvement of, and support for, family and carers
- continuity of care and smooth transitions.

Dimensions of quality

The range of different desired outcomes above demonstrates the multidimensional nature of quality. The first stage in any attempt to measure quality is to think about what dimensions of quality should be measured, and what group of people value those dimensions. Two influential taxonomies of quality of health care were published in the 1980s by Donabedian and Maxwell. These frameworks are also used for evaluation (see Chapter 8). Donabedian [7] distinguished between measures of the 'structure, process and outcome' of health care. The structure refers to the characteristics of such things as hospitals, clinics and qualified staff members, and so is relatively easy to measure. Process is the care delivered, and has the advantage that it is under the control of the health-care system, and so theoretically can be changed. Outcome is the resulting change in health status and is clearly the most important measure for public health. However, it has the disadvantage that it is influenced by many factors other than health care, and hence attribution of changes in outcome to changes in particular health processes is difficult, which can hamper attempts to improve health care.

As mentioned in Chapter 8, Maxwell described the following dimensions of quality: effectiveness, efficiency, acceptability, access, equity and relevance [8]. The Institute of Medicine produced a similar list in 2001, calling for health care to be effective, efficient, safe, timely, equitable and patient-centred [4]. Table 16.1

Table 16.1. Examples of quality measures in different dimensions of quality[9]

Measure of quality	Donabedian dimension*	IOM dimension**
Cancer mortality rates	Outcome	Effectiveness
Appropriateness of coronary revascularisation procedures	Process	Effectiveness
Practising physicians per 1,000 patients	Structure	Efficiency/capacity
Adverse events	Process	Safety
Waiting times for elective surgery	Process	Timeliness
Life expectancy geographically	Outcome	Equity
Low birth weight by deprivation	Outcome	Equity
Involvement in decision-making	Process	Patient-centredness

* Structure, process or outcome [7]. * * Effective, efficient, safe, timely, equitable and patient-centred [4].

gives examples of quality measures adapted from a recent chartbook on quality in the NHS [9].

Approaches to quality measurement

Health systems internationally are using more quantitative measures of quality, usually the rates of delivery of effective health care processes. Delivered health care is compared with the health care that should have been delivered, sometimes referred to as indicated care. Indicated care can be set out in guidelines such as those published by the National Institute for Health and Clinical Excellence (NICE) and Scottish Intercollegiate Guidelines Network (SIGN) in the UK, and the US Preventive Services Task Force (USPSTF) in the USA.

A good example of the method by which standards of care are developed is the RAND/ UCLA (University of California, Los Angeles) appropriateness method [10]. This was developed in response to the lack of randomised controlled clinical-trial data on many interventions, and the problems with interpreting sometimes contradictory trial results for use in routine care. It combines research data with clinical expertise, and involves the following stages:

- identifying clinical area(s) of care for quality assessment
- conducting a systematic review of care in the relevant clinical area(s)
- drafting quality indicators
- presenting draft quality indicators and their evidence base to a clinical panel for a modified Delphi process. The Delphi process typically involves asking panel members to rate anonymously the draft indicators for validity, over two rounds, with face-to-face discussion between rounds.
- approving a final set of indicators.

Table 16.2. Example clinical domains and indicators for UK general practitioners 2006–7 [11]

Clinical domain	No. of indicators	Example of indicator in each clinical domain
Hypertension	3	The percentage of patients with hypertension in whom there is a record of the blood pressure in the previous nine months
Asthma	4	The percentage of patients aged eight and over diagnosed as having asthma from 1 April 2006 with measures of variability or reversibility
Depression	2	In those patients with a new diagnosis of depression, recorded between the preceding 1 April to 31 March, the percentage of patients who have had an assessment of severity at the outset of treatment using an assessment tool validated for use in primary care
Chronic kidney disease (CKD)	4	The percentage of patients on the CKD register with hypertension who are treated with an angiotensin converting enzyme inhibitor (ACE-I) or angiotensin receptor blocker (ARB) (unless a contraindication or side effects are recorded)
Smoking indicators	2	The percentage of patients with any or any combination of the following conditions: coronary heart disease, stroke or transient ischemic attack (TIA), hypertension, diabetes, chronic obstructive pulmonary disease (COPD) or asthma who smoke and whose notes contain a record that smoking cessation advice or referral to a specialist service, where available, has been offered within the previous 15 months

The quality standards produced by methods such as this can be used to assess the quality of care in a single clinic or a whole health system. An example of quality assessment on a very large scale is the payment of incentives to general practitioners in the UK on the basis of their performance against quality indicators. Table 16.2 gives examples of indicators from the 2006–7 revision of the British general practitioners' contract [11].

Is there a problem with quality?

We have seen that health care is a powerful tool for improving public health. Like all powerful tools, it can have adverse as well as positive effects. Problems with health care fall into one of three broad categories: underuse, overuse and misuse, all of which are amenable to public health action [12]. Effective health care can be underused, so that people miss out on opportunities to benefit from it. It can be overused, wasting resources by delivering care to those who do not need it, or where the potential for harm exceeds the benefit. Misuse is where patients suffer avoidable complications of surgery or medication. An example of misuse is a patient who suffers a rash after receiving penicillin as treatment for an infection, despite having a known allergy to penicillin.

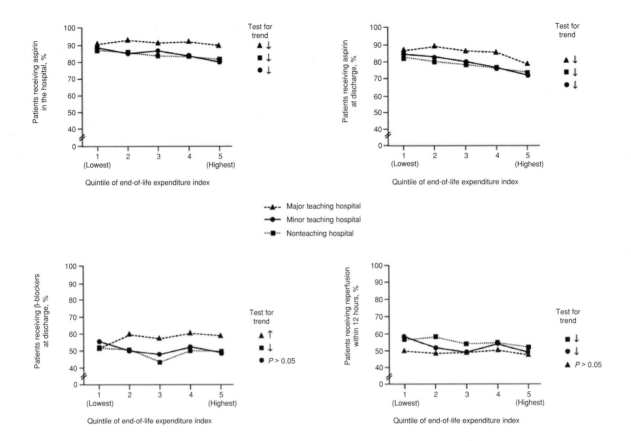

Fig. 16.1 Variations in health
care quality by hospital type and
Medicare spend. Reproduced
with permission from E. S.
Fisher, D. E. Wennberg. T. A.
Stukel *et al.*, The implications of
regional variations in Medicare
spending. Part 1: The content,
quality, and accessibility of care.
Annals of Internal Medicine,
138, 2003, 273–87.

We know effective health care is underused. Many effective interventions are only received by half the people who should receive them [9,13,14,15]. There is also great variability in the quality of care experienced by different populations, by illness, age, sex, race, wealth, geographic location or insurance coverage (Figure 16.1). This problem of inequalities or disparities has been the focus of considerable policy attention, helped by Julian Tudor Hart's devising of his famous inverse care law 'as a weapon' over thirty years ago [16] – see also chapter 14:

The availability of good medical care tends to vary inversely with the need for it in the population served. This . . . operates more completely where medical care is most exposed to market forces, and less so where such exposure is reduced. The market distribution of medical care is a primitive and historically outdated social form, and any return to it would further exaggerate the maldistribution of medical resources.

We also know that care is overused. Wennberg first documented the wide variations in care received by similar populations. He showed that health care is often driven by the availability of specialist services, rather than by the health needs of the population, with no detectable difference in health outcomes [15]. This variation in quantity of health care with no apparent relationship with quality implies that some health care is overused. People are receiving more care than they have the capacity to benefit from (Figure 16.2).

Harm resulting from misuse of health care is a major problem. Adverse drug events have been shown to cause considerable morbidity, mortality and cost in the UK and USA [17]. This patient safety problem is the flip-side of quality, and has also received much policy attention in recent years, including the creation of the National Patient Safety Agency, which aims to improve the safety and quality of care through reporting, analysing and learning from adverse incidents and 'near misses' involving NHS patients.

Four reasons have been identified for these widespread problems with quality[4]:

1. There is a growing complexity of science and technology. Our ability to deliver safe effective health care cannot keep up with the rapid advances in science and medical treatments.

2. There is an increase in chronic conditions. People are now living longer, and chronic conditions are the major cause of disability and death, and consume the majority of health care resources in developed countries.

3. Delivery systems are poorly organised. Most health care systems are still designed to deal primarily with acute health problems, and lack an effective chronic care model.

4. There are constraints on exploiting the revolution in information technology. None of these reasons for widespread quality problems lays the blame on individual clinicians making mistakes. They emphasise the important truism that quality is a property of health systems, and not simply of the health professionals in the system. Human beings will always make occasional mistakes, and experience from other industries has shown that dramatic quality improvement can occur when systems are designed that do not rely on humans avoiding mistakes. In the publication *Crossing the Quality Chasm: a New Health System of the 21st Century*, the Committee on Health Care in America [4] commented that:

The current systems of care cannot do the job. Trying harder will not work. Changing systems of care will.

Also, Mark Chassin and Robert Galvin, together with the Round Table on Health Care Quality [12] wrote that:

Our present efforts resemble a team of engineers trying to break the sound barrier by tinkering with a Model T Ford.

Fig. 16.2　Variations in health-care resource levels and spending. Reproduced with permission from E. S. Fisher, D. E. Wennberg, T. A. Stukel *et al.*, The implications of regional variations in Medicare spending. Part 1: The content, quality, and accessibility of care. *Annals of Internal Medicine*, **138**, 2003, 273–87.

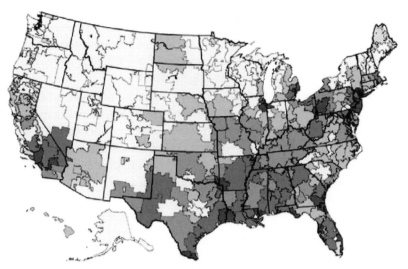

Attributes of U.S. HRRs in Different Quintiles of the EOL-EI*

Variable	Quintile of EOL-EI					Ratio (Highest to Lowest)
	1 (Lowest)	2	3	4	5 (Highest)	
EOL-EI, S[†]	9074	10 636	11 559	12 598	14 644	1.61
Per capita Medicare spending, S[‡]	3922	4439	4940	5444	6304	1.61
Hospital characteristics[§]						
Overall supply (beds per 1000), *n*	2.4	2.6	2.9	2.9	3.2	1.32
Beds in teaching hospitals, %	10.2	18.1	13.8	20.8	28.1	2.76
Beds in hospitals with >300 beds, %	31.6	37.4	38.7	43.8	57.2	1.81
Physician supply (per 10 000), *n*[§]	184.8	189.4	184.4	204.6	242.4	1.31
Medical specialists	26.9	28.8	28.6	34.8	44.4	1.65
General intemists	21.3	23.4	22.6	28.5	37.3	1.75
Family practitioner/GP	35.9	31.3	29.6	25.9	26.5	0.74
Surgeons	43.8	45.6	46	50.3	56.4	1.29
All other specialties	56.8	60.3	57.5	65.1	77.7	1.37
Medicare enrollees in HMOs, %	12.1	6.8	7.3	7.7	15.3	1.26
Residents in metropolitan areas, %	77.5	81.9	82.3	79.2	97.4	1.26

*EOL-EI = End-of-Life Expenditure Index; GP = general practitioner; HMO = health maintenance organization; HRR = hospital referral region.

[†]Average age-sex-race – adjusted per capita fee-for-service spending on hospital and physician services in the HRRs within each quintile for Medicare enrollees age 65–99 years who were in their last 6 months of life. For details, see Methods.

[‡]Average age-sex-race – adjusted 1996 annual per capita fee-for-service spending in the HRRs within each quintile on all Medicare services among enrollees age 65–99 years (9).

[§]Key attributes and average per capita supply of the specified medical resource in the HRRs within that quintile. Per capita supply is calculated per 1000 or per 10 000 residents of the general population within the HRRs (9).

　　Health care is different from other industries, but there is no reason why quality cannot improve. Some of the main approaches used to improve quality in health care are described in the next section.

Table 16.3. Approaches to quality improvement in health care

Type of approach	Example
Regulation and standards	American Board of Medical Specialties in USA, General Medical Council in UK
Education and audit	Royal Colleges, professional organisations
Market and financial	Payment of British general practitioners according to achievement of performance indicators

How can quality of care for populations be improved?

Many different approaches to quality improvement in health care have been tried in the past, with varying levels of success. They can be broadly classified into three groups, as summarised in Table 16.3.

Regulation and standards

A robust regulatory framework is important for assuring a basic standard of health care, and regulation of medical professionals is a central component of quality improvement in nearly all countries. Historically, regulation has been primarily associated with the medical profession, but is increasingly used for non-medical health professionals. Sutherland and Leatherman have described the three main purposes of professional regulation [18]: to set minimally acceptable standards of care; to provide accountability of professionals to patients and payers; and to improve quality of care by providing guidance about best practice.

In the UK, the General Medical Council regulates doctors, and is currently adapting to a new environment where greater levels of public accountability are required. The Healthcare Commission assesses the performance of health care organisations. In the USA the American Board of Medical Specialties oversees certification of doctors. The requirements are a mixture of accredited training, cognitive examination, competency-based evaluation, audit and clinical performance, and certification needs to be renewed every 6 to10 years. Certification status has been shown to be associated with higher quality of care [18]. Accreditation of US hospitals for Medicare reimbursement takes place through the Joint Commission on Accreditation of Healthcare Organisations.

Education and audit

The dominant approach for health professionals has been education and audit, with limited success. Education and audit are common requirements for

Fig. 16.3   The
plan–do–study–act cycle.

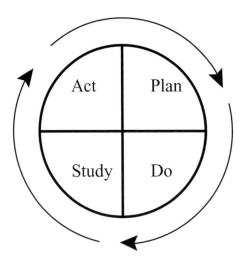

Fig. 16.3   The
plan–do–study–act cycle.

regulation, but go beyond the requirements of regulation in that they seek to go beyond a minimum standard, and strive for excellence. Education has traditionally been professionally led, and is seen by many as an obligation of professional status. Professional organisations, such as the Royal Colleges in the UK, have been influential in setting high standards and encouraging audit.

Professionals have, of course, not had a monopoly on education, and the evidence-based medicine movement and the Cochrane Collaboration have been very important in improving the quantity and quality of information on the effectiveness of health-care interventions. The plan–do–study–act (PDSA) cycle takes audit one stage further, and is widely used in health care (Figure 16.3). The PDSA cycle has four stages, designed to help with the development, testing and implementation of quality improvement plans. The stages are: first, to develop a plan and define the objective (plan); second, to carry out the plan and collect data (do), then analyse the data and summarise what was learned (study); finally to plan the next cycle with necessary modifications (act). For further information see the Institute for Healthcare Improvements website (www.ihi.org/ihi).

Market and financial

Market-based approaches have been most used in the USA, and rely on an informed consumer exercising choice. An example is the Consumer Assessment of Healthcare Providers and Systems programme. Public release of performance data alone has met with limited success in improving quality, perhaps due to lack of data to inform real choice, or perhaps because the data are not used by the public. However, data publication can be effective as part of a larger initiative. An example is the publishing of risk-adjusted mortality rates from coronary artery bypass grafting for hospitals and surgeons in New York State [19]. Importantly, the data were used to inform quality improvement efforts which were associated with state-wide reduction in mortality. Similar effects were not seen where data publication was not accompanied by improvement efforts. (Following the Bristol inquiry, cardiothoracic surgeons have pioneered similar systems in the UK.)

Payment for performance is perhaps the dominant model internationally in 2006. Examples are the payment of a substantial portion of salary to British general practitioners according to their performance against quality criteria (see Table 16.2), and financial incentives to providers from the US Centers for Medicare and Medicaid Services.

Quality improvement and health-care systems

We have seen that approaches to quality improvement can be grouped into three broad categories: regulation, education and market-based. Whichever combination of these is used, the level in the health-care system at which quality improvement approaches are applied is important. Previously, most quality improvement took place in single clinics, in patients with single diseases. Multilevel approaches to change, that impact on individuals, groups or teams, the organisation as a whole, and the larger environment and system level, have greater chances of success [20]. For example, the reduction in mortality seen in New York discussed above was effective because it was implemented at a health system level. Changes at the system level made it easier for individual hospitals and teams to drive through beneficial changes. The importance of change at a system level has already been mentioned.

The business world has given us powerful examples of quality improvement initiatives that consider the whole system, and two that have been successfully adopted into health care are 'six sigma', invented by Motorola, and Toyota's 'lean' technique. The lean technique entails assessing every process for its value to the patient, to cut waste and inefficiencies and improve patient care [21]. Six sigma describes the aspiration to reduce error rates to the extremely low level of 3.4 per million [22]. The term six sigma comes from a statistical measure of variation, the standard deviation from a normal distribution. The number of 3.4 per million comes from the limits for acceptable quality being set to include all observations within six standard deviations of the mean. The statistical terminology can be confusing, but the idea is simple: we should not accept the current common error rates of 50% in health care, nor 10% or even 1%, but strive for near perfect error rates of less than 1 in 3.4 million. Proponents of six sigma argue that these error rates are achievable in health care, just as in manufacturing; they cite anaesthesia as an example of an area that has seen dramatic improvements in safety.

Table 16.4. Sigma levels and defect rates in different industries [22]

Defects per million	Sigma level	Health-care examples	Other industry examples
3.4	6		Publishing: one misspelled word in all books in a small library
5.4		Deaths caused by anaesthesia during surgery	
230	5		Airline fatalities
6,210	4		Airline baggage handling
			Restaurant bills
10,000		1% of all hospitalised patients injured through negligence	
66,800	3		Publishing: 7.6 misspelled words per page in a book
210,000		21% of ambulatory antibiotics for colds	
	2	58% of patients with depression not diagnosed/treated adequately	
790,000	1	79% of heart-attack survivors not given beta-blockers	

Table 16.4 gives examples of the defect rates (which relate to a particular sigma level) in different industries.

The risks of quality improvement should be considered. What are the opportunity costs of quality improvement? Do the benefits outweigh the costs? Disparities in access to health care are a problem in all countries, and any quality improvement programme may worsen disparities unless the improvement has proportionally greater benefit for the relatively disadvantaged population.

Conclusion

A range of different approaches to quality improvement have been mentioned briefly in this section. All of them work some of the time, and none of them are guaranteed to work. The most important part of any quality improvement initiative is a group of committed people who consistently seek to make health care better. The particular technique chosen is probably much less important than the dedication of the people involved. As summed up by Kieran Walshe and Tim Freeman [23]:

Rather than taking up, trying, and then discarding a succession of different quality improvement techniques, organisations should probably choose one carefully and then persevere to make it work.

REFERENCES

1. T. McKeown, *The Role of Medicine: Dream, Mirage or Nemesis?*, Oxford, Blackwell, 1979.
2. J. P. Bunker, The role of medical care in contributing to health improvements within societies. *International Journal of Epidemiology*, **30**(6), 2001,1260–3.
3. I. Gemmell, R. F. Heller, P. McElduff *et al.*, Population impact of stricter adherence to recommendations for pharmacological and lifestyle interventions over one year in patients with coronary heart disease. *Journal of Epidemiology and Community Health* **59**(12), 2005,1041–6.
4. Institute of Medicine (IOM).Committee on Health Care in America, *Crossing the Quality Chasm: A New Health System for the 21st Century*, Washington DC, National Academy Press, 2001.
5. N. Steel, Thresholds for taking antihypertensive drugs in different professional and lay groups: questionnaire survey. *British Medical Journal*, **320**, 2000,1446–7.
6. A. Coulter, What do patients and the public want from primary care? *British Medical Journal*, **331**, 2005, 1199–201.
7. A. Donabedian, *Explorations in Quality Assessment and Monitoring. Vol 1. The Definition of Quality and Approaches to its Assessment*, Ann Arbor, MI, Health Administration Press, 1980.
8. R. Maxwell, Quality assessment in health. *British Medical Journal*, **288**,1984,1470–2.
9. S. Leatherman and K. Sutherland, *The Quest for Quality in the NHS. A Chartbook on Quality of Care in the UK*, Oxford, Radcliffe, 2005.
10. R. H. Brook, M. R. Chassin, A. Fink *et al.*, A method for the detailed assessment of the appropriateness of medical technologies. *International Journal of Technology Assessment in Health Care*, **2**,1986, 53–63.
11. General Practitioners Committee BMA, The NHS Confederation, Investing in General Practice. The New General Medical Services Contract. London, The NHS Confederation, 2003.
12. M. Chassin and R. W. Galvin, The National Roundtable on Health Care Quality. The urgent need to improve health care quality. *Journal of the American Medical Association*, **280**, 1998, 1000–5.
13. E. A. McGlynn, S. M. Asch, J. Adams *et al.*,The quality of health care delivered to adults in the United States. *New England Journal of Medicine*, **348**(26):2635– 45.
14. N. Steel, S. Maisey and K. Cox, Quality of healthcare. In J. Banks, E. Breeze, C. Lessof and J. Nazroo (eds.), *Retirement, Health and Relationships of the Older Population in England: The 2004 English Longitudinal Study of Ageing (Wave 2)*. London, The Institute for Fiscal Studies, 2006.
15. E. S. Fisher, D. E. Wennberg , T. A. Stukel *et al.*, The implications of regional variations in Medicare spending. Part 1: the content, quality, and accessibility of care. *Annals of Internal Medicine*, **138**(4), 2003, 273–87.
16. J. Tudor Hart, Commentary: three decades of the inverse care law [comment]. *British Medical Journal*, **320**, 2000, 18–19.
17. Committee on Quality of Health Care in America Institute of Medicine, *To Err is Human: Building a Safer Health System*. Washington, DC, National Academy Press, 2000.

18. K. Sutherland and S. Leatherman, Does certification improve medical standards? *British Medical Journal,* **333**, 2006, 439–41.

19. M. R.Chassin, Achieving and sustaining improved quality: lessons from New York State and cardiac surgery. *Health Affairs (Millwood)* **21**(4), 2002, 40–51.

20. E. B. Ferlie and S. M. Shortell, Improving the quality of health care in the United Kingdom and the United States: a framework for change. *The Milbank Quarterly* **79**(2), 2001, 281–315.

21. D. Jones and A. Mitchell, Lean thinking for the NHS. London, NHS Confederation, 2006.

22. M. R. Chassin, Is health care ready for six sigma quality? *The Milbank Quarterly* **76**(4), 1998, 565–91.

23. K. Walshe and T. Freeman, Effectiveness of quality improvement: learning from evaluations. *Quality and Safety in Health Care,* **11**(1), 2002, 85–7.

17

International development and public health
Jenny Amery

Key points

- Almost all preventable deaths of children, and of women in pregnancy and childbirth, occur in poor countries. Poor people carry the greatest burden from communicable diseases, and non-communicable diseases are increasing in poor countries.
- Reducing income poverty through economic development, debt relief and fairer trade, will improve health status, but faster progress will be made by access to health services including affordable medicines. This should be government-driven and supported internationally.
- Around half of all poor people live in countries where the state institutions are weak or ineffective, including during and after armed conflicts. International agencies have a particular responsibility to address the health needs of such populations.
- Different models of financing and organising health services are appropriate for different contexts. Robust, effective heath systems accessible to and used by poor people are key. There is no one 'right' model.
- The impact of health systems in poor countries must be strengthened by: protecting poor people from large out-of-pocket expenditure on health; improving equity of access to health services; ensuring sustainable health-care worker capacity.
- Better data systems are needed to monitor the impact of health policies and to measure health service quality.
- There has been a proliferation of agencies and initiatives working to address global health needs since the 1990s. Greater co-ordination is urgently needed to increase the impact of the many agencies and initiatives which aim to improve global health.

Essential Public Health, eds. Stephen Gillam, Jan Yates and Padmanabhan Badrinath.
Published by Cambridge University Press. © Cambridge University Press 2007.

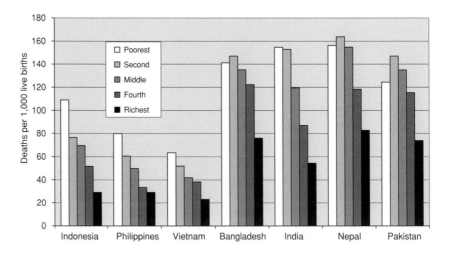

Fig. 17.1 Under-five mortality rate in eight countries in Asia by income quintile

Introduction

This chapter extends the consideration of the changing global burden of diseases begun in Chapter 1 with direct reference to the links between poverty and ill health and discusses what is required to mount an effective response to the public health challenges, particularly in poor countries. It considers the role of international development assistance and the responsibilities of the international community in improving the health of poor people. Finally, the relevance of some of the issues to UK health policy is considered.

The links between poverty and health

Poor health results from poverty: hunger, limited or no access to clean water, sanitation, housing, health and education services; in turn it contributes to poverty and impedes economic growth [1]. A person who is repeatedly ill cannot earn a decent living or contribute to the workforce. Unmet need for modern family planning methods results in early and repeated pregnancies, closely spaced births, increased risks of illness and death to child and mother. Undernourished and frequently sick children do not learn well at school and often drop out early. When a family member falls sick, poor households may have to make huge payments for health care, sell their livestock, land or other assets, become indebted to money lenders or enter bonded labour agreements, which may keep the family in poverty. Poverty and ill health cause misery and loss of hope.

There are wide differences between health outcome for the richest and poorest within poorer countries. Figure 17.1 shows the under-five mortality rate in eight countries in Asia by income quintile. The gap is widest in India and Indonesia.

Table 17.1. Population numbers (millions) and percentages in parentheses living on less than US$ 1 per day, 1990, 2002 and projected to 2015

Region	1990	2002	2015
East Asia and Pacific	472 (30)	214 (15)	14 (0.9)
Europe and central Asia	2 (0.5)	10 (3.6)	4 (0.4)
Latin America and Caribbean	49 (11)	42 (10)	29 (7)
Middle East and North Africa	6 (2)	5 (2)	3 (0.9)
South Asia	462 (41)	437 (31)	232 (13)
Sub-Saharan Africa	227 (45)	303 (46)	336 (38)
Total	1218	1011	617

Source: World Bank. Global Economic Prospects, 2006.

The global burden of disease

There have been rapid falls in mortality and overall improvements in health globally in the last half century, but many poor countries have not shared in these benefits, and have fallen behind high-income countries. The number of people living in poverty globally is falling (poverty here meaning income poverty defined by the UN Millennium Project as living on less than 1 US dollar (Purchasing Power Parity) per day), but at current rates of poverty reduction, there will still be 617 million people living on the equivalent of less than a dollar a day by 2015.

Poverty and ill health are closely linked. The premature deaths and preventable ill health of millions of poor people present a major contemporary challenge. Poor people carry the greatest burden from communicable diseases, particularly in Africa where these conditions account for over 60% of disease burden, compared to about 30% in the low-income countries of south Asia. Acquired immuno deficiency syndrome (AIDS), TB and malaria are the three biggest killers, but the so-called neglected tropical diseases such as lymphatic filariasis, onchocerciasis, guinea worm, leprosy and trachoma contribute very significantly to the total burden of disease of poor people in Africa (see Figure 17.2).

Figure 17.1 also shows the burden from non-communicable diseases which is projected to rise over the next 10 years, and is increasingly affecting poor people in poor countries. Projections to the year 2030 suggest that ischaemic heart disease, stroke, smoking-related cancers, respiratory problems and road traffic accidents will cause proportionately more deaths and AIDS will remain a major

Fig. 17.2   Burden of disease in DALYs per 100,000 population due to four broad disease categories by region. Source: WHO Global Burden of Disease data for 2002.
Disability Adjusted Life Year (DALY) is a measure of the burden of ill health that takes into account both reduced life expectancy and quality of life. It is widely used internationally despite limitations. Values vary widely according to discount rates and weighting of different age groups used. Relatively poor data are available for some countries and conditions, but no better alternative measure has yet been agreed.

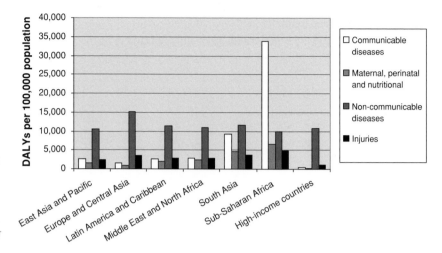

cause globally [2]. Robust public health measures in sectors other than health are required to address the key risk factors of nutrition, smoking, unsafe sex and the growing epidemic of injury and death from road traffic accidents [3, 4]. Other factors contributing to the changing pattern of disease include international migration, rapid rural-to-urban migration in most poor countries and changing family structures; also climate change and emerging microbe and vector resistance to drugs and insecticides. New diseases such as severe acute respiratory syndrome (SARS) may emerge, and there is the ongoing risk of pandemic human influenza.

Key health issues and effective interventions

(a) Preventable illness and deaths amongst children

Despite falling death rates in many countries, approximately 10.8 million children under five years of age die each year; 3.9 million deaths occur in the first 28 days of life. Six countries: India, Nigeria, China, Pakistan, the Democratic Republic of the Congo (DRC) and Ethiopia accounted for 50% of global under-five deaths in the year 2000. Ninety per cent of the deaths occurred in only 42 countries. In poorer countries, serious illnesses commonly occur sequentially or concurrently before death. For example, measles is often complicated by pneumonia or diarrhoea. Underweight and micronutrient deficiencies decrease host defences, and malnutrition is estimated to contribute to about 60% of avoidable childhood deaths [5]. Seventy-three per cent of all child deaths in sub-Saharan Africa and seventy-six per cent in South Asia are from acute respiratory infections, diarrhoeal

Table 17.2. Under-five deaths that could be prevented in the 42 countries with 90% of worldwide child deaths in 2000 through achievement of universal coverage with individual interventions

Preventive interventions	Estimated under-five deaths prevented	
	Number of deaths ($\times 10^3$)	Proportion of all deaths
Breast-feeding	1301	13%
Insecticide-treated materials	691	7%
Complementary feeding	587	6%
Zinc	459 (351)[*]	5% (4%)[*]
Clean delivery	411	4%
Hib (*Haemophilus influenzae type b*) vaccine	403	4%
Water, sanitation, hygiene	326	3%
Antenatal steroids	264	3%
Newborn temperature management	227 (0)[*]	2% (0%)[*]
Vitamin A	225 (176)[*]	2% (2%)[*]
Tetanus toxoid	161	2%
Nevirapine and replacement feeding	150	2%
Antibiotics for premature rupture of membranes	133 (0)[*]	1% (0%)[*]
Measles vaccine	103	1%
Antimalarial intermittent preventive treatment in pregnancy	22	<1%
Treatment interventions		
Oral rehydration therapy	1477	15%
Antibiotics for sepsis	583	6%
Antibiotics for pneumonia	577	6%
Antimalarials	467	5%
Zinc	394	4%
Newborn resuscitation	359 (0)[*]	4% (0%)[*]
Antibiotics for dysentery	310	3%
Vitamin A	8	<1%

[*] Numbers represent effect if both levels 1 (sufficient) and 2 (limited) evidence are included; value number in brackets shows effect if only level 1 evidence is accepted. Interventions for which only one value is cited are all classified as level 1. Source: G. Jones, R. W. Steketee, R. E. Black et al. How many child deaths can we prevent this year? *Lancet,* **362**, 2003, 65–71. Reproduced by permission of Elsevier Science.

diseases, perinatal conditions, measles, and – in Africa – malaria. The interventions to prevent these deaths are well researched.

Table 17.2 shows the percentage of deaths in under fives that could be prevented in the 42 countries with 90% of worldwide child deaths, through universal coverage of specific interventions.

Table 17.3. Maternal mortality estimates by UN regions in 2000

Region	Maternal mortality ratio	Numbers of deaths
Sub-Saharan Africa	920	247,000
Northern Africa	130	4,600
South-central Asia	520	207,000
South-eastern Asia	210	25,000
Western Asia	190	9,800
Latin America/Caribbean	190	22,000
Europe	24	1,700
World	400	529,000

(b) Maternal health

Ninety-nine per cent of deaths in pregnancy and childbirth occur in poor countries, and over two thirds in 13 countries: India, Nigeria, Pakistan, DRC, Ethiopia, Tanzania, Afghanistan, Bangladesh, Angola, China, Kenya, Indonesia and Uganda (see Table 17.3).

Overall, the lifetime risk of maternal death for a woman in high-income countries is 1 in 4,000. In middle-income countries it is 1 in 61, and in low-income countries 1 in 17. This is the largest disparity in health outcome between the richest and poorest countries. Most of these deaths could be prevented if known, cost-effective interventions were available to all women.

Maternal and child health are linked, but there are fundamental differences in effective approaches to addressing them. While evidence-based, successful approaches to child health deliver services as close to the community as possible [6], the reduction of maternal mortality requires access to hospital-based interventions to deal with life-threatening complications which mostly develop around the time of delivery. Good maternal health requires functioning health services at community, clinic and hospital levels, and effective referral systems, and is therefore considered an important marker of a functioning health system [7]. The reduction of neonatal deaths is closely linked to maternal health [8].

(c) Reproductive health

Concern at the rapid population growth in the second half of the twentieth century often resulted in population policies focussing on controlling demographic growth, at the expense of the needs and rights of individuals. At the landmark International Conference on Population and Development held in Cairo in 1994, more than 170 countries agreed that reproductive health services should be

available without coercion to all those who need them, and the conference set out a clear action plan. It defined comprehensive reproductive health care as:
- voluntary contraceptive and family planning services
- antenatal care, safe abortion, delivery, post-partum and post-abortion services (or safe motherhood services)
- services for the prevention, detection and treatment of sexually transmitted infections, including HIV.

It was recognised that many of the issues which impact on reproductive health, including women's empowerment, literacy, poverty and lack of access to health services, could not be resolved quickly, and would require new policies and in some cases new legislation. There has been considerable progress in many countries, but about one third of pregnancies worldwide each year, about 80 million, are unwanted or unplanned. There remains an unmet need for family planning worldwide, and on-going concerns about how to ensure the future supply of contraceptive methods to those who need them. Following renewed calls, the UN General Assembly agreed in September 2006 to include a new reproductive health target under Millennium Goal 5: to achieve universal access to reproductive health by 2015.

(d) Communicable diseases

Communicable diseases remain a major cause of ill health and death in poor countries, despite advances in vaccine development, diagnosis and available treatment. Most of this disease burden is from malaria, HIV, TB, and the so-called neglected tropical diseases including leishmaniasis, trypanosomiasis, Chagas disease, lymphatic filariasis, onchocerciasis (river blindness), schistomiasis, dracunculiasis, soil-transmitted helminth infections, leprosy and trachoma (which causes 6 million people to go blind each year). Globally in 2005, there were nearly 2 million deaths from TB, close to 1 million from malaria (mostly children in Africa) together with a huge morbidity, and 2.8 million deaths from AIDS, most of these in Africa.

HIV and AIDS

Human immunodeficiency virus was first reported in the early 1980s, and has become the first pandemic since that of influenza in 1918. An estimated 38.6 million people worldwide were living with HIV at the end of 2005. An estimated 4.1 million became newly infected and 2.8 million died. Overall the HIV incidence rate is thought to have peaked in the late 1990s, and stabilised, although incidence continues to rise in some countries. Sub-Saharan Africa has 10% of the world's population and more than 60% of all those living with HIV. Women are disproportionately affected especially in sub-Saharan Africa where three women are affected for every two men. People infected with HIV are particularly susceptible to TB and co-infection is very common. Recent trends suggest declining prevalence of HIV in Kenya and Zimbabwe, and in Haiti in the Caribbean, alongside significant behavioural changes including increased condom use, fewer sexual partners and delayed sexual debut. There is also emerging evidence of falling HIV prevalence and new infections in four southern states in India, attributed to effective preventions interventions [9]. Countries which have successfully slowed the progress of the epidemic include Uganda, Senegal, Thailand, Cambodia and Brazil. Top-level political commitment, and sustained implementation of effective policies to change behaviour have been key. Africa remains the global epicentre, and there is no evidence of a decline in South Africa – one of the worst-affected countries. Even where new infections are decreasing, the lag time between infection and death means the burden of disease will remain high for years to come [9].

In Asia there were some 8.3 million people living with HIV at the end of 2005, more than two thirds of them in India. Here the epidemics are driven by unsafe sexual practices, particularly commercial sex, male-to-male sex and injecting drug use; progress is hampered by stigma and discrimination. Rates of HIV infection continue to rise in eastern Europe and central Asia, with Ukraine and the Russian Federation most affected.

Acquired immunodeficiency syndrome continues to have a huge impact on population structure, family and social life, and economic growth in high-prevalence countries. It has the potential to do the same where epidemics are emerging. Stigma and discrimination prevent many people from coming forward for testing or treatment. Health services in high-prevalence countries are struggling to cope even when low-cost antiretroviral medicines are available. In parts of Africa AIDS is reversing improvements in health indicators and average life expectancy. There has been intense advocacy and action globally to address the epidemic in recent years, and progress is being made both in securing global political commitment and funding, and in implementing comprehensive programmes of prevention, care, treatment and support in countries. However, there is no room for complacency [9].

(e) Access to medicines

Even when health services reach them, medicines are often not affordable for poor people, who often have to pay out-of-pocket for them. Barriers to accessing effective medicines in poor countries include high prices; insufficient overall financing of health services and poor priority setting with too little money to fund supplies of essential drugs; inappropriate drug selection, weak procurement and distribution systems; and poor-quality or fake medicines. The WHO estimates that 15% of the world's population consumes 91% of the global production of pharmaceuticals, by value [10]. Some pharmaceutical companies are working in

Table 17.4. Summary of effective health-care interventions for reducing illness and death from HIV and AIDS, TB and malaria

Goal	Preventive intervention	Treatment
Prevent and reduce burden of HIV and AIDS	Safe sex including use of male (and female) condoms; injecting drug users have clean needles and oral substitution therapy; prompt diagnosis and treatment of sexually transmitted infections; safe, screened blood supplies; antiretroviral drugs to prevent mother-to-child transmission	Prompt treatment of opportunistic infections including TB; cotrimoxazole prophylaxis; highly active antiretroviral therapy; palliative care and support.
Prevent and reduce burden of TB	Directly observed treatment of infectious cases to reduce transmission and emergence of drug-resistant strains; testing of people with AIDS for early diagnosis of TB; preventive isoniazid therapy; BCG (Bacille Calmette Guérin) to reduce childhood TB.	Directly observed treatment to cure symptomatic cases; second-line therapies for multiple drug-resistant cases.
Prevent and reduce burden from malaria	Use of insecticide-treated bed-nets; in epidemic-prone areas indoor residual spraying and intermittent presumptive treatment of pregnant women; prompt identification of drug-resistant strains.	Rapid detection and treatment of cases with locally effective medicines, depending on drug resistance. Increasing use of Artemisin combination treatments (ACTs).

private–public partnerships to bring key medicines to poor people, for example the ivermectin donation programme as part of the initiative to eradicate onchocerciasis in Africa [11].

The World Trade Organisation agreement on trade related aspects of intellectual property rights (TRIPS) gives countries the right under the Doha TRIPS and public health decision of 2003, to protect public health, for example by importing copies of patented medicines, if their own pharmaceutical industry has insufficient capacity to produce them. International trade policy is important to increase poor people's access to medicines[12].

There are a number of public–private product-development partnerships in research and development of medicines for diseases disproportionately affecting poor people. Current approaches to vaccine research for diseases of the poor are unlikely to deliver results quickly enough. Advance market commitments (AMCs) for vaccines aim to create a competitive developing country market for future vaccines that is sufficiently large and credible to stimulate private investment in research and development and manufacturing capacity. Advance market commitments are being developed initially for the production of new vaccines for pneumococcus and malaria (for children).

How can improvements in health be delivered?

There is a complex inter-relationship between poverty and health which can be a virtuous cycle with a healthier population contributing to economic growth and prosperity, or a vicious cycle of worsening health, increasing indebtedness from health-care expenditure, marginalisation from the economy and slowing economic growth. Orthodox economic arguments highlight the need for macro-economic growth to reduce levels of poverty, but not all growth benefits poor people, and there are increasing concerns about 'jobless' growth, with millions of poor people remaining at the margins of society. Debt relief, fairer trade with access to markets for poorer countries and communities are also key, and require action from rich-country governments. Poor countries need more international aid. More predictable aid would enable countries to fund sustainable five- to ten-year health plans and invest in well-trained workforces. Greater investment is needed in new technologies: for example, better diagnostics, medicines and vaccines for HIV, TB and malaria.

However, none of these will make a significant difference without strong health services, accessible to poor people, staffed by well-trained, supervised, motivated and adequately rewarded health workers.

The framing of numerical goals and targets focuses attention, but also risks a technocratic, top-down approach to the complex challenges facing different countries and cultures [13].

Global knowledge of effective interventions alone is not sufficient to improve health. Governments have a key role, and where a government is unwilling or too weak to implement change, poverty and ill health prevail. The role of the state is, at minimum, firstly to maintain borders, provide peace and security; secondly, to create conditions that provide livelihoods and economic growth; and thirdly, to ensure provision of public goods and services such as health and education (see Box 17.1).

Much poor performance in terms of health-service delivery is due to weaknesses in institutions, budgeting and public-expenditure management, and the fact that governments are not accountable to their people [14]. Governments should be held to account for maintaining fiscal discipline, ensuring resources are allocated and spent in line with stated priorities and not lost through corruption or mismanagement, and are used to achieve maximum impact on health outcomes. Making information more accessible and promoting transparency in fees, budgets and expenditure enable corruption to be tackled more easily, but there are often strong forces at work to avoid such transparency. The 2005 Commission

> ## Box 17.1 Good governance
>
> Good governance can be summarised as:
> - The capacity of the state to raise revenue, use resources and deliver services
> - Responsiveness of public policies and institutions to the needs and rights of citizens
> - Accountability including free media access to information, opportunity to change leaders through democratic means

for Africa Report [15] concluded that without progress in improving governance, all other reforms would have limited impact.

Weak or corrupt states, engulfed in armed conflicts or run by repressive military regimes, will not have institutions capable of delivering health services. In such environments creative, context-specific responses are needed. Donors may wish to work through UN bodies, non-governmental organisations (NGOs), faith-based organisations, for-profit providers and community-based providers to meet the humanitarian needs of the people, and support the long-term development of government institutions that can eventually take on responsibility for service delivery. Exceptional responses are also required in the face of earthquakes, hurricanes, floods and other such disasters.

Organising and financing health systems

One of the reasons for low health-service coverage and poor health outcomes is low per capita expenditure on health. The Commission on Macroeconomics and Health calculated that US$ 34 per capita in 2002 prices is needed to provide a basic package of services to address the main causes of ill health and premature death in low-income countries. The package covers essential prevention and treatment for TB, malaria, HIV; childhood immunisation; vitamin A supplementation for children; integrated management of childhood diseases, including diarrhoea and acute respiratory infections; and maternal health including antenatal care and skilled attendance at delivery. This would require an additional US$ 40–52 billion by 2015 and would save some eight million lives each year. African countries pledged at Abuja, Nigeria, in 2000 to increase funding for health from around 8% on average to 15% of their budgets, but few have achieved that level to date, and 15% of a very small budget is not enough.

The method of financing health services will influence whether poor people can access them. Tax-financed universal health care is the most equitable, but may be subject to high administrative cost, poor governance, and

Box 17.2 Core public health functions

Core public health functions include:
- Collection and dissemination of evidence for public health policies
- Public health regulation and enforcement
- Pharmaceutical policy regulation and enforcement
- Epidemiological and, where appropriate, behavioural surveillance for risk factors of disease
- Prevention and control of disease
- Health promotion
- Intersectoral action for improving health
- Monitoring and evaluation of public health policy
- Development of human resources and capacity for public health

disproportionate use by the articulate and well-off. Social insurance can combine risk-pooling and distribute the financial burden according to ability to pay. Pre-payment into a community financing scheme tailored to local needs, to pool risk, has to date delivered only limited coverage. Voluntary private insurance benefits those able to pay and will often exclude people with chronic conditions. Out-of-pocket payments at the time of illness is the most regressive form of financing, yet in many low-income countries it is the source of well over half of all financing for health care. User charges levied by public and private providers of health care have had mixed impact, but almost universally result in deterring access by poor people or impoverishing those on or near the poverty line [16].

Some countries are attaining measurably better levels of service coverage with lower levels of expenditure. For example, Sri Lanka has remarkably good health outcomes and its public sector spends only US$ 15 per capita, with investment in more cost-effective interventions and greater efficiency of spend. Low-income countries where significant improvements have taken place in the health of the population without high or rapidly rising incomes, include Bangladesh, Costa Rica, Cuba, Sri Lanka and Kerala State in India. Effective policies, well implemented, can greatly improve the health of poor people. The HIV epidemic, and emergence of new diseases such as SARS have highlighted the crucial role of governments in strengthening and maintaining core public health functions [17] (see Box 17.2).

To maximise their benefit, health resources must be re-allocated towards more cost-effective services, poorer geographical regions within countries, and services that are used by poor people. The allocation and distribution of resources is an intensely political process, affected by power struggles between competing stake-holders (e.g. different parts of government, external agencies). The ability of the

> **Box 17.3 Critical issues in financing and organising of health services**
>
> - Bringing health care benefits to those who are currently not accessing services of acceptable quality, including access to essential medicines
> - Protecting people from unexpected large financial expenditures (risk protection)
> - Creating incentives for appropriate, cost-effective, high-quality health care.
> - Strengthening core public health functions
> - Regulating and assuring the quality of service providers

state to set priorities and negotiate the allocation of resources in a way which increases equity and meets the needs of stakeholders is a measure of the state's legitimacy and its commitment to procedural justice [7]–see Box 17.3.

Balancing vertical and horizontal approaches

Vertical approaches address one disease or issue at a time, and tend to be top-down and controlled by experts. The eradication of smallpox was a success, but efforts to eradicate malaria since the 1960s have failed, and total eradication of malaria is no longer the goal. Vertical approaches can divert human and financial resources, and undermine and weaken other health initiatives, despite achieving their own specific objectives. Current examples of vertical programmes include those addressing polio eradication, AIDS (in particular antiretroviral therapy), TB, malaria, and childhood immunisation.

The Alma-Ata Declaration of 1978 [18] rejected the vertical approach and called on governments to tackle common underlying causes of ill health, with the building of sustainable health care systems, locally based and locally controlled. Emphasis was given to people's participation in health.

Vertical programmes raise the profile of specific health conditions, mobilise additional resources, and often deliver short-term results against specific targets. There is increasing concern that they may undermine broader health-service delivery, through duplication of effort, distortion of national health plans and budgets, and particularly through diversion of scarce trained staff. At best, they can complement country efforts, and integrate with country planning cycles, and financial, monitoring and other systems.

In 2006 there were over 70 global health partnerships and initiatives addressing disease or other specific health needs, many with private–public financing. This is in addition to the multilateral development agencies working in health, notably the European Commission, World Bank, Regional Development Banks, WHO and UN technical agencies such as UNICEF, UNFPA, UNAIDS, private entities, such as the Bill and Melinda Gates Foundation, and many bilateral donors (See Appendix). Questions are being asked about the overall impact of this 'international health architecture'. Is it really strengthening poor countries' own capacity to deliver health services? How might such efforts be better channelled, in line with emerging evidence on the effectiveness of international aid [19]?

What else stops poor people using health services?

Complex social, cultural and political factors make it difficult to break the intergenerational poverty which affects hundreds of millions of people.

Social exclusion

Social exclusion is a process causing systematic disadvantage on the basis of ethnicity, religion, caste, descent, disability, HIV status, i.e. who you are and where you live. Excluded groups and individuals are denied equal rights and opportunities compared with others. Some people may suffer multiple forms of exclusion, for example low-caste women living in isolated rural areas [20].

Gender inequalities

Gender inequalities are a manifestation of one form of exclusion. Sex disparities are higher in south Asia than anywhere else in the world. A girl in India is greater than 40% more likely to die between her first and fifth birthday than is a boy. Child mortality would drop by 20% if girls had the same mortality rate as boys between the ages of one month and five years. The reasons for this are both environmental and behavioural. Girls are less likely to be brought for timely treatment and have less money spent on them when they are sick than boys [21].

Cost

Cost is a major obstacle. Both formal and informal charges will prevent poor people from using services, and may plunge them further into poverty if charges for drugs or treatments require selling assets or borrowing money at inflated rates.

Human resources for health

Adequate numbers of well-trained, motivated health workers are essential for effective service delivery. Many countries face a deep crisis in staffing their health services, resulting from chronic under-investment in staff and health systems. This is exacerbated by outward migration and, especially in southern African countries, by the burden of AIDS. Health services are overwhelmed with AIDS patients, and the capacity of health services to cope are further limited because of illness and death from AIDS amongst health workers and their families. Low-income countries are currently subsidising high-income ones by supplying them with trained staff. From Africa, the net outflow is equivalent to about US$ 500 million a year. Changes to international recruitment practice may help to manage the flow of migrants, but migration is the result of low pay, lack of career prospects and poor working conditions in 'source' countries, as well as the inability of the high-income 'destination' countries to train and meet their own workforce requirements [22].

Measuring progress, increasing success

The millennium development goals (MDGs) and targets collectively address the different dimensions of poverty. They are documented in the Millennium Declaration signed by 189 countries in September 2000, and progress towards them was reviewed at the World Summit in New York in September 2005 (www.un.org/millenium goals). There are 8 goals, 18 targets and 48 indicators. Countries, with the support of international agencies and donors, are intensifying efforts to make faster progress on the MDGs, particularly in Africa and south Asia. The MDG indicators measure average progress for a country, but do not reflect inequalities or widening gaps if poor people are left further behind.

Progress towards the health-related millennium development goals and respective indicators is being monitored closely, but is limited by incomplete vital registration of births and deaths, and poor-quality data. Key outcomes are listed in Table 17.5.

There is an urgent need for better data systems to guide result-based performance monitoring, better disaggregation to allow analysis of equity and distributional issues, and improved capture of health-service quality measures. Governments and international organisations do not always use the same data sources or definitions. The demand for high-quality data has grown in response to the need to monitor progress against the MDGs, to monitor and evaluate health-system interventions, to show that increased funding is having the desired impact and to hold governments and international donors to account for the money spent on health. Priorities include accurate reporting on mortality, morbidity, health status, service coverage and risk-prevalence. For this to happen in a sustainable way, efforts must be made to strengthen poor countries' own capacity to collect and analyse data. Vital registration systems (of births and deaths), household surveys, and analysis at sub national level wherever feasible, are priorities. The

Table 17.5. The Millennium development goals and health-related targets: progress at 2005 in sub-Saharan Africa and South Asia

Goal	Target by 2015	Selected indicators	Progress in sub-Saharan Africa	Progress in south Asia
1. Eradicate extreme poverty and hunger	Reduce extreme poverty by half	Proportion of people living on equivalent of less than US$1 per day	High rates – no change	On track
	Reduce hunger by half	% children under five underweight	Very high rates – little change	Progress but lagging
2. Achieve universal primary education	Universal primary schooling	Net enrolment in primary education Completion rate at Grade 5	Progress but lagging	Progress but lagging
3. Promote gender equality and empower women	Girls equal enrolment in primary, secondary and tertiary education	Ratio of girls to boys in primary, secondary and tertiary education	No significant change	Progress but lagging
4. Reduce child mortality	Reduce under-five mortality rate by two thirds	Under-five mortality rate. Infant mortality rate	Very high rates – no change	Progress but lagging
		Percentage of one year olds immunised against measles	Low – no change	Progress but lagging
5. Improve maternal health	Reduce maternal mortality ratio by three quarters	Maternal mortality ratio. Births attended by skilled health worker	Very high	Very high
6. Combat HIV/AIDS, malaria and other diseases	Halt and reverse spread of HIV and AIDS.	HIV prevalence amongst 15–24 year old pregnant women (generalised epidemics)	Stable	Increasing in vulnerable groups
	Halt and reverse spread of malaria	Prevalence and death rates associated with malaria	High	Moderate
	Halt and reverse spread of TB	Prevalence and death rates associated with TB	High, increasing	High, declining
7. Ensure environmental sustainability	Halve the proportion without access to safe drinking water		Some progress but lagging	On track
	Halve the proportion without access to sanitation		Low access – no change	Progress but lagging
8. A global partnership for development	Multiple targets on aid, trade and debt, includes access to essential drugs			

Source: Adapted from the United Nations Millennium Project Progress Report, 2005.

health metrics network has been set up to help address these issues (who.int/healthmetrics).

Making international aid for health more effective

To avoid the burden on countries of multiple-donor projects and vertical programmes, sector-wide approaches (SWAps) have been developed particularly in low-income, aid-dependent countries, to strengthen the whole health sector and provide support for country-specific priorities. Donor funds which go through the receiving country governments' own budget can increase transparency of allocation and work towards a sustainable increase in the per capita spend on health. Donors need to ensure more predictable flows of funds, and this is one of the criteria for more effective international aid, agreed in the Paris Declaration on Aid Effectiveness, March 2005, together with greater mutual accountability of both donors and recipient countries [19].

Research

Only 10% of the annual US$70 billion spent on global health research targets the diseases responsible for 90% of the world's health problems. In addition to increased global investment, new ways of stimulating research into the diseases of poverty, and the development of commodities including vaccines, diagnostics and medicines are required. Research is urgently needed on the best way of delivering health interventions, and more rigorous impact evaluations of new approaches to better understand what works and why.

Some issues of relevance to UK policy

(i) Rich and poor countries need to develop better ways of ensuring that poor and marginalised populations have access to effective health services, and of reducing inequalities in health. Accountability of governments and service providers to users and communities is key.

(ii) The increasingly global market for health workers means rich countries have a responsibility to minimise the detrimental impact of their recruitment policies on the training and supply of health workers in poor countries, and consider how they can support poor countries to develop and retain an appropriately skilled workforce.

(iii) The capacity of poor countries to prepare for, detect and manage emerging communicable diseases such as SARS and human pandemic influenza, will impact on the global spread of these diseases. Investing in the capacity of poor countries to respond to communicable diseases is of benefit to the

developed world as well as to the poorer countries. For example, the eradication of polio world wide will ultimately remove the need for vaccination
globally.

(iv) The UK government policy on health, trade, industry and intellectual property, can support best practice in the pharmaceutical industry, and help
improve access to essential medicines in poor countries.

Appendix

A typology of international organisations working on global health issues

1. Multilateral development and technical agencies

Example	Strengths	Challenges
World Health Organization	Technical norms and standard setting; global mandate	Maintain technical independence; manage the inevitable tension between rich- and poor-country demands
UNICEF (UN Childrens' Fund)	Clear mandate on child-related issues; experience at community level	Right balance between advocacy, technical support and programme implementation
UNFPA (UN Fund for Population Activities)	Global advocacy for reproductive rights and services	Small agency and thinly stretched across countries
UNDP (UN Development Programme)	Co-ordination of UN development assistance	More effective co-ordination at country level
UNAIDS (UN Agency for HIV and AIDS)	Single issue focus and advocacy	More integration of AIDS activities into overall development
World Bank – group of five organisations, part of UN	Provides loans at concessional rates and grants to poor countries; large budget; strong health technical expertise; mandated to focus on poverty reduction	Risk of overly technocratic approach; strong incentives to disburse money because it is a bank; rigid procedures
Regional Development Banks: e.g. Africa, Asia, Inter-American, Caribbean	Accountability to governing boards which are dominated by governments in the region; often specific focus, e.g. infrastructure in Asia	Variable technical capacity; may be subject to political influence
European Commission	Large budget for grant-aid; high profile for health and HIV; reforms underway to increase aid effectiveness	History of slow disbursement of funds and rigid procedures; aid is not prioritised to poorest countries; growing role in support to EU accession countries

2. Bilateral donors

Example	Strengths	Challenges
UK Department for International Development (DFID)	Good track-record of health-related development and technical capacity; clear policies on reproductive health and AIDS; proactive in donor harmonisation and improving effectiveness of aid to poor countries	Maintain quality and impact as aid budget rises to 0.7% GNI by 2013; more predictable longer-term aid flows including to 'fragile states'; ensuring its preferred approach of budget support leads to improvements in health and other social sectors; getting the right balance of support between the health sector and politically high profile diseases such as AIDS; better monitoring of impact
United States Agency for International Development (USAID)	Large budget; strong technical capacity in health	US Congress accountability rules limit extent of harmonisation with other donors or recipient country systems; increasing amounts of US aid are being channelled through routes other than USAID, e.g. PEPFAR (Presidents Emergency Programme for AIDS Response)
Nordic countries (Norway, Sweden, Denmark) and Netherlands	Health high priority; strong on harmonisation	More predictable aid flows and monitoring of impact
Japan	Second largest aid budget after USA 2004	Low public support in Japan for development funding (compared to UK)
China and India	Emerging donors in Asia and in Africa	Adopt OECD 'good donorship' practice although they are not members

3. Private philanthropic organisations

Example	Strengths	Challenges
Bill and Melinda Gates Foundation	Huge budget (endowment of $26 billion) focus on research and new technologies for disease of poor; lean administration; efficient disbursement	No money goes through government systems, risks of parallel ones. Potential risk of an overly technological approach
Clinton Foundation	Focus on AIDS, particularly treatment	Risk of parallel systems in poor countries; co-ordination is key

4. Global health partnerships (public–private)

Example	Strengths	Challenges
Global Fund for AIDS, TB and malaria (GFATM); created in 2002	A new kind of multilateral organisation with big funding from many rich governments including USA and UK; tight focus on three key diseases of poverty; funds prioritised to poor countries	To have measurable impact on the three diseases without distorting country priorities; to align its projects with country systems and not create duplicate mechanisms
Global Alliance for Vaccines and Immunisation (GAVI); established in 1999	Targetted funding for immunisation delivery and roll-out of new vaccines	Improve immunisation coverage without fragmenting efforts at country level to improve broader service delivery
African Partnership for Onchorcerciasis (river blindness) Control	Innovative partnership with pharmaceutical company providing medicines free; very successful impact in reducing burden of disease	Eradication of disease or reduction to minimal levels
International AIDS Vaccine Initiative (IAVI)	Brings key researchers together with private and public funding to accelerate development of a vaccine, especially for poor countries	Maintain momentum in face of technical challenges to effective vaccine development

5. International non-governmental organisations (NGOs)

Example	Strengths	Challenges
Médecins Sans Frontières	Effective provision of impartial health care in emergency settings	Support development of sustainable health systems while addressing urgent humanitarian needs
Care International: large US-based NGO	Large provider of services; innovative delivery in range of contexts	Co-ordinate with other health providers and strengthen national systems
Oxfam family	Strong on water and sanitation, community involvement and humanitarian relief	To achieve most effective balance between advocacy and innovative service delivery

6. Private-sector contractors and consultants

There are a significant number of limited companies and for-profit firms winning contracts to provide technical assistance, and to manage large health projects and programmes in poor countries on behalf of donor agencies. Their strengths lie in their flexibility and speed of response, and often high technical capacity, though this is variable. They have been criticised for their high fees and costs, and for absorbing significant amounts of the aid budgets from some sources.

REFERENCES

1. J. Sachs (chairman), Macroeconomics and health: investing in health for economic development. Report of the Commission on Macroeconomics and Health. Geneva, World Health Organization, 2001.
2. C. D. Mathers and D. Loncar. Updated projections of global mortality and burden of disease, 2002–2030: data sources, methods and results. Geneva, World Health Organization, 2005.
3. Disease Control Priorities Project, *The Global Burden of Disease and Risk Factors.* Washington, DC, World Bank, 2006.
4. S. Ameratunga, M. Hijar and R. Norton, Road traffic injuries: confronting disparities to address a global health priority. *Lancet*, **367**, 2006, 1533–40.
5. R. E. Black, S. S. Morris and J. Bryce, Where and why are 10 million children dying every year? *Lancet*, **361**, 2003, 2226–34.
6. J. Bryce, S. el Arifen, G. Pariyo *et al.*, Reducing child mortality: can public health deliver? *Lancet*, **362**, 2003, 159–64.
7. United Nations Millenium Project Task Force on Child Health and Maternal Health. *Who's Got the Power? Transforming Health Systems for Women and Children.* London, Earthscan, 2005.
8. J. Lawn, S. Cousens, J. Zupan, for the Lancet Neonatal Survival Steering Team, Why are 4 million newborn babies dying each year? *Lancet*, **364**, 2004, 399–401.
9. Report of the Global AIDS epidemic. Geneva, Joint United Nations Programme on HIV/AIDS (UNAIDS), 2006.
10. World Health Report: shaping the future. Geneva, World Health Organisation, 2003.
11. D. Molyneux, P. Hotez and A. Fenwick, Rapid-impact interventions; how a policy of integrated control for Africa's neglected tropical diseases could benefit the poor. *PLoS Medicine.* Nov 2005, **2**(11), 2005, 1064–70.
12. Increasing access to essential medicines in the developing world: UK government policy and plans. Department for International Development.
13. L. Freedman, Achieving the Millennium Development Goals: health systems as core social institutions. *Development*, **48**(1), 2005, 19–24.
14. M. Grindle. Good enough governance: poverty reduction and reform in developing countries (Monograph). Cambridge, MA, Kennedy School of Government, Harvard University, 2002.
15. Our Common Interest. Report of the Commission for Africa 2005. Commission for Africa. (www.commissionforafrica.org, accessed 20th November 2006)
16. N. Palmer, D. Mueller, L. Gilson *et al.* Health financing to promote access in low income settings – how much do we know? *Lancet*, **364**, 2004, 1365–70.
17. A. Wagstaff and M. Claeson, *The Millennium Development Goals for Health, Rising to the Challenges.* Washington, DC, World Bank. 2004.

18. Primary Health Care. Report of the International Conference on Primary Health Care, Alma-Ata, USSR, 6–12 September 1978. Geneva, World Health Organisation, 1978.

19. R. Manning, Organisation for Economic Cooperation and Development (OECD) Development Co-operation Report 2005. Paris, OECD, 2005.

20. N. Kabeer, Poverty, social exclusion and the MDGs: the challenge of "durable inequalities" in the Asian context. *IDS Bulletin*, **37** (3), 2006, 64–78.

21. C. Victora, A. Wagstaff, J. A. Schellerberg *et al.* Applying an equity lens to child health and mortality: more of the same is not enough. *Lancet*, **362**, 2003, 233–41.

22. World Health Report: working together for health. Geneva, World Health Organization, 2006.

Jenny Amery works for the UK Department for International Development (DFID). The views expressed are not necessarily those of DFID.

Public health – the future – be part of it . . .

David Pencheon

The only thing you can be certain about the future is that your predictions will be wrong. Or, put another way, it is easy to predict the future; it is just difficult to get it right. This short chapter is therefore not a crystal-ball exercise to describe the future (specifically of public health). It will, instead, aim to describe some general themes that are already with us, and that show every sign of being increasingly important in determining the future, and how we should be trying to influence such themes for the benefit of all. The issues raised in this chapter are what makes public health so frustrating, so fascinating, so challenging and so rewarding. Any competent and committed health professional is likely to want to address them as a clinician, as a public health professional, as a politician, or as all three!

1. What causes health today?

It does not take long for a health worker, early in their career, to realise that a huge burden of ill health in any part of the world is better addressed through prevention rather than through just cure. The next common revelation is that the vast majority of illness prevention is not done actively unto individuals in programmes such as screening and immunisation, but done in a much more empowered and profound way by giving people more protection and control over their own current and future health. This implies that we know the real causes of health and illness; not just which bacteria cause which infectious diseases, but how one's place in society determines one's life chances, and, crucially, what can be done to help oneself and others though the organised efforts of society.

The biggest changes to the causes of health and illness in societies today are ultimately determined by wider societal changes. These include the relative ageing of nearly all populations around the world; the technology that we have (and are likely to develop) in preventing and curing diseases; the perpetual tension between the average health and health inequalities; and, finally, the

Essential Public Health, eds. Stephen Gillam, Jan Yates and Padmanabhan Badrinath.
Published by Cambridge University Press. © Cambridge University Press 2007.

increasing expectations, fuelled by a global information system that shows what might be possible rather than what is currently affordable.

Many single-cause illnesses from past centuries (such as infectious diseases) are potentially preventable and curable (although many people, especially in economically poorer countries still die in obscenely large numbers). The effect on population health has been that we have seen other diseases become the main causes of illness and death: cancer, heart disease, and many other lifestyle-related conditions. Demographic changes (a relative ageing of the population) has meant that many of us live to older ages with many conditions rather than die younger of one specific cause. This is true, not only in economically wealthy countries, but also in the many countries in transition to such economic wealth. Lastly, we live on a fragile and highly interdependent planet. The effects of contagious viruses, warfare, social injustice, and carbon dioxide affect everyone on the planet.

Despite these profound and global threats, there are at least two eternal verities in the struggle for social justice and public health. The first is that social justice never happens by accident. It is the result of the relentless struggle to assess and address inequalities and inequities. The natural order, sadly, is that opportunities and services tend to be more available to those with the least need (the 'inverse care law' referred to so often throughout this text [1]). The practice of public health is a constant struggle to demonstrate this and to do all that is possible to ensure that the resources and opportunities are directed and available to those with the most need. The second is that everywhere in the world, the health of individuals and populations is won largely outside the formal health care system, especially outside the hospital system. Hospitals are hugely important, but tend to be the icing on the cake. Moreover, many commentators have viewed the concentration of resources and techniques within hospitals as being largely for the convenience of professionals, rather than for the benefit of patients. There is therefore a constant need to remind ourselves that good health depends on peace, clean water, sanitation, food, education, jobs, lack of corruption, accountability and good governance – and many of these are ultimately determined by an informed and empowered population.

There is nothing more empowering in the twenty-first century than high-quality information (for public, patients, policy makers, practitioners and politicians). However, this access to information needs to be coupled with an ability to sort the wheat from the chaff, and the opportunity to actually use the information appropriately.

Knowledge (information used in context by human beings) is an important cause of health in its own right. Moreover, that knowledge in different forms diffuses either as new technologies, professionally applied, or less formally through the population at large, changing behaviours and ultimately improving health. Knowledge is the enemy of disease, whether it comes over the radio to under-empowered women in poor villages, or whether it helps scientists share expertise globally to develop an effective vaccine for malaria.

The world is increasingly difficult to divide into developed and less-developed countries. Industrialised countries have public health challenges that sometimes differ from those of more resource-poor countries. However, many of the public health challenges will be similar (at least in type if not scale) and need to be addressed with similar approaches. Globalisation itself poses significant challenges for the public health infrastructure. Multinational companies wield huge influence where the health of their present customers may not be their biggest concern.

However, the most pressing public health concerns of the globe must be the shocking inequities in health and opportunities. Thirty thousand deaths in children before the age of five each day is a tragedy (see www.who.int/healthmetrics). That we are not clear where, why and how they all happen (a failure of systematic health information and thus, prioritised political and operational action) is a crime.

2. Causes of health: using information, evidence and knowledge – key skills for health professionals

Just as knowledge is an increasingly important cause of health, so the use of knowledge is an absolutely central competence for health professionals, especially public health professionals. The practice of public health depends on individuals, teams and organisations keeping abreast of the knowledge (e.g. of effective interventions to protect and improve health). There is an increasing pressure to move away from simplistic approaches to evidence of effectiveness to a more integrated approach where evidence of multiple types and from multiple sources are assessed and appropriately combined (e.g. evidence of need, evidence of effectiveness, public acceptability and evidence of cost-effectiveness and cost benefit, as described in Chapter 9). Politics of all types will inevitably still play a large part in decision-making. However, without being able to say: 'this is the need, this is the burden, this is how it compares and is changing, and these are the costed and publicly acceptable interventions that are potentially available', your contribution to strategy and tactics will be marginal and marginalised. These sorts of knowledge are vital to governments and organisations if they are to justify their decisions, priorities and actions to an increasingly empowered and vocal population. Such decisions will be challenged and will therefore need to be defensible, and explicit in their origin.

The evaluation, availability and affordability of information and communications technology (ICT) is having a significant effect on how professionals can and should work. However, the speed at which the public (and selected sub-populations) are being similarly empowered is equally important; ICT allows ready access to debate, information, and evidence specifically, as well as to the broader political process. If we, as members of the public, can shop, lobby, and debate round the clock, then we may not find a public health report that uses three-year-old data (and published largely as jargon only in hard copy) very engaging, very empowering or very useful.

Public health professionals serve an increasingly diverse and demanding set of people and organisations. As the public realise they are faced by bewildering choices, these decisions will be influenced by many factors. Within health, we will increasingly choose everything from our carers to our food. Such decisions are based on many factors. The role of health professionals will be to ensure that food choices are not influenced solely by the food industry. Similarly, an empowered and vocal population will look somewhere credible for unbiased information on health care professionals and health care facilities. Good hospital guides and good doctor guides will be increasingly common, and will need to be written in an unbiased way, acknowledging that different people will have different requirements and priorities for themselves and their families.

3. Developing competency in the key skills for public health

Public health professionals, like all professionals in areas which are broad and multidisciplinary, need to be jacks of all trades and masters of some. Importantly, you need to have insight and evidence of your own personal competencies, in order to be able to work well with others. The same applies to the organisations of which you are a part. You need a clear description (and ideally quantification) of personal and organisational strengths and weaknesses in order to be able to deliver effectively with others.

Individuals need breadth and depth, and to know exactly where they are for their present roles and where they need to be for future roles. This is not simply an annual process of reflection but should be a constant self-reflection and critique of fitness to practice and deliver results.

If you profess to be competent, you need to demonstrate that competency in a changing world. You will need evidence of assessment of competency to practice today, and of continual professional development to practice tomorrow.

Ask yourself the following questions regularly:

1. What did I learn today/this week?
2. Are my references databases and my contacts databases as extensive, broad and up-to-date as they could be? Can I find the right reference or the right person to ask for help (or to help) quickly?

3. Am I writing well, speaking well and thinking critically?* Any politician will tell you that it is useful to have a position on almost any issue – not to be always right, or to express expertise all of the time, but to understand more clearly the position of others. ('The pull of the tide is felt best by one whose anchor does not drag.')

4. Do I read broadly? Concentrate especially on high-quality writing from people who think differently from you, and who can justify their positions.

5. Do I always seek to understand before I seek to be understood[2]?

6. What would a member of the public think of my meeting if they were observing it?

7. Do I listen carefully to the language (especially the jargon and the acronyms) I am using, especially if in a multidisciplinary group?

8. Am I developing a deeper interest in at least one related discipline such as anthropology, economics, current affairs, ethics?

9. What would I do if I were in charge, had money or other resources?

10. Do I stop and reflect and think deeply and regularly (half an hour a day, unless you are busy in which case it should be *more . . .*)?

3. Why public health is a good place to be and a good thing to do

To improve public health you don't need the words 'public health' in your job title. Indeed, most health improvement, health protection and health service quality improvement are all done by people who would not necessarily consider themselves public health professionals. However, a formal public health training can open career opportunities to you in any and all of these areas.

The two most important resources you need are knowledge and oratory. There are countless traditional and a seemingly endless supply of new threats to public health. A motivated and skilled individual will never be short of challenging work. Public health is a worthwhile, exciting, fulfilling and noble endeavour. It is a stimulating mixture of science and politics, and, best of all, no two days are ever the same!

REFERENCES

1. J. T. Hart, The inverse care law. *Lancet*, **1** (696), 1971, 405–12.
2. S. R. Covey, *The 7 Habits of Highly Effective People*, New York, Simon and Schuster, 1990.

* Remember the true meaning of 'thinking critically'. It is as much about finding value as about finding fault.

Glossary

Absolute risk reduction (ARR) The difference in the absolute risk (rates of adverse events) between study and control populations.

Absolute risk The observed or calculated probability of an event in the population under study.

Acquired immunity Resistance acquired by a host to a pathogen as a result of previous exposure from natural infection or immunisation. It is the result of the production of antibodies (immunoglobulins) targeted to specific antigens.

Adjustment A summarising procedure for a statistical measure in which the effects of differences in composition of the populations being compared have been minimised by statistical methods.

Aetiology The study of the causes of disease.

Agent (of disease) A term used to imply the organism that causes a disease.

Antibody Protein molecule formed in response to a foreign substance (antigen). It has the capacity to bind to the antigen to allow its removal or destruction.

Antigen A foreign molecule which elicits an antibody response.

Association Statistical dependence between two or more events, characteristics, or other variables. An association may be fortuitous or may be produced by various other circumstances; the presence of an association does not necessarily imply a causal relationship.

Attributable risk The proportion of the risk of a disease which can be attributed to a named causal factor.

Audit (clinical) A planned assessment of a clinical process against predefined standards.

Bias (syn: systematic error)   Deviation of results or inferences from the truth, or processes leading to such deviation. See also selection bias.

Blind(ed) study (syn: masked study)   A study in which observer(s) and/or subjects are kept ignorant of the group to which the subjects are assigned, as in an experimental study, or of the population from which the subjects come, as in a non-experimental or observational study. Where both observer and subjects are kept ignorant, the study is termed a double-blind study. If the statistical analysis is also done in ignorance of the group to which subjects belong, the study is sometimes described as triple blind. The purpose of 'blinding' is to eliminate sources of bias.

Carriage/carrier   When a host is infected but shows no signs of disease it is termed a carrier. It may transmit infection so is a potential source of infection.

Case fatality rate   The proportion of people with a disease who die within a defined period from diagnosis.

Case–control study   Retrospective comparison of exposures of persons with disease (cases) with those of persons without the disease controls – see retrospective study.

Case-series   Report of a number of cases of disease.

Causality   The relating of causes to the effects they produce. Most of epidemiology concerns causality and several types of causes can be distinguished. It must be emphasised, however, that epidemiological evidence by itself is insufficient to establish causality, although it can provide powerful circumstantial evidence.

Clinical governance   The framework through which NHS organisations and their staff are accountable for the quality of patient care.

Cohort study   Follow-up of exposed and non-exposed defined groups, with a comparison of disease rates during the time covered.

Commensalism   A neutral relationship between host and another organism. Often used to describe the bacteria which live in the human gut harmlessly.

Co-morbidity   Co-existence of a disease or diseases in a study participant in addition to the index condition that is the subject of study.

Comparison group   Any group to which the index group is compared. Usually synonymous with control group.

Confidence interval (CI)   The range of numerical values in which we can be confident (to a computed probability, such as 90 or 95%) that the population value being estimated will be found. Confidence intervals indicate the strength of evidence; where confidence intervals are wide, they indicate less precise estimates of effect. The larger the trial's sample size, the larger the number of outcome events and the greater becomes the confidence that the true relative risk reduction is close to the value stated. Thus the confidence interval is narrow and 'precision' is increased. In a 'positive finding' study the lower boundary of the confidence interval, or lower confidence limit, should still remain important or clinically significant if the results are to be accepted. In a 'negative finding' study, the upper boundary of the confidence interval should not be clinically significant if you are to accept this result confidently.

Confounding variable, confounder   A variable that can cause or prevent the outcome of interest, is not an intermediate variable, and is associated with the factor under investigation. A confounding variable may be due to chance or bias. Unless it is possible to adjust for confounding variables, their effects cannot be distinguished from those of factor(s) being studied.

Contamination   The presence of an infectious agent on the body of a host or on inanimate articles. A contaminated host does not always become infected but may be a possible source of infection for others.

Demography   The study of human populations.

Determinant   Any definable factor that effects a change in a health condition or other characteristic.

Disability   In the context of health experience a disability is any restriction or lack (resulting from an impairment) of ability to perform an activity in the manner or within the range considered normal for a human being.

Disability adjusted life year (DALY)   A method of calculating the health impact of a disease in terms of the cases of premature death, disability and days of infirmity due to illness from a specific disease or condition.

Dose–response relationship   A relationship in which change in amount, intensity or duration of exposure is associated with a change – either an increase or decrease – in risk of a specified outcome.

Dynamic population   A population in which there is turnover of membership during the study period.

Effectiveness   A measure of the benefit resulting from an intervention for a given health problem under usual conditions of clinical care for a particular group; this form of evaluation considers both the efficacy of an intervention and its acceptance by those to whom it is offered, answering the question, 'Does the practice do more good than harm to people to whom it is offered?' See intention to treat.

Efficacy   A measure of the benefit resulting from an intervention for a given health problem under the ideal conditions of an investigation; it answers the question, 'Does the practice do more good than harm to people who fully comply with the recommendations?'

Endemic   The constant presence of a disease or infectious agent within a given geographic area or population group.

Environmental health   The theory and practice of assessing, correcting, controlling and preventing those factors in the environment that can potentially affect adversely the health of present and future generations.

Epidemic   The occurrence of disease at higher than expected levels. This could be an endemic disease at higher than usual levels or non-endemic disease at any level.

Epidemiology   The study of the distribution and determinants of health-related states or events in specified populations, and the application of this study to control of health problems.

Evaluation   A process that attempts to determine as systematically and objectively as possible the relevance, effectiveness and impact of activities in the light of their objectives.

Evidence-based health care/medicine/public health   Systematic use of evidence derived from published research and other sources for management and practice.

Exclusion criteria   Conditions which preclude entrance of candidates into an investigation even if they meet the inclusion criteria.

Fertility   The childbearing capability of a woman, couple or population.

Follow-up   Observation over a period of time of an individual, group, or initially defined population whose relevant characteristics have been assessed in order to observe changes in health status or health-related variables.

Gold standard   A method, procedure, or measurement that is widely accepted as being the best available.

Handicap   In the context of health experience a handicap is a disadvantage for a given individual, resulting from an impairment or a disability, that limits or prevents the fulfilment of a role that is normal (depending on age, sex and social and cultural factors) for that individual.

Health   The extent to which an individual or a group is able to realise aspirations and satisfy needs, and to change or cope with the environment. Health is a resource for everyday life, not the objective of living; it is a positive concept, emphasising social and personal resources as well as physical capabilities. Your health is related to how much you feel your potential to be a meaningful part of the society in which you find yourself, is adequately realised.

Health equity audit   A technique to identify how fairly services or other resources are distributed in relation to the health needs of different population groups or geographical areas.

Health improvement   The theory and practice of promoting the health of populations by influencing lifestyle and socio-economic, physical and cultural environment through methods of health promotion, directed towards populations, communities and individuals.

Health inequality   Differences observed between groups due to one group experiencing an advantage over the other group rather than to any innate differences between them.

Health inequity   The presence of unfair and avoidable or remedial differences in health among populations or groups defined socially.

Health promotion   The process of enabling people to exert control over and to improve their health. As well as covering actions aimed at strengthening people's skills and capabilities, it also includes actions directed towards changing social, environmental conditions, to prevent or to improve their impact on individual and public health.

High risk strategy   This Targets preventative interventions at people most at risk of a disease.

Host   A living organism on or in which an infectious agent can subsist.

Impairment   In the context of health experience an impairment is any loss or abnormality of psychological, physiological or anatomical structure or function.

Incidence rate   The rate at which new cases occur in a population.

Incidence   The number of new cases of illness commencing, or of persons falling ill, during a specified time period in a given population. See also prevalence.

Incubation period   The interval from exposure to onset of clinical disease.

Index case   The first case identified in an outbreak.

Infant mortality   The proportion of live births that die up to one year of age.

Infection (colonisation)   This occurs when an organism enters the body, and multiplies. It may be termed infection when damage is caused and colonisation when no damage is caused to the host. Acute infection implies a short-lived infection with a short period of infectivity. Chronic infection refers to a persistent condition with on-going replication of the organism. Latent infection refers to a persistent infection with intermittent replication of the organism.

Infectivity   The proportion of exposed, susceptible persons who become infected (for a given number of organisms).

Intention to treat analysis   A method for data analysis in a randomised clinical trial in which individual outcomes are analysed according to the group to which they have been randomised, even if they never received the treatment they were assigned. By simulating practical experience it provides a better measure of effectiveness (versus efficacy).

Interviewer bias   Systematic error due to interviewer's subconscious or conscious gathering of selective data.

Koch's (Henle-Koch's) postulates   These postulates should be met before a causal relationship can be inferred between an organism and a disease:
1. The agent must be shown to be present in every case of the disease by isolation in pure culture.
2. The agent must not be found in cases of other disease.
3. Once isolated the agent must be able to reproduce disease in experimental animals.
4. The agent must be recovered from this experimental disease.

Lead time bias   If prognosis study patients are not all enrolled at similar, well-defined points in the course of their disease, differences in outcome over time may merely reflect differences in duration of illness.
Lead time bias occurs when detection by screening seems to increase disease-free survival but this is only because disease has been detected earlier and not because screening is delaying death or disease.

Length time bias   Length time bias occurs if a screening programme is better at picking up milder forms of the disease. This means that people who develop a disease that progresses more quickly or is more likely to be fatal are less likely to be picked up by screening and their outcomes may not be included in evaluations of the programme. Thus the programme looks to be more effective than it is.

Life expectancy   The average number of additional years a person could expect to live if current mortality trends were to continue for the rest of that person's life. Generally given as a life expectancy from birth.

Likelihood ratio   Ratio of the probability that a given diagnostic test result will be expected for a patient with the target disorder rather than for a patient without the disorder.

Maternal mortality ratio   The number of deaths during pregnancy and up to 42 days after delivery, per 1,000 live births.

Morbidity   The impact of a disease which is not death. Measures of morbidity include incidence and prevalence rates.

Mortality (rate)   The number of deaths in an area as a proportion of the number of people in that area

Needs   These may be expressed by action, e.g. visiting a doctor; or felt needs, e.g. what people consider and/or say they need. The need for health care is often defined as the capacity to benefit from that care.

Negative predictive value (of a diagnostic or screening test)   The proportion of persons who test negative for a disease who, as measured by the gold standard, are identified as non-diseased.

Neonatal mortality   The proportion of live births who die within the first 28 days.

Non-specific immunity   This is the natural barriers a host has to pathogens. It includes mechanical barriers, body secretions, physical removal of organisms, phagocytosis, inflammatory response.

Normal distribution   Many biological variables show a normal distribution of ranges between individuals within a population. A probability density graph of the normal distributions takes the shape of a bell-shaped curve.

Number needed to treat (NNT)   The number of patients who must be exposed to an intervention before the clinical outcome of interest occurred; for example, the number of patients needed to treat to prevent one adverse outcome.

Odds Ratio   A measure of the degree of association; for example, the odds of exposure among the cases compared with the odds of exposure among the controls.

Odds   A proportion in which the numerator contains the number of times an event occurs and the denominator includes the number of times the event does not occur.

Outbreak   A localised epidemic. Health protection professionals often look for two or more cases linked in time and place.

P value   The probability (ranging from zero to one) that the results observed in a study (or results more extreme) could have occurred by chance.

Pandemic   A global epidemic. This is sometimes used for a very large-scale epidemic.

Perinatal mortality   The proportion of all births that die before birth or in the first week.

Policy   An overall statement of the aims of an organisation within a particular context.

Population strategy   Targets preventative interventions at the whole
population.

Positive predictive value (of a diagnostic or screening test)   The proportion of persons
who test positive for a disease who, as measured by the gold standard, are identified as
diseased.

Poverty   Absolute poverty – a family's ability to purchase essential goods (such as
housing, heating, food, clothing and transport).
Relative poverty – poverty in relation to the average income in a particular population
(such as below 50% of the national average).

Precision   The range in which the best estimates of a true value approximate the true
value. See confidence interval.

Predictive value   In screening and diagnostic tests, the probability that a person with a
positive test is a true positive (i.e., does have the disease) or that a person with a negative
test truly does not have the disease. The predictive value of a screening test is determined
by the sensitivity and specificity of the test, and by the prevalence of the condition for
which the test is used.

Prevalence   The proportion of persons with a particular disease within a given
population at a given time. Point prevalence is the prevalence at one single point in time.
Period prevalence is the proportion of persons with a particular disease over a specified
period of time.

Prevention   Primary prevention – actions designed to prevent the occurrence of the
problem, e.g. health education, immunisation.
Secondary prevention – actions designed to detect and treat the occurrence of a problem
before symptoms have developed, e.g. screening, early diagnosis.
Tertiary prevention – actions designed to limit disability once a condition is manifest, e.g.
limitation of disability, rehabilitation.

Prevention paradox   Preventive measures bringing large benefits to the community offer
little to each participating individual.

Primary care trust   Local NHS health authorities in England charged with improving
health and commissioning health care.

Primary health care   First-contact care provided by a range of health care professionals:
general practioners, nurses, dentists, pharmacists, optometrists, and complementary
therapists working in the community.

Prognosis   The possible outcomes of a disease or condition and the likelihood that each
one will occur.

Prognostic factor   Demographic, disease-specific, or co-morbid characteristics associated strongly enough with a condition's outcomes to predict accurately the eventual development of those outcomes. Compare with risk factors. Neither prognostic nor risk factors necessarily imply a cause and effect relationship.

Prospective study   Study design where one or more groups (cohorts) of individuals, who have not yet had the outcome event in question, are monitored for the number of such events which occur over time.

Public health   The science and art of preventing disease, prolonging life, and promoting health through the organised efforts and informed choices of society, organisations, public and private, communities and individuals. Public health practice is the emphasis in this book, while public health may also be considered as a discipline or a social institution.

Public health practitioner   In this book, includes anyone working in the broad field of public health, neither defined by formal qualifications nor restricted to a professional group.

Quality-adjusted life year (QALY)   A health measure which combines the quantity and quality of life. It takes one year of perfect-health life expectancy to be worth 1 and regards one year of less than perfect life expectancy as less than 1.

Randomised controlled trial   Study design where treatments, interventions or enrolment into different study groups are assigned by random allocation rather than by conscious decisions of clinicians or patients. If the sample size is large enough, this study design avoids problems of bias and confounding variables by assuring that both known and unknown determinants of outcome are evenly distributed between treatment and control groups.

Recall bias   Systematic error due to the differences in accuracy or completeness of recall to memory of past events or experiences.

Relative risk   The ratio of the probability of developing, in a specified period of time, an outcome among those receiving the treatment of interest or exposed to a risk factor, compared with the probability of developing the outcome if the risk factor or intervention is not present.

Reproducibility (repeatability, reliability)   The results of a test or measure are identical or closely similar each time it is conducted.

Retrospective study   Study design in which cases where individuals who had an outcome event in question are collected and analysed after the outcomes have occurred (see also case–control study).

Risk   The number of cases of a disease that occur in a defined period of time as a proportion of the number of people in the population at the beginning of the period.

Risk factor   Patient characteristics or factors associated with an increased probability of developing a condition or disease in the first place. Compare with prognostic factors. Neither risk nor prognostic factors necessarily imply a cause and effect relationship.

Screening   A public health service in which members of a defined population, who do not necessarily perceive they are at risk of, or are already affected by, a disease or its complications, are asked a question or offered a test. The aim is to identify those individuals who are more likely to be helped than harmed by further tests or treatment to reduce the risk of a disease or its complications.

Secular trend   A trend over time, also termed temporal trend.

Selection bias   A bias in assignment or a confounding variable that arises from study design rather than by chance. These can occur when the study and control groups are chosen so that they differ from each other by one or more factors that may affect the outcome of the study. In screening, selection bias occurs when the screening programme attracts people who are more or less likely to have the condition being screened for than the general population.

Sensitivity (of a diagnostic or screening test)   The proportion of truly diseased persons, as measured by the gold standard, who are identified as diseased by the test under study.

Social capital   Networks together with shared norms, values and understandings which facilitate co-operation within or among groups and which may thereby improve health.

Specificity (of a diagnostic or screening test)   The proportion of truly non-diseased persons, as measured by the gold standard, who are identified as non-diseased by the test under study.

Strategy   A plan of action designed to achieve a series of objectives.

Stratification   Division into groups. Stratification may also refer to a process to control for differences in confounding variables, by making separate estimates for groups of individuals who have the same values for the confounding variable.

Strength of inference   The likelihood that an observed difference between groups within a study represents a real difference rather than mere chance or the influence of confounding factors, based on both P values and confidence intervals. Strength of inference is weakened by various forms of bias and by small sample sizes.

Surveillance   The on-going, systematic collection, collation and analysis of data and the prompt dissemination of the resulting information to those who need to know so that an action can result.

Survival curve   A graph of the number of events occurring over time or the chance of being free of these events over time. The events must be discrete and the time at which they occur must be precisely known. In most clinical situations, the chance of an outcome changes with time. In most survival curves the earlier follow-up periods usually include results from more patients than the later periods and are therefore more precise.

Validity   The extent to which a variable or intervention measures what it is supposed to measure or accomplishes what it is supposed to accomplish.
The internal validity of a study refers to the integrity of the experimental design.
The external validity (generalisability) of a study refers to the appropriateness by which its results can be applied to non-study patients or populations.

Years of life lost(YLL)   Years of potential life relate to the average age at which deaths occur and the expected life span of the population. Therefore, a measure of how many potential years are lost due to early death and provides a measure of the relative importance of conditions in causing mortality.

Index